Chronic Diseases

Chronic Diseases

An Encyclopedia of Causes, Effects, and Treatments

Volume 1: A–H

JEAN KAPLAN TEICHROEW, EDITOR

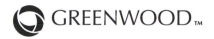

GREENWOOD™

An Imprint of ABC-CLIO, LLC
Santa Barbara, California • Denver, Colorado

Library of Congress Cataloging-in-Publication Data

Names: Teichroew, Jean Kaplan, editor.
Title: Chronic diseases : an encyclopedia of causes, effects, and treatments / Jean Kaplan Teichroew, editor.
Other titles: Chronic diseases (Teichroew)
Description: Santa Barbara, California : Greenwood, [2017] | Includes bibliographical references and index.
Identifiers: LCCN 2016025459 (print) | LCCN 2016026316 (ebook) |
    ISBN 9781440801037 (hard copy (set) : alk. paper) | ISBN 9781440846205
    (v. 1 : alk. paper) | ISBN 9781440846212 (v. 2 : alk. paper) | ISBN 9781440801044
    (set EISBN) | ISBN 9781440801044 (ebook (set))
Subjects: | MESH: Chronic Disease | Encyclopedias
Classification: LCC RC41 (print) | LCC RC41 (ebook) | NLM WT 13 | DDC 616.003—dc23
LC record available at https://lccn.loc.gov/2016025459

ISBN: 978-1-4408-0103-7 (set)
      978-1-4408-4620-5 (vol. 1)
      978-1-4408-4621-2 (vol. 2)
EISBN: 978-1-4408-0104-4

21 20 19 18 17   1 2 3 4 5

This book is also available as an eBook.

Greenwood
An Imprint of ABC-CLIO, LLC

ABC-CLIO, LLC
130 Cremona Drive, P.O. Box 1911
Santa Barbara, California 93116-1911
www.abc-clio.com

This book is printed on acid-free paper ∞
Manufactured in the United States of America

Contents

Alphabetical List of Entries

Guide to Related Topics

Following are the entries in this encyclopedia, arranged under broad topics for enhanced searching. Readers should also consult the index at the end of the encyclopedia for more specific subjects. Some entries are listed more than once.

ADDICTION

Alcoholism
Fetal Alcohol Syndrome

Substance Abuse
Tobacco Addiction

ARTHRITIS

Adult Onset Still's Disease
Gout
Juvenile Arthritis

Osteoarthritis
Reactive Arthritis

BLOOD, HEART, AND CARDIOVASCULAR DISORDERS

Aneurisms
Angina
Angiogram
Arrhythmias/Dysrhythmias
Arteriovenous Malformations
Atherosclerosis
Atrial Fibrillation
Bleeding Disorders
Blood Cancers
Blood Disorders
Blood Pressure
Bradycardia
Cardiomyopathy
Cardiovascular Disease
Cholesterol
Circulation Disorders
Congenital Heart Disease
Congestive Heart Failure
Cor Pulmonale
Deep Vein Thrombosis
Endocarditis
Familial Hypercholesterolemia
Gangrene

Heart Diseases
Heart Murmur
Heart Valve Disorders
Hemochromatosis
Hemophilia
Hyperlipidemia
Hypertension (High Blood Pressure)
Hypoglycemia
Hypotension (Low Blood Pressure)
Iron Overload Disease
Kawasaki Disease
Leukemia
Multiple Myeloma
Pericardial Disorders/Pericarditis
Peripheral Arterial Disease
Platelet Disorders
Raynaud's Phenomenon
Rheumatic Fever and Rheumatic Heart
    Disease
Tachycardia
Thrombophlebitis
Vascular Disorders
Venous Disorders

BREAST DISORDERS

Breast Cancer
Breast Diseases

Male Breast Cancer
Paget's Disease of the Breast

CANCER

Anal and Rectal Diseases
Basal Cell Carcinoma
Bile Duct Cancer
Bladder Cancer
Blood Cancers
Bone Cancer
Brain Cancer
Breast Cancer
Cancer Survivorship
Cancer
Cancers, Childhood
Cancers, Occupational
Cervical Cancer
Colon Cancer
Esophageal Cancer
Eye Cancer
Gastric Cancer
Head and Neck Cancer
Hodgkin Disease
Kidney Cancer

Laryngeal Cancer
Leukemia
Liver Cancer
Lung Cancer
Male Breast Cancer
Melanoma
Neoplasms
Non-Hodgkin Lymphoma
Oral Cancer
Ovarian Cancer
Pancreatic Cancer
Prostate Cancer
Skin Cancer
Squamous Cell Children
Testicular Cancer
Throat Cancer
Thyroid Cancer
Urethral Cancer
Uterine Cancer

CHILDREN AND YOUTH

Asthma, Children and Youth
Cancers, Childhood
Failure to Thrive
Fetal Alcohol Syndrome

Juvenile Arthritis
Overweight and Obesity in Children
Phenylketonuria
School Wellness Programs

DIABETES

Diabetes, Type 1
Diabetes, Type 2

Prediabetes
Sugar Diabetes

DIGESTIVE SYSTEM/EXCRETORY SYSTEM

Abdominal Diseases
Anal and Rectal Diseases
Bile Duct Cancer
Biliary Cirrhosis
Biliary Diseases
Bowel Incontinence
Crohn's Disease

Cyclic Vomiting Syndrome
Cystic Fibrosis
Digestive Diseases
Diverticular Disease
Esophageal Cancer
Gall Bladder Disease
Gastric Cancer

Diabetes, Type 1
Diabetes, Type 2
Failure to Thrive
Hashimoto's Disease
Immune System Disorders

Kaposi's Sarcoma
Lupus
Neoplasms
Sjögren's Syndrome

INFLAMMATORY DISORDERS

Adult Onset Still's Disease
Allergies
Amyloidosis
Ankylosing Spondylitis
Arthritis
Autoimmune Disease
Behcet's Syndrome
Buerger's Disease
Bursitis
Crohn's Disease
Felty Syndrome

Gout
Inflammation
Inflammatory Bowel Disease
Kawasaki Disease
Lupus
Myopathies
Pelvic Inflammatory Disease
Peritoneal Disorders
Polymyositis
Rheumatoid Arthritis
Thrombophlebitis

INFORMATION

Centers for Disease Control and
    Prevention (CDC)
Epidemiology
Etiology

Health Literacy
National Institutes of Health (NIH)
World Health Organization

ISSUES

Environment
Health Disparities
Minority, Chronic Disease
Pollution

Poverty
Public Health
School Wellness Programs

KIDNEY AND URINARY DISORDERS

Addison's Disease
Bladder Cancer
Bladder Diseases
Kidney Cancer
Kidney Disease
Kidney Failure
Kidney Stones

Nephritis
Urethral Cancer
Urethral Disorders
Urinary Incontinence
Urinary Tract Infections
Uterine Cancer
Uterine Diseases

LIFE STAGES

Adolescence and Chronic Disease
Aging, Healthy

Family Health

LIVER DISORDERS

Bile Duct Cancer
Biliary Cirrhosis
Biliary Diseases

Hepatitis
Liver Cancer
Liver Diseases

LYMPHATIC DISORDERS

Hodgkin Disease
Lymphatic Disorders

Lymphoma
Non-Hodgkin Lymphoma

MEN'S HEALTH

Male Breast Cancer
Men's Health

Prostate Cancer
Testicular Cancer

MENTAL HEALTH DISORDERS

Anxiety Disorders
Attention Deficit Hyperactivity Disorder
 (ADHD)
Cutting and Self-Harm
Depression
Eating Disorders
Mental Health Disorders

Obsessive Compulsive Disorder
Psychotic Disorders
PTSD (Post-Traumatic Stress Disorder)
Schizophrenia
Seasonal Affective Disorder
Stress

METABOLIC DISORDERS

Addison's Disease
Cystic Fibrosis
Diabetes, Type 1
Hypothyroidism

Metabolic Disorders
Metabolic Syndrome
Phenylketonuria
Tay-Sachs Disease

MUSCULOSKELETAL

Arthritis
Back Pain
Bursitis
Carpal Tunnel Syndrome
Ehlers-Danlos Syndrome
Joint Disorders
Juvenile Arthritis

Legg-Calve-Perthes Disease
Muscle Cramps
Musculoskeletal Disorders
Myopathies
Osteoarthritis
Reactive Arthritis
Rheumatoid Arthritis

NEUROLOGICAL DISORDERS

ALS (Amyotrophic Lateral Sclerosis)
Alzheimer's Disease
Autism
Autonomic Nervous System Disorders

Bell's Palsy
Bipolar Disorder
Brain Cancer
Brain Diseases

Carpal Tunnel Syndrome
Cerebrovascular Disease
Charcot-Marie-Tooth Disease
Chronic Fatigue Syndrome
Complex Regional Pain Syndrome
Creutzfeldt-Jakob Disease
Dementia
Epilepsy
Fetal Alcohol Syndrome
Fibromyalgia
Hansen's Disease (Leprosy)
Herpes
Lead Poisoning
Lyme Disease
Lyme Disease
Meniere's Disease
Meningitis
Mental Health Disorders

Multiple Sclerosis
Neurodegenerative Diseases
Neurofibromatosis
Neurological Diseases
Neuromuscular Disorders
Neuropathy
Pain, Chronic
Parkinson's Disease
Peripheral Nerve Disorders
Pituitary Disorders
Polio and Post-Polio Syndrome
Shingles
Sjögren's Syndrome
Sleep Disorders and Sleep Disturbances
Spinal Diseases
Stroke
Tay-Sachs Disease
Wilson's Disease

ORAL PHARYNGEAL DISORDERS

Bruxism
Oral Cancer
Oral Health
Oral Pharyngeal Disorders
Salivary Gland Disorders

Thoracic Outlet Syndrome
Throat Cancer
Throat Disorders
Tracheal Disorders

OVERWEIGHT AND OBESITY

Body Mass Index (BMI)
Diet and Nutrition
Obesity

Obesity, Morbid
Overweight and Obesity in Children

PREVENTION AND CARE

Acceptance and Commitment Therapy
Access to Health Services
Adherence
Allied Health Professionals
Alternative Medicine
Caregiving and Caregivers
Chronic Disease Management
Diet and Nutrition
Food Guides from the U.S. Department of
    Agriculture

Physical Activity
Physical Therapy
Rehabilitation
Risk Factors
Secondhand Smoke
Self-Management
Spirituality
Vaccines

REPRODUCTIVE SYSTEM DISORDERS

Atrophic Vaginitis
Dysmenorrhea

Gonorrhea
HPV (Human Papillomavirus)

Pelvic Inflammatory Disease
Reproductive Disorders
Sexually Transmitted Diseases

Testicular Cancer
Vaginal Diseases

RESPIRATORY, LUNG, AND NASAL DISORDERS

Allergies
Asthma
Asthma, Children and Youth
Black Lung Disease
Bronchiectasis
Bronchitis
COPD (Chronic Obstructive Pulmonary
   Disease)
Cystic Fibrosis
Emphysema
Inhalers
Legionnaires' Disease

Lung Cancer
Lung Diseases
Nasal Disorders
Pleural Disorders
Pneumonia
Pneumothorax
Respiratory Diseases
Secondhand Smoke
Sinusitis
Tuberculosis
Whooping Cough

SEXUALLY TRANSMITTED DISEASES

AIDS (Acquired Immune Deficiency
   Syndrome)
Gonorrhea

HPV (Human Papillomavirus)
Sexually Transmitted Diseases

SKELETAL (BONE) DISORDERS

Ankylosing Spondylitis
Bone Cancer
Bone Diseases
Osteomyelitis

Osteonecrosis
Osteoporosis
Paget's Disease of the Bone
Rickets

SKIN

Basal Cell Carcinoma
Cellulitis
Dermatitis
Eczema
Hansen's Disease (Leprosy)
Herpes

Melanoma
Psoriasis
Rosacea
Skin Cancer
Squamous Cell Carcinoma

VIRAL, BACTERIAL, AND CONTAMINANT DISORDERS

Environment
Herpes
Lead Poisoning

Malaria
Occupational Health
Parasitic Diseases

WOMEN'S HEALTH

Atrophic Vaginitis
Breast Diseases
Cervical Cancer
Dysmenorrhea
Fetal Alcohol Syndrome

Osteoporosis
Ovarian Cancer
Vaginal Diseases
Women's Health

Preface

Chronic Diseases: An Encyclopedia of Causes, Effects, and Treatment provides more than 300 entries on chronic diseases and disorders, general health topics, treatment, and social issues. Chronic diseases such as asthma, cancer, diabetes, heart disease, and stroke are the leading causes of disability and death in the United States. Chronic disease is a serious problem around the world, causing not only suffering to individuals and loved ones, but also economic problems to society at large. It can lead to painful conditions and lost days at work and prevent the ability to be employed, go to school, or enjoy a normal life. It leads to enormous health costs: According to statistics from the Centers for Disease Control and Prevention, 86 percent of all health care spending in 2010 was for people with one or more chronic medical conditions. And according to the Centers for Medicare and Medicaid, 2015 health care expenditures were expected to be $3.207 trillion total and nearly $10,000 per person (Munro 2015).

Chronic disease and *chronic disorders* are health problems that affect people over a period of time. Chronic disease is typically an illness that can be managed but never completely cured, but in some contexts, a chronic condition is defined as lasting three months or longer, whether curable or not. Many diseases and disorders have both acute and chronic forms.

Diseases and disorders are both related to the malfunction of a body system or physiological process, but *disease* is an illness that has a known cause, while a *disorder* is a set of symptoms that may or may not have a known cause. Further, disorders may also have types of symptoms that arise from a disease, or they may be symptoms with an unknown underlying cause that creates disease-like effects.

Purpose and Scope

Chronic Diseases: An Encyclopedia of Causes, Effects, and Treatment will serve as a first point of reference for users of high school, public, community, and college libraries. This work will provide the reader with an overview of the most important topics in the field of chronic disease and public health. Although there are many books, articles, and online sources that present excellent information on chronic disease and disorders, there are few sources that consolidate this knowledge into one resource and provide it for a nonprofessional readership.

The 323 entries in *Chronic Diseases* provide a basic overview of significant and common chronic diseases. They will provide an excellent starting place for those needing to obtain information on a wide variety of chronic diseases. All entries on disorders or diseases provide definitions of the condition, symptoms, causes, and treatments. Many entries also include background on history, risk factors, diagnostic procedures typically used, prevention, outcomes, and future for research and new protocols. Entries are written by a variety of contributors, including health care professionals with many years of experience, students enrolled in graduate programs in health, and science writers.

Entries range from non-life-threatening chronic diseases and disorders, such as bruxism, back pain, rosacea, and dermatitis; to painful and debilitating illnesses and conditions, such as rheumatoid arthritis, fibromyalgia, or multiple sclerosis; to those diseases and disorders that may eventually result in death, including some cancers and cardiovascular diseases. Some entries describe conditions and disorders that are part of a chronic condition, such as cellulitis or cholesterol. A number of mental disorders are included as well, including depression, anxiety, bipolar disorder, and others. Topics also include those related to prevention, treatment, or types of therapies; risks and behaviors; and general public health issues. Finally, societal issues, such as poverty, minority groups and chronic disease, health disparities, environmental issues, and pollution, among other topics in public health, are discussed.

Each entry concludes with cross references to related entries and further reading references to authoritative sources, including websites of organizations that study certain conditions, such as the American Cancer Society, and government sources, such as the Centers for Disease Control and Prevention and National Institutes of Health, among others; also included is online information provided by major medical schools and research and clinical centers. Other resources listed include periodical articles and books, most of which are geared toward readers without professional expertise in health studies. At the end of the book, there is a general selected bibliography, "Recommended Resources," of the most important books and online sources.

Access

Entries are arranged in alphabetic order, but the front of each volume will include, in addition to the alphabetic list of entries, a "Guide to Related Topics." This is a list of the entries arranged under broad topics so that readers can easily scan for diseases or disorders under certain topics, like "Lung and Respiratory-Related Disorders." Each entry also includes cross references to related entries, and there is a comprehensive index to content.

References

Centers for Disease Control and Prevention (CDC). (2016). Chronic disease overview. Retrieved from http://www.cdc.gov/chronicdisease/overview.
Munro, D. (2015, January 4). U.S. healthcare spending on track to hit $10,000 per person this year. *Forbes*. Retrieved from http://www.forbes.com/sites/danmunro/2015/01/04/u-s-healthcare-spending-on-track-to-hit-10000-per-person-this-year/#739f8293294c.

Introduction

Chronic diseases and disorders are adverse health conditions that affect an individual over the long term. There are variable definitions for the distinction between *chronic* and *acute* (short-term or sudden) conditions. The most common definition of *chronic* in terms of disease or disorder is a state of illness that can be controlled but never completely cured, although in some contexts, a chronic condition is defined as one lasting three months or longer, whether curable or not. Many diseases and disorders have both acute and chronic forms. Medical professionals may draw a further distinction between constant chronic conditions and recurrent conditions that intersperse periods of remission and relapse.

Diseases versus Disorders

Diseases and disorders both address malfunction of a body system or physiological process. Diseases are adverse health conditions that have a known etiology, or cause. A *disease* may be caused by a pathogen, exposure to a toxin or allergen, damage to a body part or system, or congenital or hereditary conditions. A *disorder* is a set of symptoms that may or may not have a known etiology. Disorders may be clusters of symptoms that arise from a disease, or they may be clusters of symptoms with an unknown underlying cause that creates disease-like effects.

Another definition of "disease versus disorder" states that diseases have a physical cause, while disorders have a psychological cause. This distinction can be foggy because the more scientists learn about the human brain, the more it appears that all psychological activity has an underlying biological basis. This distinction has led to the idea that diseases are real, or have a biological cause, while disorders are less legitimate and "all in a person's head," which can add to the distress of persons suffering from chronic disorders, as they may face additional stigma and judgment.

Chronic Communicable Diseases

Many pathogens can cause chronic disease. These pathogens may be *viruses, bacteria, fungi*, or *parasites*.

Viruses that can cause chronic disease include human immunodeficiency virus (HIV); HPV, or the human papillomavirus (which in some cases can cause genital warts or cervical cancer); and the various herpes viruses. Herpes viruses are particularly good examples of pathogens that cause both acute and chronic illness. Herpes simplex—or herpesviruses 1 and 2—causes genital herpes and oral herpes, or cold sores. Varicella zoster—or herpesvirus 3—which causes chickenpox, can also cause the chronic disease shingles. Epstein-Barr virus—or herpesvirus 4—causes mononucleosis and is associated with a host of chronic conditions, from various cancers to chronic fatigue syndrome, lupus, and multiple sclerosis. Cytomegalovirus—or herpesvirus 5—may causes minor, recurrent inflammation of the salivary glands in children and adults but may be fatal in fetuses and newborns and is associated with various chronic conditions, including epilepsy. Roseolovirus—or herpesviruses 6A, 6B, and 7—causes acute infection with a rash in children and may cause lifelong, chronic conditions ranging from periodic flu-like symptoms to epilepsy, learning disorders, multiple sclerosis, and chronic fatigue syndrome. Kaposi's sarcoma-associated herpesvirus—or herpesvirus 8—is associated with various forms of cancer and lymph disorders.

Chronic bacterial infections include Lyme disease, MRSA (methicillin-resistant *Staphylococcus aureus*), and chronic urinary tract infections. The most common chronic bacterial disease in the world is tuberculosis, a lung disease caused by *Mycobacterium tuberculosis* and related species. It currently infects about one in six people worldwide, with the vast majority of cases concentrated in developing countries.

Chronic fungal infections are usually caused by the yeast *Candida albicans*. This fungus can infect the mouth (thrush), genital and anal area (yeast infection, jock itch, diaper rash), feet (athlete's foot), nail beds, or gastrointestinal tract. Other pathogenic fungi can cause chronic meningitis; pneumonia; and liver, bone, and skin infections.

Chronic disease may be a symptom of endoparasites (parasites that live inside the body) or spread by ectoparasites (parasites on the skin). Some, like the protozoan *Plasmodium*, cause acute illness—in this case, malaria—which can lead to chronic disorders such as epilepsy. Others, like roundworms, cause chronic disease directly. Chronic diseases caused by parasitic worms include river blindness, elephantiasis, and ascariasis.

Hereditary and Congenital Chronic Diseases and Disorders

Some chronic diseases and disorders are present from birth. Chronic diseases that are inherited from an individual's parents include the lung disease cystic fibrosis, sickle-cell disease, and Tay-Sachs disease. These diseases are caused when a baby inherits versions of normal genes that carry the abnormal trait. They are passed down within families because many healthy people in the family carry a gene for the disorder.

Other chronic conditions are present at birth but are caused by abnormal development of the gametes (sex cells) or early embryo rather than by the parents' genetics. Down syndrome and 5P-minus (Lejeune's or cri-du-chat syndrome) are examples of conditions usually caused by abnormal gamete development. While neither condition is a disease in itself, both are associated with chronic disorders involving the heart and digestive system. Examples of disorders caused by abnormal embryonic development include spina bifida and congenital heart defects. These conditions develop early in pregnancy, and while risk factors exist, the exact cause may be unknown. Other chronic conditions such as fetal alcohol spectrum disorder result from intrauterine environmental exposures.

Other Chronic Disorders

Multifactorial disorders have many possible causes. Idiopathic disorders are ones for which the underlying cause is completely unknown. The same disorder may have many known potential causes or risk factors in one person but be idiopathic in another. Examples of these confusing disorders include amyotrophic lateral sclerosis (ALS, or Lou Gehrig's disease), multiple sclerosis, lupus, Alzheimer's disease, epilepsy, thyroid disease, schizophrenia, some cancers, asthma, arthritis, and muscular dystrophy.

Chronic "Lifestyle Diseases"

Many chronic illnesses are considered lifestyle diseases, or diseases caused by specific things a person does. They are especially associated with sedentary lifestyle, an unhealthy diet, tobacco use, and alcohol abuse. Chronic diseases of lifestyle include cardiovascular disease, Type 2 diabetes, and some cancers. Some multifactorial diseases such as osteoporosis and chronic obstructive pulmonary disease may include lifestyle components. There is some disagreement over what constitutes a disease, disorder, symptom, or risk factor when it comes to chronic lifestyle disease. For example, depending on who is giving the information, obesity may be considered a disorder, a symptom of an underlying condition, a risk factor for cardiovascular disease or diabetes, or a chronic disease in itself.

Underlying causes for chronic lifestyle diseases are not always understood. Many are multifactorial and may have genetic components. Lack of understanding around why some people develop these diseases, while others with similar risk factors do not, can interfere with appropriate, individualized care. It can also cause feelings of judgment and shame in afflicted persons, which can interfere with self-care and healing.

Prevention and Treatment

Many chronic diseases can be prevented; others cannot. Some of the pathogens that cause chronic disease have been eradicated or strongly controlled in industrialized countries by public health measures, personal hygiene practices, large-scale vaccination, and frequent testing (such as for tuberculosis). Others such as HIV are targeted by educational prevention campaigns, while active cases may be controlled by drug therapy.

Heritable diseases may be reduced by genetic screening and alternative family planning measures for prospective parents who carry a high genetic risk. Congenital disorders may be treated by advanced management techniques that improve quality of life for affected persons. Multifactorial and idiopathic conditions may be impossible to prevent. Some, such as ALS, are very difficult to treat; others, such as thyroid disease, are easily managed with hormone therapy, other drugs, or surgical interventions.

Lifestyle diseases are hypothetically the easiest to prevent. On the surface, it seems as if they could be eradicated by simple changes such as daily exercise and healthy diet. However, in practice, they include some of the most pervasive and difficult-to-manage illnesses. Chronic lifestyle diseases such as cardiovascular disease and tobacco-related illnesses are the leading cause of death for adults in the United States. A study published in 2013 (Ford et al.) that examined health care data and chronic disease showed that more than 70 percent of deaths in the United States and about 75 percent of health care spending costs can be attributed to chronic diseases. The study also stated that the five leading causes of death—heart disease, cancer, chronic lower respiratory disease, cerebrovascular disease, and diabetes—accounted for more than half of all deaths in 2009 and represent a high percentage of the nation's health care costs. (Ford et al. 2013).

Angela Libal

Reference

Ford, E. S., Croft, J. B., Posner, S. F., Goodman, R. A., & Giles W. H. (2013). Co-occurrence of leading lifestyle-related chronic conditions among adults in the United States, 2002–2009. *Preventing Chronic Disease.* Retrieved from http://www.cdc.gov/pcd/issues/2013/12_0316.htm; doi:http://dx.doi.org/10.5888/pcd10.120316.

A

ABDOMINAL DISEASES

Overview

The term *abdomen* refers to the region of the body located between the chest and hip areas and includes the stomach, small intestine, large intestine, liver, gall bladder, pancreas, and spleen. The stomach is the organ found between the long muscular tube that starts in the area of the throat or esophagus and the small intestine, which is a coiled muscle tube in the hip region and the organ where protein digestion starts.

Some problems that affect the stomach and other parts of the abdomen are temporary and can be relieved by over-the-counter remedies or a change in diet, such as reducing one's fat intake or trying to eat more slowly. Other problems that do not resolve easily may be more serious and should be investigated by a medical practitioner to prevent them from becoming chronic or longstanding. Examples include a peptic ulcer, pancreatic cancer, and celiac disease. Other conditions that can become longstanding are irritations or inflammation of the stomach (gastritis), colon (colonitis), liver (hepatitis), and gallbladder (cholecystitis). Others are said to be functional in nature rather than inflammatory, such as irritable bowel syndrome, which has symptoms that accompany this diagnosis but no visible signs of any disease.

All these abdominal diseases, whether structural or functional, can hinder everyday existence, especially social-, work-, and family-related aspects of life, and cause severe disability. The abdominal diseases are thus very important to prevent or identify from a medical point of view, as well as from a personal and societal point of view, because of the wide variety of abdominal diseases. In particular, it appears that if these conditions cannot be prevented, they should be diagnosed and treated accordingly as soon as possible. In some undiagnosed and/or untreated conditions, digestive problems may even lead to anorexia if individuals eat less or fail to eat because eating causes unpleasant symptoms. Abdominal diseases can also lead to a diminished life quality and influence psychological status and well-being. In this regard, some new evidence concerning the microbes that are housed in the human body suggests that problems such as obesity may be related to internal system disorders, such as fewer types of bacteria or the wrong types of bacteria, according to Stanford scientist Justin Sonnenburg. This situation is attributed to aspects of the Western diet, the use of antimicrobials ingested with meals, or the nature of how food is processed to become sterile. Other cited reasons are the low level of fiber in the Western diet and the use of food additives and highly processed calorie-dense foods that may influence the presence and function of useful microbes and bacteria (Pollan 2013).

Historical View

In 1934, lack of oxygen intake as a result of infections of the nasal region, which reduced the body's resistance and fostered congestion and inflammation of one or more components of the abdomen, was offered as a reason for the existence of many abdominal diseases. This situation was more likely to occur in the presence of poor nutrition or harmful foods. It was also thought that a lowering of the activity of the vagus nerve due to infection lowered the resistance of the person as a whole to health problems, such as abdominal diseases. It was thought that if the nasal problem was treated and a simple diet followed, the health problem would cease in almost any abdominal organ. It was reported that abdominal diseases due to mechanical obstructions also became less threatening with the timely use of these methods, although surgery was often undertaken if tumors were present. It was also a common belief in medicine that certain abdominal problems, such as peptic ulcers, were caused by spicy foods or stress, but doctors now know that a bacterial infection or some medications—not stress or diet—cause most peptic ulcers (Mayo Clinic 2013).

Symptoms

Symptoms that can indicate a problem in the abdominal region, especially if prolonged, include the following: anemia; digestive symptoms such as nausea, bloating, and constipation; severe abdominal pain; unintended weight loss; and ongoing vomiting or diarrhea. A lump in the pelvic area may be another symptom.

Clinically, however, individuals may present to a medical professional with one or more of these symptoms, and their symptom profile may vary over time.

Causes and Risk Factors

In addition to aging, which affects the body's ability to produce digestive enzymes, poor nutrition, plus several lifestyle factors such as "eating on the run," can result in one or more long-term abdominal problems. Research shows excessive use of painkillers can cause stomach problems (Garcia Rodriguez & Hernandez-Diaz 2001). Another study showed young people who are obese or excessively overweight often have different types of functional abdominal diseases, such as constipation and irritable bowel syndrome, or diverticular disease (Pilgrim, Hart, & Speakman 2013). This suggests that there is a link between some abdominal diseases and being overweight; therefore, preventing overweight, as well as introducing factors that can reduce functional types of abdominal symptoms, may help to reduce long-term-related health problems that can affect one or more components of the abdominal tract. Anxiety, chronic stress, and adverse life events may be additional factors that cause functional abdominal disorders or increase the severity of structural disorders. Additional risk factors may include environmental factors such as food-derived cancer-causing agents, including heterocyclic amines and polycyclic aromatic hydrocarbons. These are chemicals that form when muscle meat (such as beef or chicken) is cooked using pan frying or high temperature grilling.

Diagnostic Procedures

Abdominal diseases may be diagnosed by using computer-assisted ultrasound examinations. To help in making a diagnosis, the ultrasound image is compared with a data set of standard reference images, which serves as a diagnostic assistant tool. Another tool that has shown success in the diagnosis of presumed or known diseases that affect the lower abdomen or intestine is the combined use of cinematography and magnetic resonance imaging (MRI) enteroclysis examination, which appears to provide additional findings of clinical relevance to a greater degree than when it is not used. Another is known as ileocolonoscopy, which is used as the reference standard in MRI examinations. Another involves blood sampling for nutritional deficiencies and antibodies and biopsies or removal of tissue to diagnose structural or infectious problems.

Treatments

Treatments depend on the cause of the prevailing problem and may include:

Chemotherapy for various forms of cancer
Cognitive behavioral therapy for various forms of anxiety and for obesity problems
Digestive enzyme supplementation for various genetic disorders
Medical interventions for treating various symptoms such as bloating, pain, and constipation
Nutritional education for treating eating disorders, and malnutrition, as well as obesity or overweight
Radiation therapy for treating cancer related problems of the abdominal tract
Surgical interventions for treating certain forms of cancer, ulcers, colon problems, among other conditions that do not respond to conservative treatment.

Prevention

Eating healthy foods, especially raw foods, and foods that match one's digestive capacity is recommended. Exercising daily to aid in functioning of the digestive system and to keep weight down is also recommended. Limiting video and computer time to prevent overweight, stress control, and limiting excessive alcohol intake to reduce problems of digestion related to lower impairment are recommended. Treating abdominal health conditions, if they are diagnosed, is important for preventing inadequate food consumption that can lead to underweight and its related health problems.

Future

There are currently many research projects that are aiming to understand one or more aspects of digestive diseases more comprehensively. To view these, the U.S.-based website ClinicalTrials.gov lists information on both federally and privately supported clinical trials using human volunteers. Topics include the use of drugs, surgery, chemotherapy, or a combination of these to reduce abdominal health problems.

Ray Marks

See also: Celiac Disease; Digestive Diseases; Diverticular Disease; Gall Bladder Disease; Gastroesophageal Reflux Disease (GERD); Irritable Bowel Syndrome; Pancreatic Diseases; Peptic Ulcer

Further Reading

American College of Gastroenterology. Patient Education and Resource Center. (2015). Retrieved from http://patients.gi.org/.

American Gastroenterological Association. (2015). Conditions & diseases. Retrieved from http://www.gastro.org/patient-care/conditions.

Chang, L. (2004). Review article: Epidemiology and quality of life in functional gastrointestinal disorders. *Alimentary Pharmacology & Therapeutics, 20*, 31–39.

Garcia Rodriguez, L. A., & Hernandez-Diaz, S. (2001). Relative risk of upper gastrointestinal complications among users of acetaminophen and nonsteroidal anti-inflammatory drugs. *Epidemiology, 12*, 570–576.

KidsHealth. (2015). Digestive system. Retrieved from http://kidshealth.org/teen/your_body/body_basics/digestive_system.html.

Mayo Clinic. (July 16, 2013). Peptic ulcer. Retrieved from http://www.mayoclinic.org/diseases-conditions/peptic-ulcer/basics/definition/con-20028643.

National Cancer Institute. (October 19, 2015). Chemicals in meat cooked at high temperatures and cancer risk. Retrieved from http://www.cancer.gov/about-cancer/causes-prevention/risk/diet/cooked-meats-fact-sheet.

Pilgrim, S. M., Hart, A. R., & Speakman, C. T. (2013). Diverticular disease in younger patients—is it clinically more complicated and related to obesity? *Colorectal Disease, 15*(10), 1205–1210.

Pollan, M. (2013, May 19). Some of my best friends are germs. *New York Times.* Retrieved from http://www.nytimes.com/2013/05/19/magazine/say-hello-to-the-100-trillion-bacteria-that-make-up-your-microbiome.html?pagewanted=7&_r=2&ref=magazine&pagewanted=print.

ACCEPTANCE AND COMMITMENT THERAPY

The term *acceptance and commitment therapy*, also known as ACT, was named after one of its key ideas that could be helpful to people suffering from chronic health conditions that are not reversible and may be disabling. The idea behind ACT, which is a form of behavioral therapy, is that individuals will be more successful in coping with their situations of life if they accept those situations that appear to be out of their control and, instead, try to focus on actions that can enhance and improve their lives. The developers of ACT wanted to use this idea to help humans achieve a high life quality, where individuals could maximize their potential by following the ACT steps outlines to achieving this, and believed that most situations of personal suffering are due to individuals' perpetual or excessive focus on painful personal issues and experiences or their attempts to avoid dealing with painful personal or threatening situations.

Earliest Information

Created in 1986 by Steven Hayes, there is much research today to support this psychological approach, which is an outgrowth of behavioral therapy and cognitive behavioral therapy. Another pioneer in this area, Kirk Strosahl, was one of the originators of ACT and was well known for his brief interventions and highly effective outcomes, which have since been followed or adapted by others. The approach involves commitment and acceptance in addition to more traditional behavior change therapies and plans and focuses on increasing one's psychological flexibility and one's awareness of their thoughts and actions. Since 1996, about 20 studies have supported the benefits of ACT in clinical trials. The acronym ACT has been used to describe the concepts of this form of therapy where A = acceptance of life's hardships, C = choosing to behave in ways that are aligned with one's motivating values, and T = taking action to accomplish one's goals in the face of unpleasant emotions or psychological associations.

Current Application

Today, counselors and others who apply ACT to help their clients deal with challenging life issues frequently focus their therapies on helping individuals develop skills to deal with painful thoughts and feelings. They also try to help individuals reframe their beliefs, focus on issues of value to them, or help them identify these values, so those values and issues can be used as a target for setting positive goals that can change their lives for the better.

One feature of ACT is the use of an approach to increasing one's ability to cope with challenging situations, called *mindfulness*. Being *mindful* involves being aware, focused, and open, and this approach is believed to permit more positive affirmative actions and behaviors to be carried out than denial, or inattention to one's painful challenges. The state of *mindfulness* can be achieved in different ways, and one key way is through meditation. Another is by taking a step-by-step approach to letting go of painful beliefs or thoughts, allowing these feelings to exist without struggle, focusing more on the present moment and its positive elements, and being aware of surrounding stimuli and situations.

ACT is thus a new method of trying to change one's thoughts and deal more effectively with one or more challenging or upsetting situations. It can be delivered in the form of ultra-brief therapy, a brief intervention, or a medium- or long-term therapy program, depending on the problem. It can be used by a student, coach, client, patient, therapist, or health professional. It can be adapted to suit the needs of the individual and can also be used to influence groups or organizations. By following the ACT way of thinking and doing, it likely that individuals can improve their life quality—as well as their sense of vitality, well-being, and fulfillment. If practiced actively in everyday life, acceptance and commitment therapy can be highly effective for the treatment of obsessive compulsive disorder, depression, anxiety disorders, substance abuse, chronic pain, post-traumatic stress syndrome, at-risk adolescents, anorexia, terminal cancers, and even schizophrenia. For example, in individuals who experience chronic pain, results of one recent study showed ACT can help chronic pain sufferers, both young and old, without addictive or debilitating medications.

Acceptance and commitment therapy is a third-generation, or modern, form of cognitive-behavioral therapy and analysis and can potentially be of significant benefit in helping people with chronic illnesses—such as stroke, chronic heart and respiratory diseases, diabetes, obesity, epilepsy, and various forms of arthritis—to have a better quality of life and functional capacity in the absence of any medical cure for any of these illnesses but where stress, distress, anxiety, and depression may be quite common. It can also help these individuals with chronic physical diseases to meet their needs more ably. It is different from other more traditional forms of behavior therapy because it focuses on thoughts and whether they are true or not, rather than trying to reduce them, and then stresses the person's own inner values and encourages behaviors that are supportive of these values. The principle of mindfulness is important in ACT, and the focus is on controlling some forms of behavior that can be changed for the better, such as breathing in a normal way rather than in a rapid way when a thought or feeling seems to be causing this type of emotional reaction to occur regularly. The ACT approach is based on the idea that individuals can control some of their own behaviors and reactions without first having to change their feelings or thoughts or eliminating these thoughts. Individuals can thus observe and acknowledge their feelings but still act to accept these feelings and modify some of the reactions that are not helpful to their well-being by choosing to behave in ways that are aligned with their values, despite the presence of negative emotions. By doing this, they can potentially overcome negative thoughts, find ways of carrying out empowering behaviors, and have a more fulfilled life.

The six core processes in ACT, used to help achieve a rich meaningful life, are summarized here:

Contacting—actively connecting with what is happening in the present.

Defusion—letting go of painful thoughts and distancing yourself from them while trying to be an observer of your thoughts, rather than a victim of your thoughts.

Acceptance—accepting your feelings, giving them space and letting them be there, but not letting them become excessive or self-limiting.

Observance—observing yourself and becoming aware of your thoughts and beliefs.

Values—thinking about what matters most and reframing thoughts and behaviors accordingly. Identifying what you want to be remembered for.

Committed action—carrying out actions that are aligned with your goals and deepest values, even if this is not easy or straightforward, and being fully "present" in this process.

Ray Marks

See also: Anxiety Disorders; Chronic Disease Management; Depression; Obsessive Compulsive Disorder; Post-Traumatic Stress Disorder (PTSD); Schizophrenia; Substance Abuse

Further Reading

Acceptance and Commitment Therapy Introduction. (2015). Retrieved from www.drluoma .com/ACT.html.

Association for Contextual Behavioral Sciences. (2015). About ACT. Retrieved from http:// contextualpsychology.org/about_act.

Carrasco, J. (2013). Acceptance and commitment therapy. GoodTherapy.org. Retrieved from http://www.goodtherapy.org/acceptance-commitment-therapy.html.

Dewane, C. (2008). The ABC's of ACT—acceptance and commitment therapy, *Social Work Today, 8*, 36.

Harris, R. (August 2006). Embracing your demons: An overview of acceptance and commitment therapy. *Psychotherapy in Australia, 12*.

Hayes, S., Luoma, J. B., Bond, F. W., Masuda, A., & Lillis, J. (2006). Acceptance and commitment therapy (ACT): Models, processes, and outcomes. *Behaviour Research and Therapy, 44*, 1–25.

ACCESS TO HEALTH SERVICES

Health care can be thought of as involving the diagnosis, treatment, and prevention of disease, illness, injury, and other physical and mental impairments in individuals through services provided by medical or allied health care professionals (*American Heritage Dictionary of the English Language*). Therefore, access to health services can be thought of as having adequate, appropriate time with a health care professional or organization to monitor one's health and provide recommendations for both wellness screenings and treatment regimens in a timely fashion (National Research Council 1993). Health care is generally thought of as a crucial component in determining the health and well-being of populations. Despite this, access to health services varies across countries, within countries, and across individuals and is influenced by a number of factors. For example, most global organizations or governments have limited resources available to meet the health care needs of their populations. Priorities regarding access are set depending on the goals and needs of the population.

Historically, access to care was not dependent on whether one had health insurance. Visits to health care professionals were done on a fee-for-service basis; one paid the provider directly for the care provided. For the most part, these visits tended to be relatively inexpensive. The historical barriers to access to care have not changed much in that individuals without the money to pay their care out-of-pocket would most likely seek help at a clinic or hospital setting, where they were expected to pay less. This has stayed the same in today's health care. However, as the advent of managed care plans and other health insurance plans increased, access to health care services in the United States has become dependent on whether an individual has had health insurance or not, and many studies have demonstrated that not having health insurance is one of the major factors in determining access to health services (Andrulis, 1998; Ross, Bradley, & Bush 2006). However, access to high-quality health services alone requires more than just having health insurance. This is because there is a growing trend to view access as also including the availability of services, the actual utilization of health services, and the financing (or afford-ability) and quality of services received. Any of these factors can affect an individual's overall access to quality care. As well, even if individuals have health insurance, individuals may not have access to appropriate health services resources because they may also not be able to navigate the system appropriately due to other factors such as low health literacy, economic issues, educational barriers and social or cultural factors.

There are significant cost implications associated with poor access to health services for both individuals and society. Multiple studies have demonstrated that there are economic costs associated with poor access (National Research Council 2001). Individuals without access also tend to have poorer health outcomes, are less likely to follow screening guidelines, and ultimately have greater medical expenditures in the long term. Early screening and, consequently, early detection lead to better outcomes in most cases. Although not having health insurance is not the only factor involved in accessing health services, it is certainly one that cannot be ignored. Studies have found that individuals without health insurance are seven times more likely to skip medical care for cost reasons (Adams, Vickerie, & Kirzinger 2011). Within the United States, according to a 2010 national survey, it was estimated that about 50 million (or one in four) adults ages 18 to 64 went without health insurance during the past year and about 30 million (or one in six) went without health insurance for at least a year or longer (Adams et al. 2011).

Some may argue that providing health insurance to all people is not necessarily a strategy to aim for when trying to improve the access of care for all individuals. Research shows that even in countries that have implemented a national health care plan guaranteeing insurance for everyone, there are still discrepancies in who actually has access to health services. That is, universal health insurance does reduce many disparities in access to health services, but not all (Lasser, Himmelstein, & Woolhandler 2006). Some of the issues that create barriers to access in Canada are long waiting times for services and immigrants not utilizing screening resources as often as other groups. Despite having insurance, factors that are based on organizational, social, and cultural factors may play a larger role in determining access. Strategies that involve addressing these barriers may make a bigger impact than just providing health insurance.

In addition, the literature recommends that other strategies be included to start addressing the needs of individuals in today's society. People are living longer and, as a result, are living with chronic conditions rather than acute conditions. According to estimates, 40 percent of the entire U.S. population is living with one or more chronic illnesses (National Research Council 2009). Having access to health care is crucial to prevent complications due to chronic diseases and premature mortality.

However, the current health care system in the United States is still focused on acute care according to the Institute of Medicine (National Research Council 2001).

Health service strategies should provide individuals with the resources needed to deal with their chronic conditions, including treatment and early screening guidance. Finally, strategies that accommodate and account for demographic factors should certainly not be ignored. Taking into account an individual's social, ethnic, racial, cultural, and economic situation should also be embedded in strategies related to improving access to health care. As the cost of health care continues to skyrocket without any end in sight, discussion has turned to providing appropriate solutions to the health care crisis in the United States. One such effort is the idea of federally supported medical care, which President Obama enacted into law in 2010 under the Affordable Care Act and which went into effect after a rocky start in 2013. Specifically, this act reforms specific aspects of both private and public health insurance industry and expands access to insurance to more than 30 million Americans (U.S. Department of Health and Human Services 2015). The act is under fire by Republican lawmakers in Congress and by potential 2016 Republican presidential candidates.

Rachel Torres

See also: Adherence; Family Health; Health; Health Literacy; Healthy People 2020; Minorities, Chronic Disease; Prevention; School Wellness Programs; Self-Management; Social Health; Wellness; World Health Organization

Further Reading

Adams, P. F., Martinez, M. E., Vickerie, J. L., & Kirzinger, W. K. (2011). Summary health statistics for the U.S. population: National Health Interview Survey, 2010. National Center for Health Statistics. *Vital Health Statistics, 10*, 251.

American Heritage Dictionary of the English Language. (2007.) "Health care." Retrieved from https://ahdictionary.com/word/search.html?q=health+care.

Andrulis, D. P. (1998). Access to care is the centerpiece in the elimination of socioeconomic disparities in health. *Annals of Internal Medicine, 129*, 412–416.

Lasser, K. E., Himmelstein, D. U., & Woolhandler, S. (2006). Access to care, health status, and health disparities in the United States and Canada: Results of a cross-national population-based survey. *American Journal of Public Health, 96*(7), 300–307.

National Research Council. (1993). *Access to Health Care in America.* Washington, DC: The National Academies Press.

National Research Council. (2001). *Crossing the Quality Chasm: A New Health System for the 21st Century.* Washington, DC: The National Academies Press.

National Research Council. (2009). *America's Uninsured Crisis: Consequences for Health and Health Care.* Washington, DC: The National Academies Press.

Ross, J. S., Bradley, E. H., & Busch, S. H. (2006). Use of health care services by lower-income and higher-income uninsured adults. *JAMA, 295*(17), 2027–2036.

U.S. Department of Health and Human Services. (2015). Key features of the Affordable Care Act. Retrieved from http://www.hhs.gov/healthcare/facts-and-features/key-features-of-aca/index.html.

ADDISON'S DISEASE

Overview

Addison's disease is a chronic health condition where the adrenal glands—small glands that are located on top of each kidney—that produce life-supporting hormones do not function adequately. It can be life threatening due to lack of sufficient hormones produced by the adrenal glands. The three key hormones that are involved in Addison's disease, also termed *primary adrenal insufficiency* (AI) or *hypocortisolism*, and that result from disease of the adrenal gland or damage to the outer portion of the adrenal gland known as the cortex are:

a. Glucocorticoid hormones
b. Mineralcorticoid hormones
c. Sex hormones

The glucocorticoid hormones such as cortisol:

- Help maintain appropriate sugar levels in the form of blood glucose
- Help suppress the immune system's inflammatory responses
- Help the body to respond to stress
- Help maintain blood pressure and cardiovascular function
- Help regulate protein, fat, and carbohydrate metabolism.

Mineralcorticoids such as aldosterone regulate the sodium and potassium balance of the body and help to maintain blood pressure, water, and salt balance of the body.

Sex hormones such as androgen and estrogen affect sexual development and sex drive in men and women, respectively.

When damage is sustained by the adrenal cortex, output of these hormones can be reduced, especially the hormone cortisol, and the health condition that follows is termed Addison's disease. This disease is important because it currently affects one to four persons out of 100,000, regardless of age or gender. Its onset is often gradual, but it may occur suddenly and prove fatal.

There are two forms of Addison's disease. If the problem lies within the adrenal glands themselves, it is termed *primary adrenal insufficiency*. If the adrenal glands are affected by a problem starting elsewhere—the condition is termed *secondary adrenal insufficiency*.

History

When English physician Dr. Thomas Addison (1793–1860) first described this disease in London in 1855, in his classic paper entitled *On the Constitutional and Local Effects of Disease of the Supra-Renal Capsules,* the most common cause was tuberculosis (TB). This remained the leading cause until the middle of the 20th century when antibiotics reduced the incidence of TB.

Symptoms

Symptoms usually develop slowly over several months and can include:

    Appetite and weight loss
    Changes in blood pressure or heart rate
    Chronic fatigue
    Depression and irritability
    Diarrhea
    Extreme weakness
    Headache
    Irregular or no menstrual cycle in women
    Loss of appetite
    Low blood glucose and blood pressure
    Mouth sores
    Muscle and joint pain
    Muscle weakness
    Nausea or vomiting
    Paleness
    Skin hyperpigmentation
    Sow sluggish movement
    Sweating
    Unintentional weight loss

On occasion, an acute adrenal failure (Addisonian crisis) can occur, and the signs and symptoms may also include:

    Pain in the lower back, abdomen or legs
    Severe vomiting and diarrhea, leading to dehydration
    Low blood pressure
    Loss of consciousness
    High potassium (hyperkalemia)

Causes

As a result of the reduction of the incidence of tuberculosis in people, the major cause of Addison's disease has been from an autoimmune reaction in which the body's immune system mistakenly attacks cells of the adrenal cortex and slowly destroys them, a process that can take months to years.

According to Dr. Paul Margulies, writing as medical director for the National Adrenal Diseases Foundation (2007), there are also several less common causes of Addison's disease: other chronic infections besides tuberculosis, especially certain fungal infections; invasion of the adrenal by cancer cells that have spread from another part of the body, especially the breast; the CMV virus in association with AIDS; rarely, hemorrhage into the adrenals during shock; and the surgical removal of both adrenals.

Other key causes include amyloidosis or the buildup of abnormal or misfolded proteins that form deposits in various organs and tissues such as the brain, heart and kidney anticoagulant usage, genetic defects, pituitary gland problems such as tumors, stress, surgical removal of the hypothalamus, and trauma.

Secondary causes may include abrupt or gradual cessation of medications such as prednisone; loss of blood flow to the pituitary gland; radiation treatment of the pituitary gland; surgical removal of non-cancerous pituitary gland tumors; and surgical removal of the hypothalamus.

A diagnosis of Addison's disease is usually made based on medical history and laboratory tests and radiographs.

Diagnostic Tools

Diagnostic tools include the following:

- Abdominal or chest x-rays.
- Abdominal CT scans or MRI.
- ACTH stimulation test to see how hormone levels react to stress.
- Lab tests, including blood and urine tests, to evaluate a patient's electrolyte balance, glucose level, and kidney function. During an adrenal crisis, lab tests can help determine the severity of the imbalances and to monitor treatment effectiveness.
- Medical history, where the symptoms of hyperpigmentation, weakness, low blood pressure, and salt cravings may cause a doctor to suspect adrenal insufficiency, especially if these symptoms appear to worsen during periods of stress.
- Skin tests.

Treatments and Outcomes

Treatment options include replacement of the hormones that are not being produced, along with intravenous injections of saline and dextrose.

According to Dr. Margulies (2007), as long as the proper dose of replacement medication is taken daily, an "Addisonian" (someone with Addison's disease) can have a normal, crisis-free life with no physical or social restrictions.

Routine care should include regular physician visits, avoidance of dehydration, and the use of extra medication during illness. "Pregnancy is possible, but will require extra monitoring of the replacement medication. Every Addisonian should wear an identification bracelet or preferably a necklace stating that he or she has the disease, to insure proper emergency treatment. An identification card outlining treatment is also suggested. Today, people with Addison's disease should have a normal life expectancy" (Margulies 2007).

Future

Novel research at the Children's Hospital in Boston focuses on developing cell-based therapies using stem cell technology to optimize the replacement of missing hormones that cause conditions like Addison's disease. This research includes searching for tissue stem cells within the adrenal gland itself that may be useful for treating adrenal insufficiency or potentially using embryonic stem cells that may one day be converted into steroid-producing cells.

Another study is looking at the genetic factors underlying Addison's disease and the risk of the disease to family members of people with Addison's disease.

Ray Marks

See also: Adrenal Diseases; Chronic Disease Management; Immune System Disorders

Further Reading

Addison, T. (1855). *On the Constitutional and Local Effects of Disease of the Supra-renal Capsules.* London, UK: Samuel Highley.

Adrenal insufficiency and Addison's disease. (2011). Retrieved from http://endocrine.niddk.nih.gov/pubs/addison/addison.htm.

Boston Children's Hospital. (2012). Addison's disease. Retrieved from http://www.childrenshospital.org/az/Site1680/mainpageS1680P5.html.

Lab Tests on Line. (2012). Adrenal insufficiency and Addison's disease. Retrieved from http://labtestsonline.org/understanding/conditions/addisons-disease/?start=0.

Margulies, P. (2007). What is Addison's disease? National Adrenal Diseases Foundation. Retrieved from http://www.nadf.us/diseases/addisons.htm.

Mayo Clinic. (2012). Addison's disease. Retrieved from http://www.mayoclinic.com/health/addisons-disease/DS00361/METHOD=print.

MedlinePlus. U.S. National Library of Medicine. National Institutes of Health. (2011). Addison's disease. Retrieved from htpp://nlm.nih.gov/medlineplus/ency/article/000378.htm.

Munver, R., & Volfson, I. A. (2006). Adrenal insufficiency: Diagnosis and management. *Current Urology Reports, 7*, 80–85.

NADF (National Addison's Diseases Foundation). (2007). Retrieved from http://www.nadf.us/index.htm.

Patient Education. (2012). Managing adrenal insufficiency. Clinical Center. National Institutes of Health. Retrieved from http://www.cc.nih.gov/ccc/patient_education/pepubs/mngadrins.pdf.

ADHERENCE

Overview

Adherence is commonly referred to as the extent to which individuals are able to follow directions or guidelines from their health care professional. The World Health Organization formally defines adherence as "the extent to which a person's behavior—taking medication, following a diet, and/or executing lifestyle changes, corresponds with agreed recommendations from a health care provider" (World Health Organization 2003). Historically, adherence was defined as compliance. However, because the definition of compliance, or noncompliance, was not really an accurate picture of what was actually happening with patients, the term currently used is adherence (Aronson 2007). The term takes away the blame, usually associated with noncompliance, and just indicates that the patient was unable to follow through with the treatment. As the prevalence of chronic diseases increases, it is important to know how individuals are responding or acting on their treatment guidelines as well as what barriers are preventing them from fully adhering to recommendations. Health care systems around the world, and particularly in the United States, are moving toward a system that requires more direct involvement from the patient in following the prescribed treatments of their health care professionals.

Types of Adherence

Because there may be differences in how individuals follow medication guidelines versus medical screenings, many experts choose to distinguish the different types of activities related to adherence into two categories: (1) wellness and screening adherence and (2) medication and treatment adherence (What is adherence?, (n.d.). Wellness and screening adherence often includes programs that improve wellness such as smoking cessation, weight management, or general stress management. These types of programs are geared toward healthy individuals or individuals who may be considered "at-risk" (What is adherence?, (n.d.), including those who may have risk factors for a particular disease or even have a medical condition or symptoms they are unaware of or are ignoring. By taking part in screening guidelines as recommended by various health care organizations, these individuals may become aware of a medical condition in its earliest stages.

The next level of adherence is known as medication and treatment adherence. It includes following health care professionals' recommendations for medications, follow-up care, treatments, etc. Taking medication as directed may prevent the diseases or conditions from further spreading or worsening. The costs associated with treatment at this stage are much lower than when the disease has progressed. This approach of treating diseases early is well documented although, in reality, most people do not follow the guidelines. According to the World Health Organization, it is estimated that only about 50 percent of patients in developed countries follow treatment recommendations for chronic diseases (World Health Organization 2003). Studies have demonstrated that patients with chronic illnesses experience difficulty in following their recommended treatment regimens. For example, take the recommendations of the American Diabetes Association: In addition to taking their medication on regular basis, a diabetic patient may also need to be aware of other issues such as dietary restrictions, monitoring of their glucose levels, foot care, and eye examinations (Beckles et al. 1998).

Adherence Issues

Adherence issues are present in any situation where patients are required to monitor their own treatment. These issues can be placed in one of five categories: patient-related factors, provider factors, health care system factors, social and economic factors, and the characteristics of the particular disease and its therapies (World Health Organization 2003). Most of the research on adherence has been done in the area of patient-related factors. It is hard to refute the fact that many patients experience difficulties in following treatment or screening recommendations.

Patient-related factors include those that are under direct control of the patient. Factors that are often included are taking medication correctly, side effects from medications, self-management of treatment, and scheduling issues (such as shift work or traveling away from home). Finally, patient factors also include knowledge, attitudes, beliefs, self-efficacy or confidence, and expectations of the individual. In addition, *health literacy*, defined by the National Institutes of Health (NIH) as "the degree to which individuals have the capacity to obtain, process, and understand basic health information and services needed to make appropriate health decisions" (National Institutes of Health 2000) also points to the idea that patient factors can determine how an individual responds to treatment issues. However, it is important to recognize that patient-related factors are also affected by a number of other factors that are beyond the control of the patient.

Social and economic factors may also play an important role in adherence. Issues such as low level of education, poor or unstable living conditions, poverty, and low socioeconomic status could adversely affect an individual's ability to adhere to treatment regimens. Poor adherence does seem to affect all age groups but is certainly more prevalent in the elderly population (Jernigan 1984). Other studies also point to the important role that organizational variables such as provider factors or health care system factors have in treatment adherence (Albaz 1997). Factors that address the environment in which patients receive their care may play a large role in their adherence rates. How a health care system operates, the accessibility to the population, the way that services are provided, and how the health care providers deliver treatment are also issues that can play a large role in whether a patient is successful in adhering to treatment regimens.

Implications

Health care costs are skyrocketing. In fact, health care expenditures were predicted to exceed $3 trillion by 2013 (Heffler et al. 2002). Adherence to screening guidelines will increase our efforts in primary prevention by reducing risk factors, and following treatment guidelines will reduce the burden of chronic illnesses on both individuals and society. Most strategies to improve adherence have been geared toward the patient. Early research studies demonstrate interventions directly involved with how the patient "complied" with treatments. If the patient did not comply, the intervention was considered unsuccessful. Many of the current research studies have focused on factors that may affect patient-related factors and have determined that it may be a combination of several factors, each addressing one of the particular five areas. While many of the named factors affect adherence, there is also research that demonstrates that focusing on just one of the five factors does not greatly increase adherence.

Rachel Torres

See also: Access to Health Services; Health; Health Literacy; Healthy People 2020; Self-Management; Wellness; World Health Organization

Further Reading

Albaz, R. S. (1997). Factors affecting patient compliance in Saudi Arabia. *Journal of Social Science*, 25, 5–8.

Aronson, J. K. (2007). Compliance, concordance, and adherence. *British Journal of Clinical Pharmacology*, 63(4), 383–384.

Beckles, G. L., Engelgau, M. M., Narayan, K. M., Herman, W. H., Aubert, R. E., & Williamson, D. F. (1998). Population-based assessment of the level of care among adults with diabetes in the U.S. Diabetes Care, 21(9), 1432–1438.

Burt, V. L., Whelton, P., Roccella, E. J., Brown, C., Cutler, J. A., Higgins, M., Horan, M. J., & Labarthe, D. (1995). Prevalence of hypertension in the U.S. adult population. Results from the third national health and nutrition examination survey, 1988–1991. *Hypertension*, 25(3), 305–313.

Dekker, F. W., Dieleman, F. E., Kaptein, A. A., & Mulder, J. D. (1993). Compliance with pulmonary medication in general practice. *European Respiratory Journal, 6*, 886–890.

Heffler, S., Smith, S., Won, G., Clemens, M. K., Keehan, S., Zeeza, M., et al. (2002). Health spending projections for 2001–2011: The latest outlook. *Health Affairs, 21*(2), 207–218.

Jernigan, J.A. (1984). Update on drugs and the elderly. *American Family Physician, 29*, 238–247.

National Institutes of Health. (2000). *Current Bibliographies in Medicine: Health Literacy* (DHHS Publication No. CBM 2000-1). Bethesda, MD: National Institutes of Health. Available from: http://www.nlm.nih.gov/pubs/cbm/hliteracy.html.

What is adherence? (n.d.). Retrieved from http://purpleteal.com/pdf/Articlesadherence.pdf.

World Health Organization. (2003). Adherence to long-term therapies. Geneva, Switzerland. Retrieved from http://apps.who.int/iris/bitstream/10665/42682/1/9241545992.pdf.

ADOLESCENCE AND CHRONIC DISEASE

Adolescence is defined as the state or process of growing up, a stage of development which preceded maturity, and the period of life from puberty to maturity. The word adolescence is derived from the Latin word adolescere, which means growing up. Theoretically, this stage exists between childhood and adulthood and is often referred to as the teenage years. The term adolescence was first used in the 15th century yet not recognized until the 20th century (*Merriam-Webster's Dictionary* 2011). Adolescence can be affected by and introduce chronic diseases.

Historical Perspectives

Considered a pioneer in the fields of psychology and education, G. Stanley Hall (1844–1924) was the first to delve into the subject of adolescence (Hall 2012). Darwin's theory of evolution greatly influenced Hall's work; Hall believed that behavior and early physical development followed evolutionary changes and that each person develops according to his or her record of ancestry. Hall believed that a child, therefore, goes through several stages of growth, which are similar to those of animals. Hall believed that at the time of adolescence, any evolutionary influences subside and this becomes a time of individuality to emerge. During Hall's research and writing on adolescence, he was greatly influenced by German writers and musicians of the 18th century, who advocated complete freedom of expression. Reflecting this key influence, Hall referred to adolescence as a time of emotional upset and rebellion, with behavior that ranged from a quiet moodiness to extreme risk taking. He also considered adolescence as a time when there is heightened increase in senses, risk taking for new sensations, and lack of tolerance for any routine or monotony. Because of this time of increased sensitivity, self-consciousness, and being critical of self and others, Hall believed that adolescents were susceptible to depression. Despite the difficulties of adolescence, Hall also believed that adolescence was a time of new beginnings as a more civilized, more developed, higher-order human being emerges.

Current Perspectives

Many of Hall's tenets are reflected in current research and have been further developed to include more detailed descriptions. For example, the current definition of adolescence is similar to that of Hall's findings as the teenage years between 10 and 20, yet with increasing rates of early onset puberty, the preteen or "tween" years (ages 9 to 12) may also qualify as adolescence (*Psychology Today* 2016). The American Academy of Pediatrics roughly divided adolescence into three stages: early adolescence, generally ages twelve and thirteen; middle adolescence, ages fourteen to sixteen; and late adolescence, ages seventeen to twenty-one (American Academy of Pediatrics 2015). There appears to be growing recognition that adolescence is not easily confined to set ages and stresses that there is a wide range of what is considered normal adolescent ages (Kids Health 2015).

Looking at the biological development of adolescence, science is seeing it as a time of transition in terms of how the brain and body as well as the psyche develop (Roizen & Oz 2011). Also called puberty, adolescence is the time in which a child's sexual and physical characteristics mature, which occurs due to hormone changes. Current research delves deeper into the study of adolescent development as reflected in the identification of gender differences and biological processes, such as brain development. While the exact age a child enters puberty depends on a number of different things, such as genes, nutrition, and gender, during puberty, endocrine glands produce hormones that cause body changes and the development of secondary sex characteristics. In girls, the ovaries begin to increase production of estrogen and other female hormones, while in boys, the testicles increase production of testosterone. Changes in both males and females during adolescence include the production of hormones from the adrenal glands that cause increased armpit sweating, body odor, acne, and armpit and pubic hair. This process is called adrenarche. Breast development is the main sign that a girl is entering puberty, with the first menstrual period (menarche) usually following within about two years. Before the first menstrual period, a girl will normally have an increase in height and hip size; vaginal secretions; and pubic, armpit, and leg hair growth. Puberty for a girl is usually finished by age 17, yet her educational and emotional maturities continue to grow. For a boy, the first sign of puberty is enlargement of both testicles. Afterward, boys will normally experience faster growth, especially height; hair growth under the arms, on the face, and in the pubic area; increased shoulder width; growth of the genitals; nighttime ejaculations; and voice changes (Marcell 2007).

Adolescence and Chronic Illness

Similar to Hall's research is the current description of adolescence as time of both disorientation and discovery. Between being considered a child and not yet an adult, adolescents struggle with issues of independence and self-identity. Because of the increased importance of peer groups, there may be experimentation with drugs and alcohol or sexuality. About 2 million adolescents (6 percent of persons aged 10 to 18) in the United States have a chronic health condition that results in limitation of daily activities or disability. The most common of these conditions are asthma and other chronic respiratory tract diseases, diabetes, musculoskeletal disorders, and heart disease. Mental health problems, such as depression, are a leading cause of disability in this age group, as are speech, hearing, and visual impairments (Neinstein 2001).

Current Research and Implications

Pictures of the brain in action show that adolescents' brains function differently than adults when making decisions and solving problems. Their actions are guided more by the amygdale, which is responsible for instinctual reactions, including fear and aggressive behavior, and less by the frontal cortex, the area of the brain that controls reasoning and helps us think before we act, which develops later. This part of the brain is still changing and maturing well into adulthood. Research has also demonstrated that exposure to drugs and alcohol before birth, head trauma, or other types of brain injury can interfere with normal brain development during adolescence. Other specific changes in the brain during adolescence include a rapid increase in the connections between the brain cells and refinement of brain pathways. Nerve cells develop myelin, an insulating layer that helps cells communicate. All these changes are essential for the development of coordinated thought, action, and behavior. An adolescent's brain develops in a way to foster concrete to metaphoric or abstract thinking. Based on the stage of their brain development, adolescents are more likely to act on impulse, misread or misinterpret social cues and emotions, get involved in fights, and engage in dangerous or risky behavior. Adolescents are less likely to think before they act, pause to consider the potential consequences of their actions, and modify their dangerous or inappropriate behaviors. These brain differences don't mean that young people can't make good decisions or tell the difference between right and wrong. It also doesn't mean that they shouldn't be held responsible for their actions. An awareness of these differences can help parents, teachers, advocates, and policy makers understand, anticipate, and manage the behavior of adolescents. An adolescent is a person newly dealing with intense physical and social changes (American Academy of Child and Adolescent Psychiatry 2015).

To prepare for the adolescent years, education is important. For parents, thinking back on their own teen years, remembering their struggles or their embarrassment at their physical development rate, expecting some mood changes in their typically happy child, and being prepared for more conflict as he or she matures as an individual will aid this time of transition. Both parents and children who know what's coming can cope with it better. In addition to physiological growth, intellectual, psychological, and social developmental tasks are squeezed into these few years. The fundamental purpose of these tasks is to form one's own identity and to prepare for adulthood. The management of teens with a chronic illness must go beyond the strictly medical; it should include addressing issues such as development, family and social support, substance use, and reproductive health. For those adolescents dealing with chronic disease, primary care practitioners, as well as parents, have important roles to play as active team members in educating and empowering adolescents to manage as much of their chronic disease as they are capable of doing.

Karen Jeanne Coleman

See also: Childhood Cancer; Childhood Overweight; Chronic Disease Management; Diet and Nutrition; Eating Disorders; Family Health; Healthy Lifestyles and Risky Behaviors; Obsessive Compulsive Disorder; Physical Activity; School Wellness Programs; Social Health; Vaccines

Further Reading

American Academy of Child and Adolescent Psychiatry. (2011). Teen brain and decision making. Retrieved from https://www.aacap.org/AACAP/Families_and_Youth/Facts_for_Families/FFF-Guide/The-Teen-Brain-Behavior-Problem-Solving-and-Decision-Making-095.aspx.

American Academy of Child and Adolescent Psychiatry. (2015). Normal adolescent development part 1. Retrieved from https://www.aacap.org/AACAP/Families_and_Youth/Facts_for_Families/FFF-Guide/Normal-Adolescent-Development-Part-I-057.aspx.

American Academy of Pediatrics. (2015). Stages of adolescence. Retrieved from http://www.healthychildren.org/English/ages-stages/teen/Pages/Stages-of-Adolescence

Bashe, P., & Greydanus, D., ed. (2003). *American Academy of Pediatrics Caring for Your Teenager*, 2nd ed. New York, NY: Bantam.

Hall, G. S. (2012). Adolescence is a new birth. In The Psychology Book, edited by Sam Atkinson and Sarah Tomley, 46–47. London: DK.

Kids Health. (2015). A parent's guide to surviving the teen years. Retrieved from http://kidshealth.org/parent/growth/growing/adolescence.html#.

Marcell, A. V. (2007). Adolescence. In Nelson Textbook of Pediatrics, 18th ed., edited by R. M. Kliegman, R. E. Behrman, H. B. Jenson, & B. F. Stanton. Philadelphia, PA: Saunders Elsevier.

Merriam-Webster's Dictionary. (2011). "Adolescence." Retrieved from webster.com/dictionary/adolescence.

Neinstein, L. (2001). Treatment of adolescents with chronic illnesses. *Western Journal of Medicine,* 175(5): 293–295. Retrieved from http://www.ncbi.nlm.nih.gov/pmc/articles/PMC1071594.

Psychology Today. (2016). Adolescence. Retrieved from http://www.psychologytoday.com /basics/adolescence.

Roizen, M. F., & Oz., M. C. (2011). You: The Owner's Manual for Teens. New York: Free Press.

ADRENAL DISEASES

Background

Aging, diseases associated with aging, as well as other factors can cause adrenal diseases due to changes in the hormone levels produced by the adrenal glands.

The Adrenal Glands

The two adrenal glands that can be affected by chronic diseases or can contribute to the development of adrenal disease and other chronic health conditions are located on the top of each kidney, where they are normally responsible for producing and/or delivering essential hormones into the bloodstream. The structure of each adrenal gland is fairly complex, consisting of an outer shell or cortex and an inner portion termed the *medulla* that is divided into different divisions. Each division is responsible for producing different hormones.

The adrenal cortex manufactures steroid hormones such as cortisol, testosterone, estrogen, aldosterone, and progesterone among other key and intermediate hormones. Aldosterone, cortisone, and hydrocortisone are manufactured solely in the adrenal gland, and cortisone helps the body to use sugar and protein for energy; decreases the immune response; and helps the body recover from illnesses, infections, and other stresses. Aldosterone is involved in the control of the sodium/ potassium and water balance of the body in conjunction with kidney function. Along with the other hormones, it helps regulate stress responses, body fluid balance, and blood pressure. The medulla is responsible for manufacturing adrenaline and noradrenalin, important hormones that influence one's capability to deal effectively with acute stress or stressors. The two disorders most often associated with dysfunction of the adrenal glands are Addison's disease and Cushing's syndrome. Another condition that affects the function of the adrenal glands is known as adrenal fatigue, and all can cause adrenal insufficiency (AI).

In people with one of these conditions, there are commonly inadequate levels of the key hormones manufactured by the adrenal glands, such cortisone and aldosterone. In AI, there is usually a low level of cortisol, but there may also be a low level of aldosterone . When AI is present, it may be temporary, but if it is not responsive to treatment, the condition may become permanent.

Adrenal Insufficiency or Addison's Disease

Adrenal insufficiency can also be categorized as either primary or secondary. Primary AI is known as Addison's disease. Secondary AI occurs when the pituitary gland in the brain fails to produce enough adrenocorticotrophin hormone (ACTH), and this causes the adrenal glands to shrink. Some causes of temporary AI include infections, medications, medication nonadherence, and surgeries, such as pituitary gland tumor surgery for Cushing's disease or adrenal tumor removal. Permanent causes of AI include Addison's disease, usually due to a problem in the immune system and the presence of an autoimmune disease such as Type I diabetes; congenital adrenal hyperplasia (CAH) that occurs in childhood; surgical removal of the pituitary gland or the adrenal glands; or damage to the adrenal glands from infections such as HIV, tuberculosis, or fungal infections.

Cushing's Syndrome

In contrast to Addison's disease, Cushing's syndrome, another adrenal disease, results from overproduction of cortisol, or from excess use of cortisol based medications. The disease commonly results in:

Anxiety
Central obesity
Depression
High blood pressure
High blood sugar
Irritability
Decreased sexual desire and lowered fertility in men
Round reddish moonlike facial features
Severe fatigue
Weak muscles
Excessive hair growth in women

Adrenal Fatigue

In adrenal fatigue, the adrenal glands are usually overstressed, which leads to a decrease in the body's hormonal supply. This can weaken the immune system, and alter blood sugar metabolism. Individuals with this condition can feel weak, fatigued, and run down. Sleep patterns can also be disrupted.

Testing for Adrenal Disease

If there is some indication the adrenal glands are not functioning adequately, it is important to have this investigated because one's body cannot function without these hormones, and medication approaches to treatment are very limited and not without risk. This can be done by measuring the levels of the hormones produced by the adrenal gland through blood and urine samples. Another test, which involves injecting substances into the body and examining the body's reaction to these substances, can be conducted by a suitable qualified medical practitioner. One such test is called the adrenocorticotrophin hormone (ACTH) challenge test, where the body's reaction to this hormone is measured. Additional tests that may be necessary to arrive at an accurate diagnosis include injecting very highly concentrated corticosteroids into the body and measuring the bodies reaction to this; imaging studies, such as magnetic resonance imaging (MRI) and x-rays; or arteriography among others.

Treatments for Adrenal Disease

All treatments should be supervised by a physician and may differ depending on the type of disease present.

For Adrenal Insufficiency or Addison's Disease:

Medications such as replacement corticosteroids will control the symptoms of this disease.

Natural supplements—for example, dehydroepiandrosterone (DHEA), licorice, L-theanine found in green tea—or vitamin B5 or pantothenic acid may be recommended by some practitioners.

Prevention and Prognosis

As with any evidence of adrenal insufficiency, if Addison's disease is diagnosed, early treatment is very important because untreated disease can cause serious illness, or death. If the problem is due to AI and is permanent, treatment commonly involves the administration of corticosteriod medications. If necessary, medication must be taken daily, and more care than usual should be taken if illness is present or surgery is necessary. Those with the condition are advised to educate themselves about the disease and always wear a Medic-Alert or emergency ID bracelet. In all cases, lifestyle changes such as diet and exercise may also be helpful, and smoking should be avoided.

Ray Marks

See also: Addison's Disease; Anxiety; Chronic Fatigue Syndrome; Depression; Kidney Diseases; Obesity

Further Reading

Cleveland Clinic. (2014). Adrenal disorders. Retrieved from https://my.clevelandclinic.org/health/diseases_conditions/adrenal-disorders.

Mayo Clinic. (2012, December 4). Addison's disease. Retrieved from http://www.mayoclinic.org/diseases-conditions/addisons-disease/basics/definition/con-20021340.

Munver, R., & Volfson, I. A. (2006). Adrenal insufficiency: Diagnosis and management. *Current Urology Reports, 7,* 80–85.

National Adrenal Diseases Foundation. (2015). Adrenal diseases. Retrieved from http://www.nadf.us/adrenal-diseases/.

National Institute of Diabetes and Digestive and Kidney Diseases. (2014, May 14). Adrenal insufficiency and Addison's disease. Retrieved from http://www.niddk.nih.gov/health-information/health-topics/endocrine/adrenal-insufficiency-addisons-disease/Pages/fact-sheet.aspx.

ADULT ONSET STILL'S DISEASE

Background

This is a rare inflammatory, and often misunderstood, disease that can affect adults, especially women. The disease can affect the entire body—including many joints, internal organs, and other systems of the body, such as the lymph and blood systems—and can become chronic or long-standing, thus producing considerable disability. It is also possible that this condition represents a continuation of a better-known syndrome called Still's disease, or systemic-onset juvenile rheumatoid arthritis, that occurs in young people. It begins most commonly in adults below age 45, but it can also occur in later years. The disease is also known as AOSD, adult Still's disease, Wissler-Fanconi syndrome.

History

The disease was named after a British physician who first described the health condition known as systemic juvenile rheumatoid arthritis in 1896. Although the term *adult Still's disease* was not evident in the literature until 1971, it had already been described in the medical literature in the late 1800s. Most cases recorded in the literature have been Caucasian, although the condition has been described as affecting Blacks, Latinos and Asians.

The pattern of arthritis in this condition is distinctive and is often associated with fusion of the wrist bones on both sides of the body, as well as the small bones of the feet, along with characteristic daily fevers and salmon colored body rashes. Affected joints most commonly include the knees, wrists, ankle, elbow, shoulder, finger, and neck joints.

Symptoms of Adult Onset Still's Disease

Key symptoms include achy swollen joints, morning stiffness that lasts for several hours, having a sore throat, joint pain, and muscle pain.

There may also be a high fever that comes and goes once a day, most commonly in the afternoon or evening, and a salmon pink-colored skin rash that comes and goes along with fever, as well as warm joints.

Other symptoms may include abdominal pain and swelling, dry cough and breathlessness, pain when taking a deep breath, swollen glands, and unexplained weight loss.

These symptoms vary from case to case and may first only affect a few joints. In time, they can, however, give rise to chronic arthritis and other complications (such as osteoarthritis) and can include several joints, especially the hip joint.

Alternately, they can give rise to chronic adult onset Still's disease, which is characterized by periods of flare-ups of pain in several joints along with periods of remission or by increasing numbers of symptoms and complications due to lung, liver, spleen, or heart inflammation.

On occasion, in about 20 percent of cases, the symptoms may occur suddenly and then disappear and not return. For those who develop chronic articular disease, which include about 50 percent of cases, or who will experience flare-ups on several occasions over the next few years (approximately 30 percent of cases), the outcome may depend on the extent and duration of the joint involvement.

Cause

The cause of adult onset Still's disease is not known. It may be causes by a virus or infectious agent, but this has not been proven.

Diagnosis

A physician may conduct a medical examination and order blood tests to check for inflammation. Imaging tests may also be used to examine joints and organs for signs of inflammation. The earlier a diagnosis can be made, the better. The disease is usually difficult to diagnose, and other conditions have to be ruled out first, so this may be a lengthy process.

Common diagnostic approaches and tests include:

Abdominal ultrasound or CT scans
Blood tests
Biopsies
Documentation of fever patterns
Joint fluid tests
Liver function tests
Observation of patient for at least six weeks
Physical exams
X-rays of joints, chest or stomach areas

Treatment

Treatment may help to alleviate pain and disability and is aimed at controlling inflammation to prevent complications. Treatment usually involves various medications, especially steroid drugs. Joint replacement surgery may be performed. If an individual has any of the symptoms listed, a health care provider is desirable to prevent excess joint damage. If a person has adult onset Still's disease and trouble breathing, a health care provider is essential.

Ray Marks

See also: Arthritis; Joint Disorders; Juvenile Arthritis; Lymphatic Disorders; Osteoarthritis; Women's Health

Further Reading

Arthritis Foundation. (2015). Adult Still's disease. Retrieved from http://www.arthritis.org/about-arthritis/types/adult-onset-stills-disease/.

Genetic and Rare Diseases (GARD) Information Center. (2014, May 28). Adult-onset Still's disease. Retrieved from https://rarediseases.info.nih.gov/gard/436/adult-onset-stills-disease/resources/1.

International Still's Disease Foundation Inc. (2015). What is Still's disease? Retrieved from http://www.stillsdisease.org/index.php/stills-info/.

Mayo Clinic. (2013, April 3). Adult Still's disease. Retrieved from http://mayoclinic.com/health/adult-stills-disease/DS00792.

AGING, HEALTHY

Definition

From the moment of conception, a human being begins a continuous process of change, which is necessary to life. This process is called aging. Biogerontology is the biology of aging and examines the aging process from a cellular level. It is the study of the social, psychological, and biological aspects of aging. It is distinguished from geriatrics, the branch of medicine that studies the diseases of older adults. Through this study, scientists have found that cells follow a programmed phase of growth to maturity, followed by a plateau, and a finally a decline. The decline is believed by some to be in the cell division, not in the cells' ability to perform functions of life. Healthy aging would be to go through this process of change that occurs very naturally, adapting to changes that occur and arrive in old age with few deficits and or discomforts, especially chronic disease. The key to healthy aging is a healthy lifestyle, which consists of healthy foods and daily physical activity, as well as financial and mental wellness (Mayo Clinic 2016).

Current Perspectives

About 80 percent of older adults have one chronic condition, and 50 percent have at least two. Infectious diseases and injuries also take a disproportionate toll on older adults. The leading causes of death in order of frequency among adults ages 65 and older are heart disease, cancer, stroke, chronic lower respiratory diseases, Alzheimer's disease, diabetes, influenza and pneumonia, and unintentional injury. Research has shown that poor health does not have to be an inevitable consequence of aging (CDC 2015). However, chronic illnesses, once diagnosed in older adults are generally incurable, worsen over time, and endure many years. The causes of chronic illnesses are generally many and due to a combination of lifestyle, environmental agents, heredity and other undetermined factors (Ferrini & Ferrini 2008).

Nutrition

As one gets older, good nutrition plays an increasingly important role in how well a person ages. Eating a low-salt, low-fat diet with plenty of fruits, vegetables, and fiber can actually reduce age-related risks of heart disease, diabetes, stroke, osteoporosis, and other chronic diseases. Eating a wide variety of foods can pretty easily provide the body's nutritional needs. As the body ages, daily energy needs slowly decrease. Health care practitioners can help calculate a person's ideal caloric intake. Natural hormone changes make the body prone to depositing more body fat and less muscle. Eating a healthy, balanced diet and limiting the intake of saturated fat, along with increased activity and muscle strengthening can help a person stay at a healthy weight. Calcium and vitamin D supplements may be recommended during this time because bones lose mineral content more rapidly than before as a result of less estrogen being produced in postmenopausal women. Plaque buildup can naturally occur on the inside of the arteries that supply blood to the heart and brain. This plaque buildup can be slowed by eating foods such as lean meats, fruits, vegetables, and whole grains.

Financial Wellness

Taking an active role in your future by planning now for eventualities like retirement and health concerns facilitates financial wellness. This includes such things as consulting with a financial planner; avoiding free financial planning sessions that try to sell things; doing a yearly self-audit of finances beginning at age 30; taking advantage of trusted resources regarding changes in Social Security, Medicare, and Medicaid; and maintaining a positive attitude (WebMD 2016).

Mental Wellness

Mental health is comprised of the ability to engage in productive activities, fulfilling relationships, and the ability to cope successfully with change and adversity and is essential to overall health and well-being. Being active, challenging your mind, building healthy relationships, and maintaining a positive attitude helps foster mental wellness. The Centers for Disease Control and Prevention's (CDC) Healthy Aging Program is dedicated to monitoring the mental health status of the older adult population and connecting public health and aging services professionals with resources they can use to improve the health and quality of life of older Americans through its Healthy Brain Initiative. This serves as a national public health road map to maintaining cognitive health. Included in this report is a fact sheet on aging and depression in older adults, focusing on the fact that depression is not a normal part of growing older (CDC 2015). While most aging people adjust readily to the transitions and stresses of aging, assistance is available for dealing with mental disorders. These include mental health services in hospitals, nursing homes, and community mental health centers, as well as primary health care practitioners.

Fitness

Although the body begins to lose functionality and mobility in later years due to loss of muscle mass and degenerative agents in the bones and joints, these effects can be aided and counteracted by a healthy—and safe—exercise regimen. This includes exercises for strength, flexibility, cardiovascular endurance, and balance. There are many ways to enjoy physical activity throughout the aging process, and if done the right way, you'll be able to experience the benefits for years to come. The bottom line is that you are never too old to exercise (Hospital for Special Surgery 2012). However, health care practitioners, physical therapists, and athletic trainers and coaches need to address the practical issues that must be considered when working with this population, including exercise adherence, safety measures, and potential substance abuse of commonly used medications. There is substantial evidence documenting the many health benefits associated with all types of physical activity for adults of all ages (Resnick 2012). Thus, in the best interest of older adults, the philosophy of care provided to them should include evaluating their underlying capability, helping them achieve and maintain their highest functional level, and increasing the time they spend in physical activity. This has been referred to as a function-focused care (FFC) philosophy. This philosophy of care improves quality of life and enables older individuals to remain in the least restrictive setting, such as at home or in assisted living rather than in a nursing home (Resnick 2012).

Future and Implications of an Aging Society

By 2030, the number of U.S. adults aged 65 or older will more than double to about 71 million. The rapidly increasing number of older Americans has far-reaching implications for our nation's public health system and will place unprecedented demands on the provision of health care and aging-related services (CDC 2015). An essential component to keeping older adults healthy is preventing chronic diseases and reducing associated complications. There are no shortcuts to healthy aging. The earlier in life a person starts to think about how he or she wants to age, the better. By taking a few commonsense precautions, a person is assisting the healthy aging process. These include wearing seatbelts, flossing teeth, avoiding risky behaviors like drugs and alcohol, and experimenting with sex. Taking precautions against violence and accidents will also aid healthy aging, as well as seeking help for depression and times of low self-esteem. Older adults who practice healthy behaviors, take advantage of clinical preventive services, and continue to engage with family and friends are more likely to remain healthy, live independently, and incur fewer health-related costs.

Karen Jeanne Coleman

See also: Access to Health Services; Centers for Disease Control (CDC); Chronic Disease Management; Diet and Nutrition; Healthy Lifestyles and Risky Behaviors; Physical Activity; Social Health; Vitamin D; Wellness

Further Reading

Centers for Disease Control and Prevention. (2015). Aging. Retrieved from http://www.cdc .gov/chronicdisease/resources/publications/aag/aging.htm.
Ferrini, A., & Ferrini, R. (2008). *Health in the Later Years*, 4th ed. Boston: McGraw-Hill.

Hospital for Special Surgery. (2012). Exercise and healthy aging. Retrieved from http://www
.hss.edu/conditions_exercise-healthy-aging.asp.
Mayo Clinic. (2016). Healthy aging: Over 50. Last modified, March 2016. Retrieved from
http://www.mayoclinic.com/health/healthy-aging/MY00374.
Resnick, B. (March–April 2012). Changing the philosophy of care—A function-focused care
approach. *Aging Well*, 5(2), 34. Retrieved from http://www.agingwellmag.com/archive
/031912p34.html.
WebMD. (2016). Healthy Aging: What Can You Control? Retrieved from http://www.webmd
.com/healthy-aging/features/healthy-aging.

AIDS (ACQUIRED IMMUNE DEFICIENCY SYNDROME)

An Overview of Facts

AIDS is caused by the human immunodeficiency virus (HIV). AIDS is a global disease and it defined by a drastic immune deficiency syndrome of all infected individuals. As soon as the individual's immune system begins to malfunction, one can experience at least 26 known diseases and symptoms (Stine 2012). Previously, AIDS had been a certain death sentence that would occur within one to three years. Now, with the drugs available to fight the virus and other conditions, those diagnosed with AIDS can manage it as a chronic disease and have a near-normal life expectancy.

History of AIDS

AIDS was first described in the United States in June 1981. Hospitals in Los Angeles, California, reported treating five young men, who were all homosexuals, for confirmed pneumocystis pneumonia (PCP) (Stine 2012). Subsequently, there were reports from the CDC (Centers for Disease Control and Prevention), and doctors from across the country were reporting diseases such as cytomegalo virus (CMV), Kaposi sarcoma (a rare form of cancer), and an array of opportunistic infections linked to the malfunctioning of the immune system, including PCP, an infection of the lung; cytomegalo virus (CMV), an infection of the eye; and candidiasis, a fungal infection of the mouth, extending through the esophagus.

More than 30 years since the first reported cases, AIDS has posed undoubted challenges to the scientific community and the world.

Symptoms

Conditions and resulting symptoms of AIDS have included but are not limited to:

- Thrush: White patches in the mouth
- Tuberculosis: Fever, shortness of breath, bloody cough, and weight loss
- Pneumocystic pneumonia (PCP): Fever, shortness of breath, and dry cough
- Herpes zoster: Painful blisters specific to areas on the body

- Karposi sarcoma: Black/purplish nodes on the skin
- Cytomegalo virus (CMV): Abnormal vision, headaches, lethargy, disorientation, abdominal pain
- Toxoplasmosis: Headache, seizure, fever, weakness on one side of the body
- Herpes simplex: Blisters on skin, especially around the genitals, mouth, and rectum
- Wasting syndrome: Loss of more than 10 percent of body weight, very often associated with diarrhea and fever
- Peripheral neurotherapy: Tingling and pained sensation in the feet
- Mycobacterium avium (MAV) complex: Fever, diarrhea, abdominal pain
- Associated dementia: Inability to control basic motor functions, apathy, loss of memory
- Constitutional symptoms: Fatigue, fever, night sweats, weight loss, and chronic diarrhea

Treatment

Numerous drugs have been used to combat conditions related to AIDs. At present, there are more than 25 medications approved, which come from six classes of drugs, according to how they fight HIV. The six drug classes all work to prevent the replication, or spread, of the virus: (1) non-nucleoside reverse transcriptase inhibitors (NNRTIs), (2) nucleoside reverse transcriptase inhibitors (NRTIs), (3) protease inhibitors (PIs), (4) fusion inhibitors, (5) CCR5 antagonists (CCR5s) (also called entry inhibitors), and (6) integrase strand transfer inhibitors (INSTIs) (Overview of HIV Treatments 2015).

The type of regimen of drugs that a person with AIDS will take depends on a number of factors but is based mainly on the conditions that the person has, side effects, drug resistance, and how convenient the treatment might be, among other factors.

Although there is still no cure for AIDS, the progress of the illness has been remarkably slowed by the drugs that are currently prescribed, keeping those with AIDS in good health and leading to a long life.

Outcomes

The antiretroviral drugs have made the treatment of AIDS very dynamic. It is clear that when patients have complied in a strict treatment regimen that works for them, they show evidence of overwhelming reductions in their viral loads. The impact of antiretroviral drugs in the reduction of perinatal (mother-to-child) transmission of HIV has clearly been one of the highlights of treatment, with 20 to 30 percent chance of infection down to the current reduction rate of 1 to 2 percent. In the 1980s, young adults diagnosed with AIDS survived less than one year, whereas today, a person with the similar condition is expected to live up to age 70 (Stine 2012). Studies have shown a reduction in infection among men engaging in sexual activity with other men who are currently receiving antiretroviral medications (Stine 2012). The overall management of opportunistic infections has significantly brought down the number of hospital admissions of patients with AIDS and, thereby, has also increased the quality of life and stability for the patients. Although, there are many variables associated with the long-term survival rates of AIDS patients currently, we need to underscore that the most remarkable evidence is the progress made in antiretroviral treatment.

Future

The current biomedical research on AIDS needs to focus for the future on how to prevent infection. This will entail studying the virus that causes AIDS more extensively so that specific medications can be developed for each strain as the virus mutates.

Creation of effective vaccines has been very challenging, again, due to the high mutation rate of the virus, the virus establishing a latent state in some cells, and finally, the virus having an ability to spread through cell-to-cell contact (Fan et al. 2004). The need for vaccines should be the main focus for the future in terms of producing better outcomes. It is clear that antiretroviral studies may help AIDS patients produce antibodies against the virus; however, vaccines will help the body produce cell-meditated immunity (CMI), and CMI has been shown to be very effective in the eradication of viruses, such as smallpox (Stine 2012).

The other areas of current research and treatments needing improvement include specializing the existing antiretroviral treatments so that they can become more efficient in reducing viral replication and drug treatment failures due to viral mutation. It is clinically evident that we must come up with ways of restoring the immune system. The advantages of restoring the body's immune system cannot be overstated in terms of patient management and patient outcome. Future biomedical research could also focus on improving the existing treatments of opportunistic infections and associated malignancies.

We also need to find a way to streamline and enhance the phases of clinical trials with regard to new drugs for AIDS management. The Food and Drug Administration's monitoring of drug licensing and numerous laboratory human and animal tests prior to approval of a drug for treatment can be odious, time consuming, and extremely expensive. Having structured, less intrusive phases could more attractive to biomedical researchers.

The need for AIDS prevention must be addressed not only from the treatment point of view, but also from the social context, meaning we have to address educating the general public. Educational strategies must target high-risk populations such as the homosexuals, injecting drug users, and individuals who engage in unprotected sex with multiple partners. Preventive strategies must make these individuals aware of the consequences of their behavior and allow them to modify their behavior, thereby reducing the number of newly infected individuals.

The education strategy for prevention should also take into consideration the economic disparities among different groups, cultural diversity, compassion, religious beliefs, discriminations, and prejudices. This will facilitate trust from the public and, thereby, foster the acceptance of any type of social interventions geared toward the public.

Currently, we see many individuals who were frightened initially by AIDS and who modified their lifestyles so as not to put themselves or others at further risk in terms of contracting the virus. Most of these people have let their guards down for various reasons; therefore, future research or prevention should place emphasis on the general public moving forward and not sliding back to their detrimental behaviors, which put them at risk in the first place.

Finally, self-esteem and individual responsibility may play the most vital role in the global prevention of AIDS.

David Ajuluchukwu

See also: Autoimmune Disease; Centers for Disease Control and Prevention (CDC); Vaccines

Further Reading

Bartlett, J. G., & Finkbeine, A. K. (2001). *The Guide to Living with HIV Infection*. Baltimore, MD: Johns Hopkins University Press.

Fan, H. Y., Conner, R. F., & Villarreal, L. P. (2004). *AIDS Science and Society*, 4th ed. Burlington, MA: Jones and Bartlett.

Holtgrave, D. R., & Pinkerton, S. D. (2009). Updated annual HIV transmission rates in the United States 1977–2006. *Journal of Acquired Immune Deficiency Syndrome* (online edition).

Ledergerber, B., & Hasse, B. (2010). Frequency and determinants of unprotected sex among HIV-infected persons: The Swiss HIV Cohort study. *Clinics in Infectious Diseases, 51,* 1314–1322.

Morbidity and Mortality Weekly Report. (2009). Guidelines for Prevention and Treatment of Opportunistic Infections in HIV-Infected Adults and Adolescents. *58* [RR-4].

Overview of HIV treatments (2015, August 13). AIDS.gov. Retrieved from https://www.aids.gov/hiv-aids-basics/just-diagnosed-with-hiv-aids/treatment-options/overview-of-hiv-treatments/.

Stine, G. J. (2012). *AIDS Update 2012*. New York: McGraw-Hill.

ALCOHOLISM

Alcohol consumption is very common in North American society and can vary from moderate use to abuse to harmful use. Alcohol consumption becomes problematic when an individual consumes more than two standard drinks a day for men and one for women and older people. People with alcohol use disorders drink to excess, placing themselves and others in danger. According to the National Institute on Alcohol Abuse and Alcoholism, 1 in 12 American adults is an alcohol abuser or has alcoholism at any given time in their life (NIAAA 2007). A review of literature by Marc A. Schuckit (2009) found that alcohol use disorders are common in all developed countries with lower, but still substantial, rates in developing countries. Men are more likely to develop alcoholism than women, although women are at greater risk of developing medical complications, such as liver disease. Globally, alcoholism is responsible for a large portion of the health care burden.

Alcoholism, also known as alcohol dependence, is a chronic disease and can have a negative impact on a person's physiology over time. Alcoholism is characterized by a dependence on alcohol and a loss of control over one's own drinking. People with alcoholism continue to drink even though they know it's causing problems in their relationships, health, work, or finances. Alcoholism can cause irritability, depressive episodes, violent behavior, insomnia, and use of other drugs. Over time, continued abuse of alcohol shortens the onset of heart disease, stroke, and cancers and can have temporary cognitive deficits and increase sleep problems. Current research and studies report that alcohol-use disorders shorten lifespans of affected people by more than a decade.

A number of treatments are available to support a person recovering from alcoholism these approaches include; counseling, self-help groups, and medication.

History

Much change has occurred over the past 30 years in what we know about alcoholism. Alcoholism was believed to be a disease affecting people in their middle ages; little was known about the genetic basis of alcohol dependence or the changes that occur to the nervous system with prolonged heavy drinking.

Through epidemiological studies, research, and national surveys, alcoholism has become known as one of the largest burdens to health, affecting individuals across different age groups, genders, and socioeconomic status. Current research has identified genes that increase an individuals' risk for developing alcohol dependence, as well as genes that protect against alcohol problems. With this knowledge, families have the opportunity to take a more proactive approach to prevention and/or treatment.

Causes

Studies and research into problematic drinking have found that a number of factors contribute to alcohol-use disorders. These causes include genetics, psychological and social factors. The degree and combination to which these causes affect an individual can vary.

The psychological traits of a person—such as impulsiveness, low self-esteem, and a need for approval—can promote problematic drinking. In addition, a number of theories exist in relation to the use of alcohol to reduce feelings of stress, tension and pain. Sadock and Sadock find that these theories are partially built on the observation of individuals without alcohol-use disorders who still report using alcohol in social settings—for example, to relieve stress and anxiety (2009, 392).

With regard to social factors influencing the development of alcoholism or alcohol-use disorders, a person's environment plays a large factor. Availability of alcohol, attitudes toward drinking and being intoxicated, peer pressure, levels of stress, coping strategies, and laws are all influencing factors of a person's environment that can lead to excess use of alcohol.

Symptoms

Alcohol-use disorders have a myriad of symptoms that can have negative effects on a persons' well-being from their physiology to family, social, and work lives. Symptoms of alcoholism can appear differently in each individual, and not every symptom needs to be present in order for an alcohol-use disorder to exist. Symptoms can include:

- Feeling a strong need or compulsion to drink
- Developing a tolerance that requires an individual to drink larger amounts to feel the same effect
- Drinking alone or hiding the consumption of alcohol
- Not remembering actions or conversations, also referred to as "blacking out"
- Intentionally becoming intoxicated to feel good
- Severe anxiety and depression
- Irritability when a usual drinking time nears

Alcoholism or alcohol dependence is characterized by an addiction (compulsion) to drink and physical withdrawal symptoms (i.e., nausea, sweating, and shaking) when not drinking. Withdrawal can be very dangerous to an individual's health, and medical attention may need to be sought.

Diagnosis

The diagnosis of alcoholism is complicated by denial and a high co-morbidity rate (another disease or disorder existing at the same time). The diagnosis is determined through the criteria listed in the *Diagnostic and Statistical Manual of Mental Disorders* (*DSM-5*). Examples of criteria within the *DSM-5* for alcoholism include the need for regular use of alcohol to function throughout the day and long periods of sobriety interrupted by binges of heavy drinking (remaining intoxicated for an entire day for a minimum of two days).

The criteria required for diagnosis of alcoholism include a pattern of alcohol abuse during a 12-month period. A doctor would be looking for problems in three of more of the following areas: tolerance, withdrawal symptoms, how much someone drinks compared to his or her intended amount, ongoing desire, amount of time spent drinking, and giving up important activities or continuing to use alcohol.

Treatment

Because many people with alcoholism do not recognize they have a problem, the rate at which people seek treatment is relatively low compared to how many people alcoholism affects. There are a number of treatments available to address alcoholism and a combination of approaches might be used depending on individual circumstances.

Treatment often starts with a focus on helping an individual realize that his or her drinking is problematic and that it is, in fact, a disease. This phase of treatment involves support and counseling from a health professional; motivational interviewing and brief interventions are two recognized therapeutic techniques used. These two therapeutic techniques can assist in enhancing an individual's motivation for change and in providing education about the dangers of heavy drinking and benefits of change.

Treatment with medications, such as benzodiazepines, may also be prescribed when a person is experiencing withdrawal symptoms. Grand mal seizures, mild anxiety, insomnia, and autonomic dysfunction are examples of symptoms a person in withdrawal may experience. Due to the significance of some of these symptoms, an individual may need to be monitored in a health care setting.

Rehab is a term commonly used when speaking about alcoholism; it refers to rehabilitation and can include a range of supports that are directed toward helping maintain motivation, changing attitudes toward recovery, and diminishing the risk of relapse. Rehabilitation programs can comprise group programs, like Alcoholics Anonymous; outpatient and inpatient treatments; and residential-based care.

Expected Outcome

The number of deaths attributed directly and indirectly to alcohol abuse in North America are quite high. Approximately, 200, 000 deaths a year are directly related to alcohol use disorders, and after heart disease and cancer, alcohol related disorders are the third largest health problem (Sadock & Sadock 2007, 391).

Without proper support, alcoholism can have adverse effects on an individual's physical, social, and psychological self, as well as a negative impact on the person's family and environment. Driving while intoxicated, for instance, has a significant impact on the individual with the disorder, his or her family and greater society. With current options individuals suffering from alcoholism can improve with treatment. Research suggests a better treatment outcome with more comprehensive interventions.

Research

Research into the disease of alcoholism has made significant progress in the past 30 years. Research has currently identified genes that increase an individual's risk for developing an alcohol disorder and has fostered more informed decisions about treatment options.

Future research lies in the direction of research focused on examining the efficacy of pharmacological therapies and targeted behavioral approaches for individuals who develop alcohol dependence.

Andrea D'Souza

See also: Anxiety; Cancer; Depression; Fetal Alcohol Syndrome; Heart Disease; Hemachromatosis; Liver Diseases; Mental Disorders; Social Health; Stroke; Substance Abuse

Further Reading

Alcoholics Anonymous. (2002). *The Big Book,* 4th ed. New York: Alcoholics Anonymous World Services, Inc.

Kuhar, M. (2011). *The addicted brain: Why we abuse drugs, alcohol, and medicine.* Upper Saddle River, NJ: Pearson FT Press.

Mayo Clinic. (2015). Alcoholism. Retrieved from http://www.mayoclinic.com/health/alcoholism/DS00340.

Nathan, P., Wallace, J., Zweben, J., & Horvath, T. (n.d). Understanding alcohol use disorders and their treatment. Retrieved from http://www.apa.org/helpcentre/alcohol-disorders.aspx.

National Association for Children of Alcoholics, 10920 Connecticut Ave, Suite 100, Kensington, MD 20895, 888-554-2627.

National Institute on Alcohol Abuse and Alcoholism. (2007). FAQs for the general public. Retrieved from http://www.niaaa.nih.gov/FAQs/General-English/Pages/default.aspx#whatis.

Sadock, B. J., & Sadock, V. A. (2007). Kaplan and Sadock's Synopsis of Psychiatry: Behavioral Sciences/Clinical Psychiatry, 10th ed. Philadelphia, PA: LWW.

Sadock, B. J., Sadock, V. A., & Ruiz, P. (2009). *Kaplan and Sadock's Comprehensive Textbook of Psychiatry*, 9th ed. Philadelphia, PA: LWW.

Schuckit, M. A. (2009). Alcohol-use disorders. *Lancet, 373*(9662), 492–501.

ALLERGIES

Allergies are immune reactions to substances that do not cause direct harm within the body and that do not cause adverse reactions in most people. They may be triggered by virtually any foreign substance that enters the airway, bloodstream, or digestive tract or that touches the skin or mucous membranes. Sensitivities are similar to allergies in that normally benign substances trigger an adverse physiological response in susceptible persons; unlike allergies, however, sensitivities are not primarily an immune response. Neither allergies nor most sensitivities are present at birth; rather, they may arise at any point during an individual's development and at any age.

How Allergies Develop

The development of the immune system is like a conversation between an individual's body and his or her environment. This conversation begins at birth and continues for the entire course of a person's life. The immune system is always interacting with substances that enter or come into contact with the body. In normal, adaptive immune function, immune cells are on the lookout for invading pathogens—microbes and parasites that can invade and colonize the body and cause harm. When the immune system detects a pathogen, it creates antibodies to proteins on the pathogen's surface. One type, the IgM antibody, tags pathogenic particles for attack by immune cells. Another, the IgE antibody, prepares the body to respond to future exposure to a pathogen.

Most allergies develop when the immune system creates IgE antibodies that target a nonpathogenic substance, such as pollen or a protein within a food. Some of these antibodies attach to white blood cells, called basophils, and others attach to mast cells, or immune cells located on many tissues within the body. This creates an immune "memory" for the allergen. The first time a person is exposed to an allergen, there are no symptoms because the person is not yet allergic. It is only after the immune system creates IgE antibodies that a substance becomes an allergen and can trigger an allergic reaction. Allergic reactions caused by IgE antibodies typically occur within minutes of exposure to an allergen, happen even when the allergen dose is very small, and carry the highest risk of severe reaction.

Allergies may also be cell-mediated. Cell-mediated allergies are incompletely understood, but they are believed to occur when T cells are primed to recognize and attack a specific allergen, without associated antibodies. Cell-mediated allergies cause delayed allergic reactions, which may occur up to 48 hours after exposure.

The body naturally produces antibodies to all foreign invaders, so most people are likely to develop some level of allergic reaction to at least some substances, usually pollens and dusts that are inhaled. Many are never diagnosed because most airborne particle allergies cause allergic rhinitis, with identical symptoms to the common cold.

Natural protections in the small intestine usually keep the body from attacking nontoxic food substances. These protections develop special, nonreactive antibodies to food proteins or prevent the formation of antibodies to such proteins. When the immune system overrides these protections, a food allergy develops. Food allergies are distinct from the far more common food sensitivities and intolerances.

Allergies versus Sensitivities

It is common to call any adverse physical reaction to a normally nontoxic substance an allergy, but only responses caused by the immune system are true allergies. There are many forms of sensitivity that mimic true allergies, but they are usually not as severe as true allergic reactions and typically require larger doses of the offending item to trigger a reaction.

Sensitivities are usually limited to one region of the body. For example, skin sensitivity will cause dermatitis, but not a systemic immune response. Food sensitivities and intolerances usually cause gastrointestinal distress. Unlike true allergies, they do not pose a risk for anaphylaxis, shock, and death, even when they involve some immune reaction. Celiac disease, for example, causes inflammation as well as gastrointestinal distress when an affected person is exposed to the grain protein gluten, but exposure will not cause anaphylaxis.

Food intolerances are the most common form of sensitivity. Metabolic food intolerances, such as lactose intolerance and favism, result when an individual's body fails to produce a specific enzyme to break down a specific food component (in lactose intolerance, lactase to break down milk sugar; in favism, an enzyme that breaks down oxidants in fava beans and fava flower pollen). These intolerances are very common among certain ethnicities and age groups, and unlike allergies and other sensitivities, they can be genetically inherited.

Idiosyncratic food intolerances result from complex reactions in the digestive cells and mucosa and arise unpredictably within some individuals for reasons that are not completely understood. Still other intolerances result from an underlying condition, such as a metabolic or digestive tract disease. Pathogenic diseases may also cause chronic food intolerance as a side effect. These intolerances are immune-mediated and occur when the body makes antibodies to both the pathogen and the food it arrived on.

Symptoms

True allergies affect the skin and mucosa, respiratory system, gastrointestinal tract, and cardiovascular system. Symptoms may range from mild to severe, and severity may vary with different levels of allergen, between episodes of allergic exposure, and are based on the underlying health and stress levels of the individual. In most cases, it is not possible to predict whether an individual is at risk of a severe, life-threatening allergic reaction during any given episode—a true allergy that has seemed mild in the past can become severe at any point in the future and may arise unexpectedly at any point in an individual's life.

Allergic response is caused primarily by the release of histamine from immune cells and usually begins in the mucosa and respiratory tract. It may include itching, tingling, burning and watery eyes, runny nose, congestion, and sneezing. Areas with direct allergen contact may swell, have a burning sensation, and turn red. Mild allergic attacks are limited to these symptoms. Moderate allergic attacks progress to hives (raised, burning, itching, rashes on the skin), eczema (itching, burning, bumpy skin rash that may progress to open sores and flakey scales), gastrointestinal distress (including nausea, vomiting, cramps, constipation, and diarrhea), and shortness of breath. Severe allergic reactions include swelling of the face, lips, tongue, and throat; airway and chest constriction; wheezing, gasping, and choking; and lightheadedness, lowered blood pressure, heart palpitations, loss of consciousness, and cardiac arrest. This severe reaction, called *anaphylaxis*, can happen within minutes of exposure, even when previous attacks have been mild. Any time an allergic reaction progresses to moderate—or even mild, if the person has had a severe allergic reaction in the past—the sufferer should seek immediate medical attention.

Like true allergies, sensitivities can cause itching, burning, sneezing, congestion, and gastrointestinal distress, but they do not progress to major respiratory and cardiovascular symptoms or anaphylaxis.

Related Conditions

A number of medical conditions behave like allergies and sensitivities but are neither. In some cases, this is because the reactants cause direct toxic effects. In others, the reactions are side effects of another allergic condition, and in still others, the reasons are individual and unknown.

Anaphylactoid response is an anaphylaxis-like reaction that is caused not by the immune system, but by the direct effects of a compound in a sensitive individual. Unlike an allergy, this response happens upon first exposure to a substance. In anaphylactoid response, a chemical compound directly "attacks" the body's basophils and mast cells, breaks them open, and releases histamine, causing an immune cascade that leads to shock. It has been recorded most often with anesthesia, antibiotics, and narcotic drugs, and the reasons some people have this response remain unknown.

In pharmacological reactions, a sensitive individual has a reaction to a small amount of an additive or chemical within a food that is typical of exposure to a large amount of the substance in an individual who is not sensitive. The most common triggers for pharmacological reactions are monosodium glutamate (MSG, a flavor enhancer and preservative most commonly found in salty prepared foods), sulfites (added to some foods as a preservative, naturally occurring in others), and yellow and red artificial food colors. Sensitive individuals may experience itching, hives, flushing, headache, chest tightness, shortness of breath, and asthma attacks.

Persons with chemical sensitivities have reactions similar to pharmacological reactions, but such reactions are usually caused by airborne pollutants. The most common culprit is sulfur dioxide, a fossil fuel combustion byproduct, that can trigger hives, bronchospasm, asthma, vasculitis (inflammation of blood vessels), and gastrointestinal distress. Other common triggers include nitrogen oxide, ozone, cigarette smoke, formaldehyde, and solvents.

Histamine toxicity is a severe allergic-like reaction caused by a specific type of food poisoning. In histamine poisoning, large amounts of histamine build up on improperly refrigerated fatty fish (usually mackerel, tuna, or mahi-mahi). When consumed, the histamine causes a direct reaction similar to anaphylaxis.

Both allergies and sensitivities can predispose sufferers to chronic inflammatory conditions, including asthma, eczema, sinusitis, irritable bowel syndrome, and some types of ear infections and autoimmune disorders.

Diagnosis and Treatment

Diagnosis of allergies involves confirming that a person has an immune response to a particular substance. Most diagnosis happens after a person has a moderate to severe allergic reaction and begins with a detailed patient history. Then, an allergist tests for possible culprits with skin sensitivity tests and sometimes with blood tests.

The only medically legitimate allergy skin test is the skin-prick test, in which the clinician introduces small amounts of purified allergen proteins into the skin via injection or with an abrasive plastic pad. This method can test many potential allergens simultaneously. A positive reaction causes a raised, red welt. The only medically established allergen blood test is the RAST (radioallergosorbent test), which measures blood levels of IgE antibodies to specific potential allergens. Neither patient history nor positive test results alone are considered adequate for diagnosing an allergy—a patient must have both positive tests and a history of allergic reactions to a particular substance to establish a positive diagnosis.

In cases of food allergies and sensitivities, allergists may use elimination diets and food challenges in the diagnostic process. A limited elimination diet is used when a culprit food is already suspected. The patient completely avoids the suspect food for a certain amount of time, then eats some and waits for a reaction. A radical elimination diet is used when a patient has symptoms, but no particular culprit is suspected. The individual's diet is limited to a very small number of hypoallergenic foods for a certain length of time (usually a month or longer), then other foods are slowly added back one by one, and the patient is monitored for reaction. Radical elimination diets can be dangerous and should only be conducted under medical supervision. Food challenges are when a clinician orally administers small amounts of purified food extract in a medical setting and monitors the patient for allergic reaction. These are quite dangerous and must be conducted in a medical facility equipped to provide emergency intervention for anaphylaxis.

Diagnosis of sensitivities involves hunting down the culprit by a process of elimination and ruling out other causes through laboratory tests. Skin prick tests and RAST may be used to rule out true allergies, though skin prick tests may be reactive in sensitive individuals. Testing may include nasal smears and upper respiratory tract tests, neurological tests, a complete blood panel, and tests of major organ function. When other causes are ruled out, the clinician may continue to test for sensitivities through a detailed food-and-symptom diary, elimination diet, and food challenges.

Treatment for allergies and sensitivities may vary based on the allergen or reactant and the severity of past symptoms. The first line of defense is to avoid the offending item by not touching it, eating it, or breathing it in. The second is to control symptoms by taking medications such as antihistamines (for allergies) or enzymatic drugs (for some food intolerances) to control symptoms. The third is to always be prepared for an anaphylactic attack in the case of true allergies. Persons with these allergies are counseled to always carry EpiPen autoinjectors—single-use syringes of epinephrine to slow down anaphylactic emergencies—and advised to wear medical alert tags so first responders and medical personnel will know about the allergy if the patient is unconscious.

In some cases, true allergies can be treated with immunotherapy. In immunotherapy, the patient is given gradually increasing doses of the allergen under careful supervision in an allergist's office. The process is somewhat like vaccination, wherein the immune system is "trained" to respond a certain way to future exposures.

Are Allergies on the Rise?

In 2011, nearly one in five children in the United States were reported to have a respiratory allergy, and rates of food and skin allergies had both nearly doubled since 1997. All evidence indicates that allergy and allergic disease rates are continuing to rise. A number of hypotheses attempt to account for this increase. Each one is supported by medical evidence, and it is likely that each one plays a role.

The Hygiene Hypothesis

The hygiene hypothesis states that limited exposure to pathogens and nontoxic foreign matter during infancy prevents a child's immune system from learning to distinguish between harmful and harmless substances. This hypothesis accuses the modern, American, hyper-clean environment of infants and toddlers—ubiquitous hand sanitizer, antibacterial soaps and wipes, few animals, no eating off the floor, no playing in the dirt, etc.—of preventing normal development of a healthy immune system.

This accusation is supported by studies that show lower rates of allergic disease in people who grew up on farms, or who were otherwise in close contact with animals, than in those who did not. The hypothesis states that, among other things, the presence of innately harmful proteins, called endotoxins, on pathogenic organisms causes immune priming—a tendency to discriminate between foreign bodies that have these toxins and ones such as common allergens that do not.

Interestingly, early childhood infection with helminth worms is specifically correlated with a lack of allergic disease in later life, but the sterility of the overall environment is problematic, with or without intestinal worms. The prevalence of food and respiratory allergy in children sharply increase as family income and education levels rise.

Antibiotic and Acetaminophen Early Exposure

Antibiotics are used to treat a variety of intestinal, urinary, and respiratory illnesses in infants. Acetaminophen (brand name Tylenol) is considered the only safe painkiller for pregnant women and very young infants, and it is the treatment of choice for distress associated with infant vaccinations. However, some studies have shown a correlation between the use of antibiotics and acetaminophen in infancy and childhood development of asthma, one of the most common allergic diseases. The suggested mechanism is a change in bacterial flora that occurs when these drugs are ingested, and that may alter how the immune system responds to foreign objects.

Infant Feeding Methods

Human breast milk introduces antibodies and active immune cells to a child's system. The guts of human babies evolved to consume human milk exclusively for the first several months of life. Breast milk is considered so essential for healthy development that the World Health Organization states that all infants should be exclusively breastfed (no other food or drink, not even water) for the first six months of life and that all children continue to breastfeed until two years of age and beyond. Feeding a baby infant formula changes the bacterial flora within the gut and also changes the porosity (permeability to molecules of various sizes and composition) of the small intestine. Some research suggests that the development of food allergies, intolerances, and sensitivities is related to unusual absorption of macromolecules through the small intestine mucosa in infancy and early childhood.

Surgical Birth

As of 2012, more than one-third of infants born in U.S. hospitals were born via cesarean section (C-section), and in some hospitals the rate is well over half—at a time when the World Health Organization states that cesarean rates should never be more than 15 percent. Studies of short- and long-term variations between the health of children born by cesarean and those born naturally have noted that surgically born children have lower levels of normal flora on their skin and in their respiratory and digestive tracts. These flora are passed from mother to child during vaginal birth and may confer an immune advantage when children are exposed to both pathogens and allergens.

Obesity, Outdoor Activity, and Vitamin D Deficiency

Increased childhood obesity and decreased activity—especially outdoor activity—are associated with the current rise in asthma incidence. This association may be twofold: children who do not regularly play outside delay exposure to common outdoor allergens like pollen, and they spend prolonged periods breathing low-quality indoor air. Vitamin D deficiency is also associated with the development of allergies and allergic diseases. Exposure to sunlight without sunscreen is essential for vitamin D production, and vitamin D mediates healthy development of the respiratory and immune systems. Exposure to direct sunlight also decreases the severity of allergic dermatitis, including eczema, in some sufferers. This effect on allergic skin disease may be related to vitamin D synthesis.

Delayed Exposure to Allergenic Foods

Since the early 2000s, pediatricians have counseled parents of newborns to delay introduction of a few foods—especially peanuts, shellfish, eggs, tree nuts, cow's milk, soy, and wheat—until a child is between one and three years old. Some obstetricians and lactation consultants even instructed pregnant and nursing mothers to avoid eating these foods themselves for fear that early exposure could create an allergy.

Many parents received a recommendation to wait until age three to introduce peanuts, and it is this overzealous delay in exposure that is now being blamed for a dramatic increase in dangerous peanut allergy rates. Peanut allergy cases have more than tripled since the recommendation to delay exposure began. There are currently no recommendations to delay introduction of solids for allergenic reasons past the age of six months.

Angela Libal

See also: Asthma; Autoimmune Disease; Celiac Disease; Dermatitis; Eczema; Immune System Disorders; Inflammation; Irritable Bowel Syndrome; Psoriasis; Secondhand Smoke; Vitamin D

Further Reading

James, J. M., Burks, W., & Eigenmann, P. (2012). *Food Allergy*. Philadelphia, PA: Elsevier.

MedlinePlus. (2016). Allergy. U.S. National Library of Medicine. Retrieved from https://www.nlm.nih.gov/medlineplus/allergy.html.

Miller, S. (2011). *Allergic Girl: Adventures in Living Well with Food Allergies*. Hoboken, NJ: John Wiley & Sons, 2011.

Sears, W., & Sears, W. (2015). *The Allergy Book: Solving Your Family's Nasal Allergies, Asthma, Food Sensitivities, and Related Health and Behavioral Problems*. New York: Little, Brown & Company.

Zellerbach, M. (2000). *The Allergy Sourcebook*. New York: McGraw-Hill.

ALLIED HEALTH PROFESSIONALS

Allied health professions (also called health-related professions) is a term used to refer to a group of specialized health professions that provide support services during the delivery of health care in virtually every sector of the health care industry. While there is no industry-standard definition of an allied health professional, most work collaboratively with physicians, nurses, dentists, and others to enhance and complement patient care by providing a wide array of specialty services.

The Association of Schools of Allied Health Professionals provides the following definition (ASAHP): "Allied health professionals are involved with the delivery of services pertaining to the identification, evaluation, and prevention of diseases and disorders; dietary and nutrition services; rehabilitation and health systems management, among others."

As defined in the Patient Protection and Affordable Care Act (HR 3590), an allied health professional is a person who is employed in a health care setting after having graduated with an allied health professions degree or certificate. While the length of education varies based on job title, many allied health professionals receive highly specialized training as they develop the specific skill set needed for their career. Many of these training programs are situated within academic programs at colleges and universities. Most allied health professionals must receive certification or licensure through a professional accrediting body or must be registered by law before they are able to practice. Practice guidelines vary considerably between countries.

Representing more than 60 percent of the health care workforce in the United States, it is estimated that there are 6 million allied health care providers working in more than 200 health occupations and specialties. Because there is no standard classification system for allied health professions, there remains a lack of clarity over which careers are considered allied health professions. The ASAHP, for example, lists 20 specific career categories, while the American Medical Association's (AMA) *Health Care Careers Directory* selects only 15 to highlight.

The scope of work of allied health professionals varies greatly and is largely based on type of service provided and the amount of education and training received. While some allied health professionals work independently, others work on teams to provide direct or indirect patient care. Two broad classifications of allied health professionals are offered by the American Dental Association on its *Explore Health Careers* website—technicians (or assistants) and therapists/technologists. Technicians generally work under the supervision of a therapist or technologist and include individuals trained as respiratory therapist technicians, occupational and physical therapy assistants, medical laboratory technicians, and radiological technicians. Training programs for technicians are usually completed in less than two years as individuals are trained to perform procedures for very specific disease identification, treatment, or management purposes.

Therapists and technologists receive more comprehensive, intensive training in which they learn essential skills to perform procedures, communicate with patients, and diagnose conditions. Therapists and technologists—including physical and occupational therapists, athletic trainers, and respiratory therapists—receive training on how to develop treatment plans collaboratively with physicians and other primary health care providers. Therapists and technologists also monitor patient responses throughout treatment and make adjustments to treatment protocol when necessary.

The U.S. Department of Labor lists four major categories of allied health professionals: diagnostic professionals, medical services professionals, nondirect care professionals, and rehabilitation professionals.

Diagnostic professionals assist physicians in the diagnosis and treatment of disease, conduct diagnostic laboratory work, and/or produce diagnostic images. Diagnostic professionals include cardiovascular technologists and technicians, medical/clinical lab technicians, and radiological technologists.

Medical services professionals provide direct patient care in clinical settings and at emergency response scenes. Medical services professionals include dental assistants, emergency medical technicians, paramedics, and medical assistants.

Nondirect care professionals perform routine tasks not directly related to patient care, including dental laboratory work, labeling prescription bottles, and adjusting medical appliances, among many other tasks. Nondirect care professionals include dental lab technicians, orthotic and prosthetic technicians, and pharmacy technicians.

Rehabilitation professionals work directly with patients during treatment and follow-up care to improve the patient's ability to resume normal function, including being able to perform the tasks of daily living, breathing rehabilitation, and speech and language improvement. Rehabilitation professionals include occupational therapists, speech-language therapists, and respiratory therapists.

Allied health professionals work with patients with both acute and chronic illness. Patients with complex chronic disease or co-occurring chronic illness may often have contact with several allied health professionals during the course of their treatment. For example, a stroke patient may have images of their blood vessels taken by a diagnostic laboratory technician, have their blood pressure and temperature monitored by a medical assistant, and receive ongoing aftercare from an occupational therapist.

Allied health professionals work with patients with a variety of chronic diseases. Cardiovascular technicians and technologists, for example, work closely with physicians to perform diagnostic tests for patients with heart disease, angina, peripheral vascular disease, and arrhythmias. The diagnostic tests they perform include echocardiography, Doppler ultrasound, and electrocardiography. Specially trained cardiology technologists assist physicians with invasive diagnostic procedures, including catheterization and angioplasty.

While urban areas, large hospitals, and academic medical centers generally have access to a wide array of allied health professionals, there are critical shortages of these professionals in community health centers, walk-in clinics, and private practice settings, particularly in rural areas. The U.S. Bureau of Labor Statistics predicts projected growth and acute workforce shortages in several allied health professions, including medical assistants, pharmacy technicians, paramedics, and diagnostic medical sonographers, among others.

William D. Kernan

See also: Physical Therapy; Rehabilitation

Further Reading

American Dental Association. (2009, September 14). Allied health professions overview. Retrieved from http://explorehealthcareers.org/en/Field/1/Allied_Health_Professions.

American Medical Association. (2011). Careers in health care: Health care careers directory. Retrieved from http://www.ama-assn.org/ama/pub/education-careers.page.

Association of Schools of Allied Health Professions (ASAHP), 4400 Jenifer Street, NW, Suite 333, Washington, DC 20015, (202) 237–6481, www.asahp.org.

Explore Health Careers: American Dental Association, www.explorehealthcareers.org.

Health Professions Network (HPN), PO Box 2007, Midlothian, VA, (804) 639–9211, www.healthpronet.org.

Kacen, A. (2005). *Opportunities in Allied Health Careers.* New York: McGraw-Hill.

Sultz, H. A., & Young, K. M. (2011). *Health Care USA: Understanding Its Organization and Delivery.* Burlington, MA: Jones & Bartlett Learning.

UCSF Center for the Health Professions. (2009). Advancing the allied health workforce in California. Retrieved from http://www.futurehealth.ucsf.edu/Public/Center-Research/Home.aspx?pid=88.

U.S. Department of Labor, Employment and Training Administration. (July 2010). Allied health access: How to develop programs for youth in allied health careers. Retrieved from http://wdr.doleta.gov/directives/attach/TEN/ten2010/ten10-10a1.pdf.

ALS (AMYOTROPHIC LATERAL SCLEROSIS)

Amyotrophic lateral sclerosis (ALS) is a rapidly progressive disease of the nervous system that affects movement of the arms and legs due to damage of nerve cells located within the brain and spinal cord and causes considerable disability, and/or premature death. The disease is also known as Lou Gehrig's disease and usually affects individuals older than 50, but this may not always be the case, and younger people can be affected. It affects more men than women and can run in families: In about 10 percent of cases, there is a genetic defect that causes ALS. Other causes are not yet known, however. But chemical imbalances, immune system problems, and protein mishandling may be involved, and these possibilities are being explored. There may also be environmental factors that trigger the process in susceptible individuals, such as smoking, lead exposure, and a military-related factor.

Other names for the disease are upper and lower motor neuron disease and motor neuron disease.

History

Charcot described amyotrophic lateral sclerosis in 1874. But despite progress, this creeping paralysis, known colloquially as Lou Gehrig's disease, is still not visibly affected by available therapies.

Symptoms of ALS

Some of the initial symptoms of ALS include a loss of muscle strength and coordination, which is mild at first but worsens gradually over time as nerve cells or neurons that supply the muscles that move the arms and legs begin to die or waste away. As a result, the nerve cells that supply voluntary muscles become more and more unable to send messages to key muscles of the body, including the swallowing muscles. A person who has been diagnosed with ALS may have problems with everyday activities such as walking or running, lifting, or climbing stairs, as well as writing, plus leg and hand weakness and clumsiness. They may also develop speech problems; their muscles may twitch spontaneously; and there may be muscle cramps in the shoulders, arms, and tongue.

After a while, the muscles may be unable to move the arms, legs, or other body parts, however, and the muscles in the chest may become affected, speech can become slurred, and there may be voice changes. When this occurs, it is very challenging and often impossible for the person to breathe without assistance, and the head can drop due to weakness of the neck muscles. There may also be some problems with memory, word-fluency, and decision making even though the senses, such as vision, are generally not affected.

Once diagnosed, a person with ALS is expected to live three to five years on average. About 25 percent, however, may live longer than five years.

Causes

- Genetics
- Possible autoimmune relationship exists
- Environmental causes

Many neurologists order tests for the measurement of mercury, lead, and arsenic in blood and urine. However, there is doubt that mercury or arsenic has ever caused ALS. Lead intoxication once caused a syndrome involving both upper and lower motor neurons, but the syndrome disappeared once occupational exposure to lead began to be monitored. There has not been a convincing report of lead-induced motor neuron disease for 25 years.

Viral Infection and Prion Disease as Causes

Persistent viral infection might cause sporadic ALS. Berger et al. (2000) detected enterovirus RNA in the spinal cords of patients with ALS, but that observation was not confirmed according to Rowland and Schneider (2001).

Diagnosing ALS

ALS is challenging to diagnose because it may resemble other neurological diseases:

- In addition to standard medical examinations, including testing the individual's reflexes and strength, the doctor may order an electromyogram to measure the electrical activity in the muscles.
- Doctors may also order a nerve conduction test to measure the functioning of the nerve signals.
- Magnetic resonance imaging may provide a good picture of the brain and spinal cord.
- Blood and urine tests and muscle biopsies and spinal taps, as well as genetic tests, are other tests that may be helpful.

Treatment Approaches

There are no remedies that will cure ALS. There are some medications, however, that can be used to try to slow down the rate of deterioration of the nerve cells and to prevent muscle-related problems that interfere with daily activities, as well as pain and possible panic attacks. Medications may be indicated for helping to deal with swallowing problems; a surgical intervention that involves passing a tube surgically directly into the stomach is often needed to prevent choking.

Other forms of treatment are physical therapy, occupational therapy, speech therapy, general rehabilitation, braces, walkers, wheelchairs, and mechanical ventilation. Nutritionists may also be involved in the treatment of the ALS patient in order to prevent severe weight loss.

Prevention

There are no known ways of preventing ALS. However, some of the secondary disability associated with the disease, such as emotional distress, can be reduced through the provision of support. Genetic testing may, however, show if there is a risk of this disease in a particular case and may help in giving individuals and their families more time to adjust to the possibility of developing this problem and deriving the best solution to dealing effectively with this.

If a person has symptoms of ALS such as swallowing problems or weakness, he or she should see a doctor.

Because it is widely believed that everyone with a diagnosis of ALS becomes depressed, antidepressant drugs are often prescribed.

If a person has this condition, he or she should receive periodic attention from the doctor, especially if the symptoms become worse or new symptoms develop.

Research

Progress in research has been made during to date according to Rowland and Schneider (2001), but it has not yet resulted in any effective therapy. Nevertheless, there is some reason for hope. Genetic analysis has identified a primary cause of ALS. Mutations in a single gene can potentially initiate a cycle that leads to the selective degeneration of motor neurons. Although the cascade of events that leads to the death of motor neurons is complex, it is believed the isolation of genes responsible for other familial forms of ALS should reveal points in the pathway at which therapeutic intervention may be possible. It is possible that stem-cell therapy may be of protective value, slowing or preventing further neuronal degeneration. The challenge is to understand how these mutations cause disease.

Ray Marks

See also: Autoimmune Disease; Family Health; Immune System Disorders; Lead Poisoning; Men's Health; Neurodegenerative Diseases; Neurological Diseases; Secondhand Smoke; Swallowing Disorders

Further Reading

ALS Association. (2015). About ALS. Retrieved from http://www.alsa.org/about-als/.

Berger, M. M., Kopp, N., Vital, C., Redl, B., Aymard, M., & Lina. B. (2000). Detection and cellular localization of enterovirus RNA sequences in spinal cord of patients with ALS. *Neurology, 54*(1), 20–25.

Mitsumoto, H. (2009). *Amyotrophic lateral sclerosis.* New York, NY: Demos Health Publishing.

Mayo Clinic Staff. (2014). Amyotrophic lateral sclerosis. Retrieved from http://www.mayoclinic.org/diseases-conditions/amyotrophic-lateral-sclerosis/basics/definition/con-20024397.

MDA. (2015). Amyotrophic lateral sclerosis overview. Retrieved from http://www.mda.org/disease/amyotrophic-lateral-sclerosis/overview.

National Institute of Neurological Disorders and Stroke. (October 18, 2015). NINDS Amyotrophic lateral sclerosis (ALS) information page. Retrieved from http://www.ninds.nih.gov/disorders/amyotrophiclateralsclerosis/ALS.htm.

Rowland, L. P., & Schneider, M. A. (2001). Amyotrophic lateral sclerosis. *New England Journal of Medicine, 344,* 1688–1700. doi:10.1056/NEJM200105313442207.

ALTERNATIVE MEDICINE

Complementary and alternative medicine (CAM), as defined by the U.S. National Institutes of Health (NIH), refers to those health care practices, products, and systems that fall outside the scope of the conventional Western medical practice of physicians, nurses, dentists, and other allied health professionals. The National Center for Complementary and Alternative Medicine (NCCAM), a division of NIH, differentiates alternative medicine from complementary medicine based on its intended use. Whereas *alternative medicine* refers to the use of CAM practices (also commonly referred to as "modalities") as a substitute for conventional medical treatment, *complementary medicine* refers to the use of CAM in combination with conventional medicine. According to Eisenberg and colleagues (1998), in the United States, most use of CAM is complementary. While there are multiple health care practices, systems, and products that are considered to be a part of CAM, the field is ever changing and very broad in scope. When sufficient, high-quality scientific evidence exists to support the effectiveness and safety of a CAM modality, it is often used in combination with conventional medicine. This is referred to as "integrative medicine" or "integrated medicine." As CAM therapies are demonstrated to be safe and effective, they are adopted into conventional Western medicine, thus perpetuating an imprecise definition of CAM.

Many CAM modalities date back hundreds, even thousands, of years, stemming from the traditional healing practices and beliefs systems of ancient civilizations. Traditional Chinese Medicine (TCM), for example, can be traced back to 2697 BCE, while Ayurvedic medicine dates back more than 5,000 years. The ancient healing arts of the Tibetans and Native Americans are also commonly considered among CAM practices. Other CAM modalities are comparatively recent, new-age developments. Homeopathy, for example, dates back only several hundred years to the late 1700s, while biofeedback therapy was first described in the 1960s.

Today, CAM modalities are delivered by a wide array of practitioners, many of whom use a "holistic" philosophy to treat illness and disease. In addition to using the low-tech, "hands-on" techniques that were learned through close mentorship and practice, many CAM practitioners supplement their treatment with nutritional, emotional, social, and spiritual support. Training varies based on the type of CAM modality being studied, and in some cases, training programs are regulated by a professional association or regulating body. In some instances, CAM practitioners must be licensed or credentialed in order to practice.

Interest in and the use the use of CAM modalities has grown considerably in recent decades. Eisenberg and colleagues (1998) reported on the results of two national surveys, which found that use of CAM among adults had increased 8 percentage points from 1990 to 1997 and the number of visits to CAM practitioners had jumped from 400 million per year to more than 600 million. The amount spent on CAM during these years rose from $14 billion annually to $27 billion. In the more recent 2007 National Health Interview Survey, it was found that among American adults, approximately 4 in 10 had used a CAM therapy in the previous 12 months. This same survey showed increased use of several CAM modalities, including acupuncture, deep breathing exercises, massage therapy, meditation, naturopathy, and yoga.

While the use of CAM practices has increased steadily in the past few decades, questions of effectiveness and safety abound. In part due to the fact that many CAM practices have traditionally been practiced for centuries, to date there are relatively few published, well-designed scientific research studies about the efficacy of most CAM modalities. Most existing scientific evidence comes from small clinical trials, of which many used relatively weak methodological designs. Criticism of CAM often focuses on the lack of scientific evidence about three main issues—claims of whether the modality works for the conditions for which individuals seek treatment, how the modality works, and if the modality is safe. Critics further note concern over the quality and depth of training received by practitioners and potential harmful interactions between CAM modalities and traditional medicine (particularly pharmaceutical interactions). There is great interest among the research community to further study the efficacy of CAM practices. In the United States, the National Center for Complementary and Alternative Medicine has articulated its mission as "to define, through rigorous scientific investigation, the usefulness and safety of complementary and alternative medicine interventions and their roles in improving health and health care."

As they seek new ways to improve their health and prevent (or treat) disease, individuals who use CAM practices report doing so for a variety of reasons. Proponents of CAM modalities list several benefits, including the notion that CAM modalities are consistent with a holistic health philosophy and are often less expensive than medical treatments. Users of CAM also report that CAM practitioners spend more time listening to the patient and involving the patient in decisions about their health.

There is no formal taxonomy of CAM modalities, although several have been proposed. Because there is some uncertainty as to which practices are considered CAM and because some CAM practices may fit into several different classifications, categorizing CAM modalities has proven difficult. NCCAM suggests the following seven broad categories of CAM modalities:

Natural products. Used by human beings for centuries in traditional healing practices, natural products include herbal medicines, micronutrients, live microorganisms ("probiotics"), and other botanical products generally sold today as over-the-counter products and marketed as dietary supplements. While there are hundreds of CAM natural products purported to have medicinal value, current popular products in this category include fish oil, flaxseed, glucosamine, echinacea, St. John's wort, gingko biloba, garlic, and ginseng. Barnes and colleagues (2007) reported that 17.7 percent of American adults had used nonvitamin, nonmineral, natural products in the previous year, making these products the most used CAM modality.

Mind-body medicine. The idea that the mind is central to the healing process of the body during the treatment of illness can be traced back thousands of years to ancient medicinal practices used throughout Asia. A similar belief was held by Hippocrates—he maintained the notion that in addition to the physical body, healing included moral and spiritual aspects. Mind-body practices attempt to improve physical well-being and promote health by using the mind in a directed, meaningful manner. These modalities recognize the interaction of the brain and the body, and popular CAM mind-body practices include meditation, yoga, deep-breathing techniques, guided imagery exercises, progressive muscle relaxation, and hypnotherapy. Tai chi and qi gong can also be classified as mind-body medicine.

Manipulative and body-based practices. Various forms of massage were used by many ancient civilizations throughout Asia, Africa, and Europe. The Greeks used spinal manipulation to relieve a number of joint-related ailments and complaints. More recently, these techniques have become the foundation of physical therapy and the osteopathic and chiropractic medical fields of today. Massage therapy, a broad term used to refer to a number of different techniques used to manipulate the muscles and other soft tissues, is also a common CAM modality used today. The practice of these manipulative and body-based techniques is among the most regulated of the CAM modalities, with practitioners needing years of formal training and licensure to practice. With more than 18 million adults seeking chiropractic care/manipulation annually, it is the most commonly used CAM modality within this category.

Movement therapies. Movement-based approaches to health promotion include Rolfing Structural Integration, the Feldenkrais method, and the Alexander technique, among others. Pilates, a movement therapy that has been popularized in fitness centers, is the most commonly used movement therapy in the United States.

Traditional healing. The work of traditional healers is also considered a form of CAM. Traditional healing practices, often based on indigenous knowledge passed down through generations, are still practiced in virtually all regions of the world. In the United States, the most commonly sought after traditional healers are Sobadors, Native American healers, and Shamans.

Energy work. An entire category of CAM modalities involves the belief that within human beings are subtle fields of energy that can manipulated to rid the body of illness and enhance health. Examples of such practices include reiki, therapeutic touch, and qi gong. Magnet therapy and light therapy are also forms of energy work involving the manipulation of electromagnetic fields. More than 1 million adults use some form of energy treatment each year in the United States.

Whole medical systems. Throughout history, diverse cultures have developed entire systems of diagnostic and treatment protocol for a wide variety of physical and psychological ailments. These systems are generally grounded in theory and have a well-developed standard of practice. The Ayurvedic and traditional Chinese medicine medical systems are long-standing examples of such CAM practices. Other whole medical systems have developed more recently, including naturopathy and homeopathy.

Scant evidence currently exists for the efficacy of the use of CAM for the treatment of chronic disease, although it has been reported that patients with chronic health conditions show a high rate of CAM usage, particularly those who attain little symptom relief from conventional medical treatments. Patients who report using CAM most often list the following medical conditions for which they seek treatment: back pain, head/chest colds, joint pain and stiffness, arthritis, insomnia, anxiety, and depression. Although reported in much smaller numbers, symptom relief from cancer, cardiovascular diseases, and lung diseases and the treatment of high cholesterol is also reported among CAM users. Several recent reviews (Staud 2011; Ernst & Hung 2011; Team et al. 2011) enumerate the reasons the effectiveness of many CAM therapies is still relatively unknown: CAM usage is often not disclosed, impeding the ability of physicians to provide evidence-informed disease management; most studies of CAM usage have not used the methodologically rigorous trial designs used to demonstrate the effectiveness of current standards of practice; and the expectations of CAM users are poorly studied.

William D. Kernan

See also: Access to Health Services; Healthy Lifestyles and Risky Behavior; Physical Activity; Physical Therapy; Rehabilitation; Wellness

Further Reading

Barnes, P. M., Bloom, B., & Nahin, R. (2007, December 10). Complementary and alternative medicine use among adults and children: United States. *CDC National Health Statistics Report*, *12*, 1–24.

Centers for Disease Control and Prevention. (2007). National Health Interview Survey. Retrieved from http://www.cdc.gov/nchs/nhis/nhis_2007_data_release.htm.

Ernst, E., & Hung, S. K. (2011). Great expectations: What do patients using complementary and alternative medicine hope for? *Patient*, *4*(2), 89–101.

Eisenberg, D. M., Davis, R. B., Ettner, S. L., Appel, S., Wilkey, S., Van Rompay, M., et al. (1998). Trends in alternative medicine use in the United States, 1990–1997: Results of a follow-up national survey. *Journal of the American Medical Association*, *280*(18), 1569–1575.

Jonas, W. B., & Levin, J. S. (1999). Essential of complementary and alternative medicine. Baltimore, MD: Lippincott, Williams, & Wilkens.

National Center for Complementary and Alternative Medicine (NCCAM), National Institutes of Health, 9000 Rockville Plaza, Bethesda, Maryland, http://nccam.nih.gov.

National Center for Complementary and Alternative Medicine, National Institutes of Health. (2015, March). Complementary, alternative, or integrative health: What's in a name? CAM basics: What is complementary and alternative medicine? Retrieved from https://nccih.nih.gov/health/integrative-health.

Staud, R. (2011). Effectiveness of CAM therapy: Understanding the evidence. *Rheumatic Disease Clinics of North America*, *37*, 9–17.

Team, V., Canaway, R., & Manderson, L. (2011). Integration of complementary and alternative medicine information and advice in chronic disease management guidelines. *Australian Journal of Primary Health*, *17*, 142–149.

ALZHEIMER'S DISEASE

Overview

The most common cause of mental decline, Alzheimer's disease damages the brain irreversibly. It develops slowly; over time, it causes loss of memory and eventually affects the ability to speak, think, learn, and carry out daily activities, including living independently. It is the most common type of dementia, a condition that can severely reduce cognitive function.

About 10 percent of those with Alzheimer's are older than 65, with 50 percent older than 85. Although most people with the disease are older adults, it is not a normal symptom of aging, and it is not limited to old age. Women are more likely than are men to develop the disease due to longevity and genetics. People with Down syndrome often develop the disease, and those who have suffered a severe or repeated head trauma have a greater risk of Alzheimer's disease. The rare form of early-onset Alzheimer's affects people in their forties and fifties.

Caused by brain cells that degenerate and then die, Alzheimer's disease has no cure. Treatments can stabilize or lessen symptoms, but they're temporary.

History

The disease is named after Alois Alzheimer, a German psychiatrist who studied brains in the early 20th century. He examined the brain tissues of a woman who had died after suffering from loss of memory, unusual behavior, and language problems. Her brain showed what are now called amyloid plaques and neurofibrillary tangles. These and the loss of connections between nerve cells have been identified as the main features of the disease.

Symptoms

The earliest symptoms of Alzheimer's disease are associated with memory problems, especially remembering newly learned information, and mild confusion. A person experiencing these symptoms may not be aware of them, even when others are. Usually the information, skills, and habits learned earlier in a person's life are among the last lost to the disease, which progresses at different rates.

As the disease progresses, people experience a decline in other cognitive areas, such as finding the right word; vision problems; becoming disoriented; as well as difficulty with simple problem-solving, reasoning, planning tasks, and organizing thoughts.

As it becomes more severe, the disease leads to greater problems associated with mobility and motor skills; interpreting surroundings; concentrating, particularly on numbers and other abstract concepts; incontinence; and trouble speaking and eating. Common behavioral changes include anxiety, depression, mood swings, irritability, and distrust; restlessness and sleeplessness; withdrawing socially; losing inhibition; and experiencing delusions and hallucinations.

Causes

While the precise cause of Alzheimer's is still unknown, scientists have discovered the presence of two items that distinguish the brains of those with the disease. The first are amyloid plaques, or deposits of beta amyloid, a protein that builds up around brain cells and disturbs communication between them. Second are neurofibrillary tangles, made of the protein tau. This protein twists and clumps together, causing nerve cells to die. The effect is similar to the amyloid plaques: Cell communication is compromised. Although some experts are unsure if these proteins are the cause or side effects of this disease, they know that they are not evident in the brains of those who do not have Alzheimer's.

Risk Factors

The greatest known risk factor is age, along with a combination of genetics and health and environmental factors that are likely to increase the risk over time. For most people, symptoms become apparent around reaching age 65. The likelihood of developing Alzheimer's doubles about every five years after that, and the risk reaches almost 50 percent after age 85.

The gene apolipoprotein E-e4 (APOE-e4) has been identified as a risk factor that most likely increases developing Alzheimer's. But carrying this gene doesn't always lead to getting the disease, and some people become ill who do not carry it. Scientists have yet to determine precisely how it increases risk, but they estimate that it may cause 20 to 25 percent of cases.

A genetic mutation is usually the cause of the rare early-onset form of the disease. Studying DNA samples, scientists have discovered that some families carry a mutation in selected genes on chromosomes 1, 14, and 21. Children have a 50 percent chance of developing early-onset Alzheimer's if one parent has one mutation. People with Down syndrome often develop Alzheimer's, possibly because they have an extra copy of chromosome 21.

Some evidence points to risk factors similar to those for heart disease, including no physical exercise, high blood pressure and high cholesterol, a diet low in fruits and vegetables, and smoking.

Diagnosis

No one test can diagnose Alzheimer's definitively, but considering all potential causes leads to a diagnosis. A physician takes a medical history and conducts physical and neurological exams. An individual exhibiting symptoms will perform tasks to assess mental health and the ability to complete daily activities. Blood tests may rule out other conditions that cause similar symptoms, as will brain imaging and other lab tests. If requested by the family, a physician may examine the post-mortem brain to confirm an Alzheimer's diagnosis.

Treatment

Alzheimer's disease has no medical cure, but medication and other remedies can help slow or relieve symptoms for a limited period of time.

Two types of medications may be prescribed for cognitive symptoms, depending on the severity of the disease's progression. They help reduce or stabilize symptoms by regulating the chemicals that brain cells use to communicate, but they are not effective for everyone and they have side effects.

The behavioral changes associated with the disease have been shown to improve with exercise; a low-fat diet rich in fruits, vegetables, and omega-3 fatty acids; and a brain kept active with intellectual stimulation and social activities. Scheduling activities, avoiding confusion, and writing down lists and directions are among the coping mechanisms helpful for a person with Alzheimer's.

Prevention

No proven method exists to prevent its development, but scientists theorize that using the brain increases its cellular connections and protects against the changes related to Alzheimer's. Activities that likely reduce risk include a high level of education, a stimulating job, and frequent social activities, as well as reading, playing music and games, and other tasks that are mentally challenging.

Methods to reduce the risk of heart disease also suggest that they also lower the risk of developing Alzheimer's. Recommendations for living a healthy lifestyle include exercising and eating well, maintaining a recommended weight and healthy levels of blood pressure and cholesterol, and avoiding tobacco or excess alcohol.

Prognosis and Outcome

On average, a person with Alzheimer's lives about 8 to 10 years after developing symptoms. The disease is the sixth leading cause of death in the United States.

Future

Researchers continue to look for new treatments and interventions for the symptoms of Alzheimer's disease and improve the quality of life for patients. Clinical trials are studying immunization, drug, and physical therapies, as well as cognitive training. Scientists have intensified their genetics research for additional risk-factor genes.

Jean Kaplan Teichroew

See also: Aging, Healthy; Anxiety; Brain Diseases; Dementia; Depression; Diet and Nutrition; Physical Activity

Further Reading

Alzheimer's Association. (June 19, 2015). What is Alzheimer's? Retrieved from http://www.alz.org/.

Mayo Clinic. (2015). *Mayo Clinic on Alzheimer's Disease.* Rochester, MN: Mayo Store.

My Doctor Online. The Permanente Medical Group. (May 2014). Alzheimer's disease and dementia. Retrieved from https://mydoctor.kaiserpermanente.org/ncal/mdo/presentation/conditions/conditionpage.jsp?condition=Condition_Alzheimers_Disease_and_Dementia.xml.

NIH National Institute on Aging. (June 9, 2015). Alzheimer's disease fact sheet. Retrieved from https://www.nia.nih.gov/alzheimers/publication/alzheimers-disease-fact-sheet.

Poirier, J., & Gauthier, S. (2014). *Alzheimer's Disease: The Complete Introduction (Your Health).* Toronto: Dundurn.

AMYLOIDOSIS

Amyloidosis is the buildup of amyloid, an abnormal protein formed in the bone marrow—often in the kidneys, heart, nervous and digestive systems—that prevents them from functioning as they should. The most common type is AL amyloidosis, caused when bone marrow produces abnormal antibodies that cannot be broken down, and it can occur in anyone. AA amyloidosis is the reaction to tuberculosis, rheumatoid arthritis, osteomyelitis, or other chronic inflammatory diseases; infection; or certain cancers, most commonly affecting the spleen, kidneys, liver, adrenal glands, and lymph nodes. Familial amyloidosis is a hereditary form that usually affects the nervous and digestive systems. Other types include dialysis-related amyloidosis, which generally affects people on long-term dialysis, and wild-type ATTR, which almost exclusively in men.

Symptoms depend on where in the body amyloid builds up. But general symptoms range from skin changes to diarrhea to fatigue and dizziness to tongue swelling, numbness, or tingling in the hands or feet. There is no cure, but medications, chemotherapy and stem cell transplantation, and organ transplantation are treatments that help manage symptoms. The condition can be life-threatening if the cause is an underlying disease, especially if it causes kidney or heart failure. But it is considered rare; fewer than 4,500 people in the United States are diagnosed every year. Most people who are diagnosed are between 50 and 80 years old; about two-thirds are male.

Symptoms

Some people may not have symptoms of amyloidosis until it reaches an advanced state. Symptoms vary depending on the severity and location of amyloid deposits in the body; they may include an enlarged liver or tongue; difficulty swallowing; irregular heartbeat; bowel obstruction; diarrhea, sometimes with constipation or blood; anemia; weight loss; dizziness; weakness, feeling faint, severe fatigue, or shortness of breath; skin changes, including bruising around the eyes or elsewhere; burning sensation and other disruption in the nervous system; joint pain; swelling of the ankles and legs; and numbness or tingling in the hands or feet.

Causes and Risk Factors

It is unknown precisely why amyloid is created and builds up in bodily organs, but it is recognized as a bone marrow disorder. Amyloidosis develops when the bone marrow cells produce antibodies that they can't break down, leading to a buildup in the blood that is eventually deposited in tissues.

Amyloidosis can develop when a person has multiple myeloma, Hodgkin's disease, or the intestinal disorder known as familial Mediterranean fever. Other factors that increase the risk of developing amyloidosis are age (older than 50), gender (men are almost 70 percent of those with AL amyloidosis), chronic infection or inflammatory disease, family history of amyloidosis, and kidney dialysis for more than five years.

Diagnosis

Diagnostic testing for AL amyloidosis involves blood and urine tests, which can detect signs of amyloid proteins. An echocardiogram, or ultrasound of the heart, may show amyloid deposits in that organ. Biopsies of bone marrow, tissues, or samples from the skin, nerves, kidneys, liver, or gums can positively confirm a diagnosis.

Treatments

There is no cure for amyloidosis, so treatment focuses on treating symptoms and organ damage as well as reducing or stopping the production of amyloids. Specific treatment depends on the type of amyloidosis and the number of organs affected. Treatment options for AL amyloidosis include chemotherapy to stop the growth of amyloid-producing cells and peripheral blood stem cell transplant in which stem cells are collected and stored during high-dose chemotherapy before they are returned to the body. Medications include drugs to treat some cancers and control heart rate, corticosteroids to reduce inflammation, pain relievers, diuretics to reduce fluid retention, and blood thinners. AA amyloidosis, associated with other diseases, requires treatment for those underlying illnesses, which may cause it to disappear. Amyloidosis of the kidney may require transplantation, or dialysis, even if amyloid eventually builds up in the donor kidney. Transplantation may be performed for amyloid heart disease; myocardial amyloidosis is the most common cause of death due to arrhythmias or intractable heart failure. In some cases of familial amyloidosis, liver transplantation removes the source that produces the abnormal protein.

Proper nutrition is important for adequate energy, but scientists have not found that diet or nutrition can cause or prevent AA amyloidosis of the kidneys or dialysis-related amyloidosis, but a low-salt diet may be recommended if the kidneys have been affected or a modified diet for those with gastrointestinal amyloidosis.

Prognosis and Outcomes

The severity of amyloidosis depends on the organs affected. It can be life-threatening if it causes kidney or heart failure. Early diagnosis and treatment improves survival; without treatment, many die within two years of diagnosis.

Ray Marks

See also: Anemia; Hodgkin Disease; Inflammation; Kidney Diseases; Liver Diseases; Multiple Myeloma; Osteomyelitis; Rheumatoid Arthritis; Swallowing Disorders; Tuberculosis

Further Reading

Amyloidosis Foundation. (2015). Facts: A is for . . . amyloidosis. Retrieved from http://www .amyloidosis.org/facts/.

Cedars-Sinai. (2015). Amyloidosis. Retrieved from http://www.cedars-sinai.edu/Patients /Health-Conditions/Amyloidosis.aspx?utm_source=adcenter&utm_medium=cpc &utm_campaign=Heart_Transplants_National.

Mayo Clinic. (2015). Amyloidosis. Retrieved from http://www.mayoclinic.org/diseases -conditions/amyloidosis/basics/definition/con-20024354.

MedlinePlus. (2015). Amyloidosis. Retrieved from https://www.nlm.nih.gov/medlineplus/amyloidosis.html.

National Institute of Diabetes and Digestive and Kidney Diseases. (2014). Amyloidosis and kidney disease. Retrieved from http://www.niddk.nih.gov/health-information/health-topics/kidney-disease/amyloidosis-and-kidney-disease/Pages/facts.aspx.

ANAL AND RECTAL DISEASES

Definition

Anal and rectal diseases affect the lower part of the large intestine and can include conditions such as bowel incontinence, hemorrhoids, abscesses, ulcerative colitis, and cancer of the rectum or anus, also known as colorectal cancer. Because the rectum's opening is the anus (where stool passes out of the body), the rectal area is prone to infection, bacteria, and viruses, which makes problems with the rectum common.

Rectal diseases can differ in potential for harm, and it is useful to know the symptoms for some common rectal problems that can be treated with diet or other lifestyle changes. However, it is always important to be examined by a doctor to ensure that the problem is not serious.

People at risk for colorectal cancer and common disease of the anal and rectal area include:

- Those with a personal or family history of benign colorectal polyps
- Those with a personal or family history of colorectal cancer
- Those with a personal or family history of ovarian, endometrial, or breast cancer
- Those of African American and Hispanic descent
- Men and women over the age of 50

Symptoms, Diagnosis, and Treatment

Symptoms of a problem in this part of the body may include bleeding, itching, and pain (pain in and around the anus or rectum—the perianal region—is a common complaint and can be severe because of the many nerve endings in the perianal region). Many conditions that cause anal pain may also cause rectal bleeding. Other symptoms may include change in the bowel habit, change in stool size, unexplained weight loss, fatigue, feeling of incomplete evacuation, abdominal bloating, flatulence, and anemia.

Diagnostic tools include physical and medical examinations, colonoscopy, and lower gastrointestinal tract radiography.

Treatments vary widely depending on the particular problem. They may include chemotherapy, diet, exercise, medication, radiation, or surgery.

Prevention

Prevention and dietary suggestions include eating well-balanced meals and eliminating foods prone to causing diarrhea, including caffeine, alcohol, milk; beans, cabbage, broccoli, and the artificial sweeteners sorbitol and xylitol. Adding fiber to the diet and increasing water consumption may also help. Eating slowly and in a stress-free environment may be helpful.

Ray Marks

See also: Breast Cancer; Colon Cancer; Diet and Nutrition; Inflammatory Bowel Disease; Ovarian Cancer; Ulcerative Colitis

Further Reading

American College of Gastroenterology. Patient Education and Resource Center. (2015.) Retrieved from http://patients.gi.org/.

Enders, G. (2015). *Gut: The Inside story of our body's most underrated organ.* Vancouver, BC: Greystone Books.

Health Direct of Australia. (2014). Rectal diseases. Retrieved from http://www.healthinsite.gov.au/topics/rectal_diseases.

MedlinePlus. (2015). Anal and rectal diseases. U.S. National Library of Medicine: National Institutes of Health. Retrieved from https://www.nlm.nih.gov/medlineplus/analdisorders.html.

ANEMIA

Anemia is the term used to describe a medical condition or state where the blood, which is made up of a fluid called plasma, plus cells, does not have a sufficient number of healthy red blood cells or where the red blood cell count or hemoglobin molecule, which is the functional unit of the red blood cell, is low or below normal levels. This causes health problems because red blood cells transport oxygen to the organs of the body such as the lungs. There are different forms of anemia, but all are likely to result in similar symptoms such as fatigue if the organs do not obtain enough oxygen to function.

This condition is the most common condition affecting the blood that occurs in the United States and can affect up to 3.5 million people at any point in time, especially women and those with one or more chronic diseases. Rates in other countries may be higher than the United States.

Women are vulnerable to anemia because, during their child-bearing years, they often lose blood during their menstrual cycle, and during pregnancy, there is an increased demand for blood and red blood cells.

Older people are also at risk for anemia if they follow poor diets and have medical conditions.

Types

Among the 400 or more types of anemia there is:

- Anemia due to alcoholism
- Anemia from excess bleeding or blood loss
- Aplastic anemia due to the effects of viral infections, chemotherapy, or other medications on bone marrow

- Anemia from chronic infections
- Anemia related to medications such as chemotherapy drugs, HIV medications, some antibiotics, and antihistamines
- Iron-deficiency anemia
- Vitamin-deficiency anemia
- Bone marrow and stem cell related anemia problems, including:
  - Aplastic anemia due to a marked reduction in stem cells or the absence of these
  - Thalassemia due to inability of red blood cells to grow and mature
  - Anemia due to lead poisoning
- Anemias associated with the health conditions of advanced kidney disease, some forms of cancer, autoimmune diseases, malaria, viral hepatitis, and gastrointestinal ulcers
- Anemia related to poor nutrition
- Anemia related to pregnancy
- Hemolytic anemia, where red blood cells rupture, which could be hereditary or due to damage from medications or abnormal heart valves
- Pernicious anemia due to poor absorption or deficiency of vitamin B12
- Sickle cell anemia, a hereditary disease
- Thalassemia, which is hereditary

Acute anemia is a condition that occurs rapidly, and it can be distressing if it is unexpected.

Chronic anemia develops over a longer period of time and usually progresses more slowly.

If anemia is mild, it may cause no symptoms; however, the symptoms might arise if the anemia becomes more severe.

Causes

Red blood cells are produced in the bone marrow, and when they are mature, they are released into the blood stream. Other factors, however, are required for the formation of healthy red blood cells, such as adequate iron mineral levels and healthy kidneys.

Anemia is thus primarily caused by two mechanisms and is often a sign of a disease rather than a disease itself: (1) either a decrease in the production of red blood cells or hemoglobin or the production of too few blood cells or (2) a loss of blood, the destruction of blood cells, or having blood cells that may not function correctly.

For example, anemia can be caused by the impact of day-to-day stress of the circulatory system on the red blood cell, which is usually very fragile. Other stressors that can cause similar problems include infections, drugs, certain foods, and venom from snakes or spiders.

Anemia can also occur at birth, rather than being acquired over time, and the problem is then termed *hemolytic disease or anemia* if it started in the fetus when the mother was pregnant or if the red blood cells rupture prematurely. Anemia can also occur later on in life, following heart surgery, severe burns, chemical exposure, severe blood pressure problems, and clotting disorders. In rare cases, red blood cells can be trapped by an enlarged spleen and are destroyed prematurely or before their lifespan of 120 days is up. On occasion, anemia may occur spontaneously without any observable cause.

Inherited causes of anemia include sickle cell anemia and thalassemia. Other causes include:

- Gastrointestinal conditions such as hemorrhoids, gastritis, digestive conditions such as Crohn's disease,* and cancer
- Excess use of nonsteroidal anti-inflammatory drugs such as aspirin or Motrin
- Childbirth if bleeding is excessive
- Multiple pregnancies
- Toxins from advanced liver or kidney disease
- Iron-poor diets, especially in infants, children, and teens*
- The demands of pregnancy and breastfeeding, which can lower a women's iron reserves*
- Frequent blood donation*
- Excessive endurance training*
- Certain drugs, foods, and caffeinated drinks*
- Vitamin B-12 or folate deficiency (or deficiency of both)**
- Crohn's disease, HIV infection, or surgical removal of stomach or intestine**
- Eating little or no meat; overcooked or too few vegetables**
- Alcohol abuse**

Diagnosis

Whether an individual is anemic and what kind of anemia he or she has is commonly based on the volume of red blood cells in the blood. If the volume is low, the anemia is termed *microcytic* anemia; if it in the normal range it is called *normocytic* anemia, and if the volume is high it is termed *macrocytic* anemia. Doctors frequently describe someone having a low blood count as anemic.

If a doctor suspects that a person has anemia, she or he may try to identify if this is from an excess loss of blood or from a decrease in the production of red blood cells in the bone marrow.

Symptoms

These include:

Chest pain, angina, or heart attack
Decreased energy
Dizziness
Fainting or passing out
Fatigue
Light-headedness
Looking pale

---

* Can cause iron-deficiency anemia
** Vitamin-deficiency anemia

Palpitations
Rapid heart rate
Shortness of breath
Weakness

Signs of anemia include:

Changes in stool color or blood in stools
Enlargement of the spleen
Heart murmur
Low blood pressure
Pale or cold skin
Rapid breathing
Rapid heart rate
Yellow skin or jaundice

Diagnosis

Anemia is usually diagnosed by a blood sample, as well as by a physical examination and medical history. Some other investigative tests include bone marrow biopsies, kidney function tests, liver function tests, and blood level tests and iron level tests.

Summary

There are many types of anemia. Because these have different causes, their treatments are often different. The most common type of anemia, iron-deficiency anemia, can be treated by using iron supplements and dietary changes as well as by limiting alcohol use. Most types can be avoided by regularly visiting a medical practitioner or visiting when problems arise. Some forms of anemia are readily treated, others may require long-term treatment, and patients should follow their provider's health recommendations to either avoid anemia or to control this in the case of long-lasting problems.

Ray Marks

See also: Alcoholism; Autoimmune Disease; Crohn's Disease; Diet and Nutrition; Kidney Diseases; Liver Diseases; Malaria; Sickle-Cell Disease

Further Reading

American Society of Hematology. (2015). Anemia. Retrieved from http://www.hematology.org/Patients/Anemia/.

Mayo Clinic. (2014). Anemia. Retrieved from http://www.mayoclinic.org/diseases-conditions/anemia/basics/definition/con-20026209.

Medical News Today. (2015). Anemia: Causes, symptoms and treatments. Retrieved from http://www.medicalnewstoday.com/articles/158800.php.

MedlinePlus. (2015). Anemia. Retrieved from https://www.nlm.nih.gov/medlineplus/anemia.html.

National Heart, Lung, and Blood Institute. (2012, May 18). What is anemia? Retrieved from http://www.nhlbi.nih.gov/health/health-topics/topics/anemia/.

ANEURISMS

What Is an Aneurism?

The term *aneurism* refers to an abnormal widening, bulge, or a "ballooning" in the wall of an artery. An artery is a blood vessel that conveys oxygenated blood or blood containing oxygen from the heart to other parts of the body. An aneurism can form in any size artery, and an aneurism that becomes too large may be fatal because it can rupture or burst and cause massive bleeding or increase the risk of clotting. Other specific problems may occur, depending on the site of the aneurism and the organ(s) involved.

There are many areas of the body in which aneurisms can occur:

- Near the heart
- In the heart (ventricular aneurism)
- In the brain (brain or cerebral aneurism)
- In the main artery leading from the heart such as the aorta (aortic aneurism)
- In the chest (thoracic aneurism)
- Below the stomach (abdominal aneurism)
- Below the kidneys (abdominal aortic aneurism)
- In other parts of the body (peripheral aneurism)

Aneurisms arise especially if part of an artery wall is weak and can cause unexpected problems because their presence may not cause any observable symptoms or signs, even if they exist. They may be developing and growing slowly, however, without any symptoms; if they become too big, the artery may burst. If they are found in good time, however, it may be possible to treat them and prevent them from bursting at a later time.

An aneurism can occur in any artery in the body, but it commonly occurs in the aorta, the largest artery in the body, which leads from the heart into the abdomen. Aortic aneurisms are most commonly found in the abdominal cavity (known as abdominal aortic aneurisms) but may also occur in the chest or thoracic cavity (known as thoracic aortic aneurisms). Most commonly, people who develop aortic aneurisms are Caucasian, male, and older than 60 years.

Prevalence Rates

As summarized by a posting at *Better Medicine*, the Centers for Disease Control and Prevention has found that abdominal aortic aneurisms occur in 1.3 percent of men aged 45 to 54 years of age and 12.5 percent of men between 75 and 84 years of age in the United States.

Brain aneurisms are estimated to occur in approximately 30,000 people in the United States according to data at this site, and peripheral artery aneurisms are found to most commonly occur in the popliteal artery (behind the knees), mesenteric artery (intestine), femoral artery (groin), and splenic artery (spleen).

The most common type of aneurism is, however, the abdominal aortic aneurism.

Symptoms

Symptoms vary depending on the type and location of the aneurism.

There may be shortness of breath, a croaky voice, backache, left shoulder pain, and swallowing problems if the aorta is affected.

Abdominal aneurisms can cause pain or tenderness below the stomach or a throbbing sensation in the abdomen, can reduce one's hunger or upset one's stomach, and its rupture can cause shock. Thus, pain frequently spreads toward the back if the aneurism continues to grow and presses on the spine or chest organs. This can cause coughing, loss of voice, and breathing difficulties, as well as swallowing problems.

Cerebral aneurisms may result in trouble talking or seeing, headaches, pain in the neck and face, problems with the eyes, blurred or double vision, nausea, vomiting, seizures, tremors, confusion, light sensitivity, drooping eyelids, stiff neck, and numbness of the face, and they may cause a stroke.

Causes

Any condition that damages or weakens the walls of the artery can lead to an aneurism. Some of these conditions include atherosclerosis or buildup of fatty plaque in the arteries, advanced age, high blood pressure, high cholesterol, male gender, and smoking. Other causes include injuries, infection or deep wounds of the blood vessels, hereditary factors, and birth deformities. Pregnancy is often associated with the development and rupture of splenic artery aneurisms.

The disease may have a genetic basis and may run in families. The individuals most at risk are white men older than 55 years of age. Aneurysms are among the top 10 causes of death in this age group. People older than 65 are also at risk.

Diagnosis

Aneurisms can be detected by physical examinations that employ one or more of the following diagnostic tools:

- Angiograms
- Arteriography
- Chest or stomach x-rays
- Catheter angiography
- Chest/heart computed tomography (CT) scan
- Ultrasound
- Chest MRI
- A cerebrospinal fluid test (in cases of brain aneurisms)
- CT angiography
- Duplex ultrasound
- Magnetic resonance angiography

Sometimes, an aortic aneurism can be discovered by the general practitioner when performing a routine abdominal examination. He or she may feel a lump that pulses at the same rate as the patient's heartbeat; it is often located high up in the abdomen, slightly to the right.

Treatment Approaches

Treatment options depend on the site, size, and location of the problem and include catheter embolization; surgical aneurism endovascular repair or stent graft; observing the growth of the aneurism closely, through regular check-ups, possibly every six months; and carrying out surgery if the aneurism becomes five centimeters or two inches wide and continues to grow.

Patients may also be given medicines that lower blood pressure.

Giving up tobacco, keeping blood pressure under control, keeping cholesterol levels under control, eating a healthy diet, keeping a good ideal body weight for one's height, and improving physical fitness though exercise are also recommended.

Routine ultrasound imaging or screenings for those in high-risk groups or older age groups is also recommended.

An expanding or enlarging aneurism in the aorta often requires emergency treatment, and surgery is generally recommended. Again, the type of surgery and when it is needed will depend on the symptoms and the size and type of aneurism.

Prognosis or Expected Outcomes

If an aneurism bursts in the chest, there is only about a 20 percent chance of survival, even if emergency medical treatment is administered immediately. A ruptured abdominal aneurism will cause massive bleeding leading to shock and even death. A brain aneurism causes serious bleeding into the brain tissues and is a life-threatening emergency.

Occasionally, a piece from inside an aneurism may become dislodged and form a clot or thrombosis; if this lodges in a small artery, it can block the artery, which can be very serious if this artery supplies the heart, lung, or brain.

Owing to this situation, aneurisms are usually treated with the utmost seriousness, and medical neglect of an aneurism is not an option. Prevention is the first step. But once an aneurism is detected, individuals should place themselves under a doctor's care.

Prevention

A high percentage of aneurisms are caused by vascular disease; preventing the development of the vascular disease, called arteriosclerosis, may be helpful in preventing aneurisms.

The strategies recommended here include quitting smoking, keeping one's blood pressure under control; keeping one's cholesterol under control; eating healthy, well-balanced meals, rich in fruits and vegetables; keeping one's body weight within the ideal limits; getting seven hours of sleep per night; and being physically active if this is indicated and acceptable to the health provider.

Risk of aneurysm can be further reduced by:

- Eating a heart-healthy diet that includes potassium and fiber, and drinking plenty of water
- Exercising at least 30 minutes per day
- Limiting alcohol consumption to one drink per day for women and two per day for men
- Limiting the amount of sodium (salt) consumed to less than 1,500 mg per day
- Reducing stress

Ray Marks

See also: Anxiety; Atherosclerosis; Diet and Nutrition; Men's Health; Physical Activity; Stress; Stroke; Swallowing Disorders; Women's Health

Further Reading

American Heart Association. (2015). What is an aneurism? Retrieved from http://www.heart .org/HEARTORG/Conditions/More/What-is-an-Aneurism_UCM_454435_Article .jsp#.VjJM0mtKjwo.

Brain Aneurism Foundation. (2015). Understanding: Brain aneurism basics. Retrieved from http://www.bafound.org/brain-aneurism-basics.

Khurana, V. G., & Spetzler, R. (2006). *The Brain Aneurism.* Bloomington, IN: Author House.

Mayo Clinic. (2014). Aneurisms. Retrieved from http://www.mayoclinic.org/diseases -conditions/aneurism/basics/definition/con-20032411.

Medical News Today. (2011). Aneurism: Causes, symptoms and treatments. Retrieved from http://www.medicalnewstoday.com/articles/156993.php.

National Heart, Lung, and Blood Institute. (April 1, 2011). What is an aneurism? Retrieved from http://www.nhlbi.nih.gov/health/health-topics/topics/arm.

Texas Heart Institute Heart Information Center. (2015). Aneurisms and dissections. Retrieved from http://www.texasheart.org/HIC/Topics/Cond/Aneurism.cfm.

ANGINA

Overview

Angina (an-JI-nuh), also known as angina pectoris, is defined as chest pain due to narrowed arteries caused by coronary artery disease (CAD). As a result of CAD, there is a lack of blood flow to the heart that can result in angina, or feelings of pressure, heaviness, or tightness in a person's chest.

History

Angina was first described by the Indian surgeon, Sushruta, in 600 BCE. His descriptions of the chest pain as burning near the heart and short-term pain are still valid today (Dwivedi & Dwivedi 2007). It was William Heberden (1710–1801), a British physician and scholar, who defined the chest pain as angina pectoris in his chapter on "Commentaries on the History and Cure of Diseases" in *Medication*

Table 1   Three Types of Angina

Types of Angina	Description	Treatment
Stable angina	Triggered by physical activity	Beta blockers, nitrates, and rest
Unstable angina	Can occur at any time; is frequent, recurrent, less responsive to medication; can lead to a heart attack, or myocardial infarction	If pain lasts more than 5 minutes, call 911
Variant angina	Less common form of angina, not consistently related to physical activity	Calcium channel blockers

Source: Author.

Transaction, published in 1767 (Heberden 1802). Heberden defined stable angina as well as the variant form.

Types

There are three different types of angina: stable angina, unstable angina, and variant angina, as shown in Table 1.

Stable angina is the most common form and is triggered by physical exertion, stress, smoking, and changes in temperature. The pain lasts five minutes or less and may go away with medication and/or rest. Unstable angina occurs when blood flow to the heart is blocked or reduced by a blood clot at a narrowing of a coronary artery, which is also called atherosclerosis. It is extremely dangerous because it can occur without warning and may lead to a heart attack, also known as myocardial infarction. It is usually more severe than stable angina. Variant or Prinzmetal's angina is much less common. According to the Mayo Clinic, this type of angina accounts for 2 percent of all angina cases (Mayo Clinic 2015). It is characterized by a spasm that occurs in a coronary artery rather than by atherosclerosis. In this case, the artery is temporarily narrowed, reducing the flow of blood to the heart, and is less often associated with permanent damage.

Symptoms

Symptoms of angina are feelings of pressure, heaviness, or tightness in a person's chest. The chest pain may extend to a person's arms, neck, jaw, shoulder, or back. Angina can be felt for only once or may recur. Severity may also vary. If someone experiences angina for more than five minutes or the pain does not go away after taking medication, it may be a sign that the person is having a heart attack. Call for help right away.

The most common cause of angina is CAD, wherein blood flow to the heart is reduced by a buildup of cholesterol in the coronary arteries. High blood pressure,

Table 2   Types of Angina Medications

Medications	Description	Example
Blood thinners (or anticoagulants)	Decreases ability of blood to clot in artery; enables blood to flow to the heart	Aspirin, Clopidogrel
Angiotensin converting enzyme (ACE) inhibitors	Lowers blood pressure	Lisinopril
Nitrates	Relaxes and opens blood vessels to enable blood to flow through	Nitroglycerin
Beta blockers	Lowers blood pressure; enables blood to flow	Propranolol
Statins	Help to lower cholesterol	Atorvastin
Calcium channel blockers (or calcium antagonists)	Widens blood vessels and enables blood to flow; increased blood flow will reduce or prevent angina	Nifedipine

Source: Author.

elevated blood lipids, cigarette smoking, high body mass index (BMI), depression, chronic anger, sedentary lifestyle, obesity, diabetes, older age, and family history are risk factors.

Treatment

A cardiologist may recommend modifications to lifestyle, medications, angioplasty, or surgical treatment to treat angina. The type of treatment depends on the diagnosis and health of the patient. Treatment is meant to reduce the frequency and severity of the chest pain. Changes to lifestyle include increasing exercise, adjusting to a low-fat, low-cholesterol, and low-sodium diet, incorporating stress management into daily life, and quitting smoking.

Medications that may be prescribed include those shown in Table 2.

If surgery is necessary, angioplasty, which is a procedure that opens up a blocked artery, may be advised. With angioplasty, a balloon is inflated at a blockage site to help blood move normally, and a metallic stent is inserted to keep the artery open (NewYork-Presbyterian 2008). Lastly, major cardiac surgeries may include coronary artery bypass surgery, where a vein or artery from the patient's body is used to bypass a blocked or narrowed coronary artery. This surgery increases blood flow to the heart and reduces or eliminates angina.

Megan Aronson

See also: Atherosclerosis; Coronary Artery Disease; Diabetes; Heart Diseases; Myocardial Infarction; Physical Activity; Stress

Further Reading

Dwivedi, G., & Dwivedi, S. (2007). "Sushruta—the clinician—teacher par excellence." *Indian Journal of Chest Disease and Allied Sciences, 49*(4), 243–244.

Heberden, W. (1802). Commentaries on the history and cure of disease. Reprinted from some account of a disorder of the breast (1772). *Medical Transactions, 2,* 59–67. London: Royal College of Physicians.

Jevon, P. (2012). *Angina and Heart Attack.* New York: Oxford University Press.

Mayo Clinic. (2015). Angina. Retrieved from http://www.mayoclinic.com/health/angina/DS00994.

NewYork-Presbyterian. (2008). Coronary artery disease. Retrieved from http://www.nyp.org/heart/services/coronary-artery-disease.

ANGIOGRAM

What Is It?

An angiogram is a special type of x-ray that uses a dye and camera to take pictures of the blood flow in either an artery or vein. These can be located at any site of the body including the arms, legs, chest, or head.

Most commonly, the angiogram is used to examine arteries near the heart—hence, the term *coronary angiogram.*

During the process, a long, thin, flexible tube or catheter is placed into a blood vessel located in the groin or just above the elbow. The catheter is guided to the site under investigation; then dye is injected into the vessel so the site under investigation can be seen clearly on the x-rays. These pictures can be made into a regular x-ray and can be stored on a computer.

Another form of angiogram involves the use of a magnetic resonance imaging or a computed tomography option, which are both less invasive. Some magnetic resonance imaging tests and all computed tomography tests require dye to be injected, and computed tomography involves radiation.

Patients remain awake during the test and may be asked to help move in certain directions. They may experience tilting of the table they are lying on and be asked to hold their breath.

The test is usually considered safe and low risk. It is usually painless because a local anesthetic is given. It usually takes from 30 to 40 minutes.

Applications

Angiograms can be useful for detecting aneurisms; detecting coronary artery disease and its severity; detecting problems with blood vessels, such as injury or damage; showing the pattern of blood flow to a tumor; or showing the condition of the renal arteries before a kidney transplant.

It can also detect the source of bleeding; prepare people for surgery on diseased blood vessels of the lower legs; or be applied to open a blocked vessel, deliver medicine to a tumor, or stop intestinal bleeding.

Angiography is generally safe, but among the risks of the procedure, depending on where the angiogram is performed and on the health of the patient, are allergic reactions to dye or medication, arrhythmias, blood clots; cardiac arrest, excess bleeding, heart attack, infection, kidney damage, perforation or piercing of the heart or artery, radiation exposure, stroke, or trauma.

Ray Marks

See also: Aneurisms; Angina; Arrhythmias/Dysrhythmias; Coronary Artery Disease; Heart Diseases; Kidney Diseases; Stroke

Further Reading

Society for Vascular Surgery. (2011). Angiogram. Retrieved from http://www.vascularweb .org/vascularhealth/pages/angiogram.aspx.

ANKYLOSING SPONDYLITIS

The term *ankylosing spondylitis* (AS) is used to describe a form of arthritis that mainly affects the joints of the spine, although it may also affect other joints. The Centers for Disease Control and Prevention National Arthritis Data Workgroup estimates AS and its related diseases affect at least 2.4 million people in the United States. It is a disease that falls under the title "axial spondylarthritis."

The term *spondylitis* means inflammation of the bones of the spine called vertebrae; *ankylosing* refers to the fusing of these bones or their immobility. The combined term, *ankylosing spondylitis*, is used to describe this health condition because the joints most affected by AS usually become inflamed and can fuse.

The disease commonly starts when individuals are in their adolescence or early adulthood, but it can occur earlier or later. Typically, the inflammation of the affected joints produces a lot of pain and disability. This is because, although this pain can come and go or may be quite mild, people with this condition can sometimes experience very rapid onset of AS and severe pain over many body parts over long time periods that never goes away.

If the condition does not improve, the bones of the spine that are affected, as well as other joints, may become stiff and finally ankylose, or fuse together, to form a rigid column of bone instead of the bones remaining as separate mobile structures. In this case, the affected individual may have very limited mobility in that region; if the spine is affected, their posture may become stooped, and they may appear to have a forward curvature or a hunched-forward type of posture of their spine.

Because AS is commonly a chronic or long-standing condition that does not respond to treatments readily, it can result in considerable disability in many cases, especially among men, although women and children can be affected as well. The disease is thus very similar to other arthritic diseases because it can often be very acute and painful; at other times, it may be less painful. This makes it especially challenging to deal with if the symptoms are severe when they occur.

The disease usually starts with intermittent or gradual periods of low back pain and stiffness, followed by periods with no back pain. At first, the pain may occur only on one side, but it often spreads to the other side. This pain may be worse at night and in the early morning or wake a person from sleep. The pain is often relieved by activity or exercise; however, even though the pain may begin in one area, it often spreads to affect other areas.

If AS is severe, and the affected joints stiffen and fuse, it may be very difficult for the person to move, and it may become hard for that person to breathe if the disease becomes severe because the ribs are attached to the spine and can stiffen and restrict lung capacity and function.

People with AS may often be fatigued; they may have a fever, moderate anemia, and a loss of appetite and may generally feel less than comfortable.

Key body areas affected by AS, other than the spine, are:

- The shoulders, knees, and ankles
- Ribs
- Heels
- Hips
- Small joints of the hands and feet
- The sacroiliac joints or joints between the spine and pelvis

On occasion, the disease can affect the eyes and cause and inflammation of the iris. There may be a slight fever, loss of appetite, weight loss, and fractures of the bones in the spine that can damage surrounding nerves and the spinal cord, and in rare instances, the lungs and heart can be affected detrimentally.

Causes of AS

It is possible AS has a genetic cause. There may also be environmental factors, bacterial factors, and unknown factors that influence the disease onset directly or by interacting with genetic factors.

Risk factors for AS include:

- Being male
- Having a positive HLA-B27 gene
- Having a family history of AS
- Having a history of frequent gastrointestinal infections

Tests Used to Diagnose AS

The doctor may conduct a physical examination and may order, blood tests, genetic tests, x-rays or an MRI of the spine and pelvis, or computerized tomography (a CAT or CT scan).

Treatments

There is no cure for AS, and treatment is aimed at reducing the symptoms and minimizing disability and deformity. Treatments include medications that may reduce inflammation or slow the disease, and what would be best for an individual should be discussed with the physician.

Surgery may be employed if pain or joint damage is severe. However, it is important for people with this condition to visit their practitioners at least once a year, even if it is incurable, and to obtain support and health recommendations from well-trained physical therapists and occupational therapists about exercise, pain control, posture, and using devices or making adaptions to the workplace or home.

Lifestyle and home remedies include giving up smoking, if relevant. There is much information on various websites and support groups that sufferers can belong to that they should be aware of and find helpful.

If you have back pain that comes and goes or does not let up, if you have continual stiffness in your back or hips, or if you already have AS and are developing new symptoms, please make sure to visit your health care provider.

In addition, if your chest hurts when you breathe or you develop eye pain, light sensitivity, or blurred vision, please see your provider immediately.

Ray Marks

See also: Arthritis; Back Pain; Inflammation; Physical Activity; Spinal Diseases

Further Reading

American College of Rheumatology. (2013). Spondyloarthritis. Retrieved from http://www .rheumatology.org/I-Am-A/Patient-Caregiver/Diseases-Conditions/Spondyloarthritis.
Arthritis Foundation. (2015). Spondyloarthritis. Retrieved from http://www.arthritis.org /about-arthritis/types/spondyloarthritis/.
Mayo Clinic. (2011). Ankylosing Spondylitis. Retrieved from http://www.mayoclinic.com /health/anklyosing-spondylitis/DS00483.
National Institute of Arthritis and Musculoskeletal and Skin Diseases. (2013). Ankylosing spondylitis. Retrieved from http://www.niams.nih.gov/Health_Info/Ankylosing _Spondylitis/default.asp.
Spondylitis Association of America. (2015). Learn about ankylosing spondylitis. Retrieved from http://www.spondylitis.org/Learn-About-Spondyloarthritis.
Weisman, M. H. (2011). *Ankylosing Spondylitis*. New York: Oxford University Press.

ANXIETY DISORDERS

Some degree of anxiety is normal and healthy. It prepares people for important decisions and events and warns them of danger and when to take action, but it can also be persistent, seemingly uncontrollable, overwhelming, and debilitating. Anxiety disorders are a group of related serious mental illnesses characterized by persistent and excessive fear or worry in situations that are not threatening or an irrational dread of everyday situations. People who have an anxiety disorder experience intense anxiety that lasts hours or days or does not disappear; it also occurs frequently and can worsen over time. Anxiety disorders can interfere with daily functioning, including at work and school and in relationships.

Anxiety disorders are the most common mental illness in the United States: More than 40 million adults and one in eight children in the United States are affected, and women are more likely to develop an anxiety disorder. A combination of genetics, brain chemistry, personality, and life events contribute to the causes of the disorders. Nearly half of those diagnosed with an anxiety disorder are also diagnosed with depression. Anxiety disorders are highly treatable with forms of talk therapy and medications.

Types of Anxiety Disorders

The term *anxiety disorder* includes the following illnesses:

- Generalized anxiety disorder, or GAD, is the persistent, excessive, and unrealistic worry about a variety of everyday problems for six months or longer, even when there is no apparent reason for concern.
- Panic disorder describes people who experience spontaneous sudden panic attacks and are preoccupied with the fear of a recurring attack and the feeling of being out of control during a panic attack. Panic attacks occur unexpectedly, occasionally during sleep.
- Agoraphobia is the avoidance of situations or places in which a person has previously had a panic attack, especially in anticipation of it occurring again.
- Social anxiety disorder is the extreme fear of being judged or scrutinized by others in social or performance situations, including making a phone call or eating in public. More than shyness, it involves extreme embarrassment and self-consciousness.
- Selective mutism is the consistent failure to speak in school and other situations but not at home with close family members.
- Separation anxiety disorder is characterized by an excessive level of anxiety related to being separated from parents or others in parental roles.
- Specific phobias are excessive and unreasonable fears in the presence of or in anticipation of specific objects, places, or situations; common phobias are of animals, insects, germs, heights, thunder, driving, public transportation, flying, dental or medical procedures, and elevators.

Symptoms

The symptoms that characterize anxiety disorders are excessive worry and irrational fear and dread. Although each disorder has some unique symptoms, those common to the disorders in general include feeling uneasy, nervous, and powerless; weakness or tiredness; a sense of impending danger or panic; an increased heart rate, rapid breathing, shortness of breath, or heart palpitations; sleep difficulties; sweating; nausea or dizziness; dry mouth; trembling; muscle tension; tingling or numbness in the hands or feet; irritability; and trouble concentrating or being calm.

Causes and Risk Factors

Scientists have identified parts of the brain that are involved in fear and anxiety, although the precise causes of anxiety disorders are unknown. Similar to other mental illnesses, research suggests that they may develop from a complex set of risk factors, including genetics, brain chemistry, environmental stress, medical factors, personality, traumatic life events, and alcohol or substance abuse. Anxiety disorders often run in families, which may increase the risk of development; women are more likely to experience an anxiety disorder. It is common for someone with an anxiety disorder to also suffer from depression; almost half of those diagnosed with depression are also diagnosed with an anxiety disorder.

Diagnosis

Therapists, psychiatrists, and other mental health providers make a diagnosis of an anxiety disorder based on specific criteria listed in the *Diagnostic and Statistical Manual of Mental Disorders (DSM-5)*, which is the standard classification of mental disorders used by mental health providers in the United States. The criteria are specific for each anxiety disorder, and they include the number and severity of anxiety symptoms, as well as the length of time a person experiences them. No laboratory tests exist to diagnose anxiety disorders.

Treatments

Anxiety disorders are highly treatable. Several standard approaches are effective, either alone or in combination. Psychotherapy, also known as talk therapy, has a variety of forms. Cognitive-behavioral therapy (CBT) is well established as a highly effective and lasting treatment for anxiety disorders. It focuses on identifying, understanding, and changing thinking and behavior patterns. Depending on the individual, its benefits may be seen in about few months. Other types of therapy include acceptance and commitment therapy (ACT), dialectical behavioral therapy (DBT), and interpersonal therapy (IPT).

Medication treatment for anxiety disorders may be prescribed in conjunction with therapy. It can be a short- or long-term treatment option, depending on the severity of symptoms, other medical conditions, and a person's individual needs and circumstances. Four major classes of medications are commonly used: selective serotonin reuptake inhibitors (SSRIs) relieve symptoms by blocking the reabsorption, or reuptake, of serotonin by certain nerve cells in the brain; serotonin-norepinephrine reuptake inhibitors (SNRIs) increase the levels of the neurotransmitters serotonin and norepinephrine by inhibiting their reabsorption into cells in the brain; benzodiazepines, frequently used for short-term management of anxiety, are highly effective in promoting relaxation and reducing muscle tension and other physical symptoms; and tricyclic antidepressants are often effectively prescribed in place of benzodiazepines, but they can cause significant side effects.

A growing body of scientific evidence shows that some nonmedical treatments, when used along with conventional treatments, may produce modest, short-term reduction of anxiety in some people; among these are breathing and relaxation techniques, meditation and mindfulness, yoga, and acupuncture.

Prevention

Anxiety disorders are not preventable, but it is possible to reduce some risk factors, as well as ways to manage symptoms, including limiting caffeine and alcohol, eating well-balanced meals, learning what triggers anxiety, getting enough sleep, participating in regular exercise and activities, talking to friends and family, and seeking professional help when needed.

Prognosis and Outcomes

The vast majority of people with an anxiety disorder can be helped with professional treatment. Untreated anxiety disorders can impair daily functioning and be disabling, and they also put people at higher risk of experiencing physical health problems. Success of treatment depends on it being tailored specifically for an individual. It may also be complicated if people have more than one anxiety disorder, depression, substance abuse, or other coexisting conditions. With treatment, individuals with anxiety disorders can manage the symptoms of anxiety disorders and lead healthy lives.

Future

Research continues into the role of genetics in the development of anxiety disorders, as well as the effects of environmental factors, the long-term impact of stressful life events, and the identification of new and novel treatments for anxiety and related disorders using medications and therapies.

Andrea D'Souza

See also: Alcoholism; Depression; Substance Abuse; Mental Disorders; Social Health; Stress; Substance Abuse

Further Reading

American Psychological Association. (2015). Anxiety disorders. Retrieved from http://www .apa.org/health-reform/anxiety-disorders.html.

Anxiety and Depression Association of America. (2015). Understanding the facts. Retrieved from http://www.adaa.org/understanding-anxiety.

Mayo Clinic. (2014). Anxiety. Retrieved from http://www.mayoclinic.org/diseases-conditions /anxiety/basics/definition/con-20026282.

National Alliance on Mental Illness (NAMI). (2015). Anxiety disorders. Retrieved from https://www.nami.org/Learn-More/Mental-Health-Conditions/Anxiety-Disorders.

National Institute of Mental Health. (2015). What are anxiety disorders? Retrieved from http://www.nimh.nih.gov/health/publications/anxiety-disorders/nimhanxiety.pdf.

Stein, M., & Walker, J. (2009). *Triumph over Shyness: Conquering Social Anxiety Disorder,* 2nd ed. Silver Spring, MD: ADAA.

Wilson, R. (2009). *Don't Panic. Edition: Taking Control of Anxiety Attacks,* 3rd ed. New York: Harper Perennial.

ARRHYTHMIAS/DYSRHYTHMIAS

Description

An arrhythmia is an irregular, slow, or too rapid heartbeat. It is frequently harmless, and it can be common to have mild palpitations or irregular heartbeats. If this occurs, there is no need for treatment, and people can lead healthy lives. If this condition becomes more severe, it is also possible to be treated and lead a successful life.

During an arrhythmia, the electrical signals that control heartbeat may be delayed or blocked, which disrupts signals that control the normal heartbeat. As a result, the heart may not be able to pump blood to the body in sufficient amounts. If this occurs, the lack of blood flow to vital organs such as the heart, brain, and lungs can cause damage of these and other organs.

There are many types of arrhythmias, and the outlook for people who have these depends on their severity. Some arrhythmias are potentially fatal, causing sudden death. In one type of inherited arrhythmia that occurs in children, the person may also become deaf.

Fast rhythms are called *tachycardia*. Slow rhythms are called *bradycardia*.

Symptoms of Arrhythmias

Anxiety
Chest pain
Paleness
Palpitations
Shortness of breath
Sweating
Weakness, dizziness, lightheadedness

Causes

Most arrhythmias are caused by underlying heart disease. Strong emotional stress or anger can also cause arrhythmias. Smoking, excess caffeine intake, and thyroid disease can cause arrhythmias, as can other health problems, especially those that weaken the heart such as heart failure. Arrhythmias are also common with aging, and most serious arrhythmias affect people older than 60. Arrhythmias can occur in children and young adults, and certain drugs such as cocaine or blood chemical imbalances such as potassium can cause arrhythmias, as can high blood pressure and rheumatic heart disease.

Sometimes the cause of the arrhythmia is not known.

Diagnosis

This is usually based on medical and family history; a physical exam; and results of specific tests and procedures such as an electrocardiogram, blood tests, chest x-ray, and ultrasound waves. Another test is a stress test as well as a nuclear heart scanning test. Angiograms and implanted loop recorders can be used to detect abnormal heart rhythms.

Treatment

Medications can slow a rapidly beating heart or change an abnormal rhythm to a normal rhythm. Medicines can also control the underlying condition, where this is relevant.

Some conditions are treated with pacemakers or a form of electric shock called defibrillation. An implantable defibrillator may be used to continuously restore a normal heartbeat.

Other approaches involve inserting a catheter into the heart to destroy areas generating abnormal heart rhythms, coronary artery bypass, or maze surgery where the surgeon makes small cuts or burns in the upper chambers of the heart or atria. Another approach is to surgically cut the vagal nerve that helps control the heart rate.

Keeping well physically—including having a healthy diet low in salt, sugar, fats, and refined grains—is recommended. A heart healthy diet as well as a physically active lifestyle; quitting smoking; and maintaining a healthy weight, blood pressure, and cholesterol levels are also recommended. Stress management, meditation, and relaxation can also help.

You may have to avoid taking some over-the-counter remedies for cold or coughs because they can cause your heart rate to accelerate.

Ray Marks

See also: Aging; Anxiety; Bradycardia; Healthy; Heart Diseases; Stress; Tachycardia; Thyroid Disease

Further Reading

American Heart Association. (2011). About arrhythmia. Retrieved from http://www.heart .org/HEARTORG/Conditions/Arrhythmia/AboutArrhythmia/About-Arrhythmia_UCM _002010_Article.jsp.

American Heart Association. (2011). Types of arrhythmia in children. Retrieved from http:// www.heart.org/HEARTORG/Conditions/Arrhythmia/AboutArrhythmia/Types-of -Arrhythmia-in-Children_UCM_302023_Article.jsp.

American Heart Association. (2011). What is an arrhythmia? American Stroke Association. Learn and Live. Retrieved from http://www.heart.org/idc/groups/heart-public/@wcm /@hcm/documents/downloadable/ucm_300290.pdf.

Cohen, T. J. (2010). *A Patient's Guide to Heart Rhythm Problems*. Johns Hopkins University Press.

National Heart Lung and Blood Institute. (2001). Explore arrhythmia. Retrieved from http:// www.nhlbi.nih.gov/health/health-topics/topics/arr.

ARTERIOVENOUS MALFORMATIONS

Definition

Arteriovenous malformations are defects in the blood circulation system thought to arise during fetal development or soon after birth, and these defects within the blood circulation system can occur in many different parts of the body. The presence of these defects may not pose any problem for the individual, even though they interfere with the blood circulation. However, in about 12 percent of those affected, the problem may be associated with symptoms that may vary, depending on the affected site. There is also a chance of hemorrhage or bleeding episodes. A small number of these cases may experience disability and about one percent of cases may die prematurely in any given year.

All races and both genders can be affected to equal extents. The cause is unknown.

Sites that can be affected include the brain, the spinal cord, various organs, and the eye.

Diagnosis

Common diagnostic approaches and tests include angiograms and ultrasound.

Researchers are studying groups of these cases to try to better understand who will be susceptible to hemorrhage.

Symptoms and Treatment

Symptoms include abnormal sensation, back pain, difficulty carrying out tasks that require planning, dizziness, headache, loss of coordination and walking disturbances, memory lapses or loss, mental confusion, muscle weakness, pain, paralysis, seizures, speech problems, and visual disturbances.

Symptoms may occur at any time and may start to be more apparent after age 20.

Treatments include medications to relieve symptoms, surgery, catheter embolization, focused irradiation therapy, and gamma-knife radiosurgery.

Ray Marks

See also: Angiogram; Blood Disorders; Spinal Diseases

Further Reading

American Association of Neurological Surgeons. (2015). Patient information: Arteriovenous malformations. Retrieved from http://www.aans.org/Patient%20Information/Conditions%20and%20Treatments/Arteriovenous%20Malformations.aspx.

American Stroke Association. (2014). What is an arteriovenous malformation (AVM)? Retrieved from http://www.strokeassociation.org/STROKEORG/AboutStroke/Typesof Stroke/HemorrhagicBleeds/What-Is-an-Arteriovenous-Malformation-AVM_UCM _310099_Article.jsp#.VjJSD2tKiM8.

Boston Children's Hospital. (2015). Arteriovenous malformations (AVMs) in children. Retrieved from http://www.childrenshospital.org/conditions-and-treatments/conditions/arteriovenous-malformations-avms/overview.

Mayo Clinic. (2015). Brain AVM (arteriovenous malformation). Retrieved from http://www.mayoclinic.org/diseases-conditions/brain-avm/home/ovc-20129992.

National Institute of Neurological Disorders and Stroke. (2015). NINDS arteriovenous malformation information page. Retrieved from http://www.ninds.nih.gov/disorders/avms/avms.htm.

ARTHRITIS

Arthritis refers to a group of diseases that involve painful inflammation and stiffness of the musculoskeletal system, especially the joints. It is the leading cause of disability in adults in the United States (CDC 2016). The word *arthritis* comes from the Greek word "arthron," meaning "joint," and the Latin term "itis," meaning "inflammation." There are more than 100 different types of arthritis, and they vary in prevalence from common to rare. In the United States, as many as 50 million adults (22 percent) have been doctor-diagnosed with arthritis, with the condition being the second most frequent reason for consulting a doctor (CDC 2016). The most common forms of arthritis are osteoarthritis (OA) and rheumatoid arthritis (RA).

One of the first diseases to be clinically recognized, arthritis was described in ancient Egyptian medical texts, by ancient Greek scholars, and in an Ayurvedic medical text from around 123 CE. Ayurvedic medicine is a form of Hindu traditional medicine on the Indian subcontinent. Hippocrates, the ancient Greek physician traditionally thought of as the father of medicine, and medieval Europeans explained the cause of joint problems as bad humors, or body fluids, dripping into affected joints. Archeological remains also show some evidence of arthritis existing in Neanderthals and other early humans (Brehm 2015).

Osteoarthritis

Osteoarthritis or "degenerative arthritis" is characterized by the breakdown of cartilage in a joint, often caused by trauma or overuse. It eventually leads to abnormal bone changes and the failure of the joint's mobility. Cartilage is a flexible connective tissue that protects joints, helping to maintain stability and flexibility. Cartilage does not contain blood vessels, which helps to explain why the rate of cartilage growth and repair is relatively slow. Osteoarthritis also might affect the synovium—a fluid-filled sac that surrounds the joint and provides nutrients and oxygen to the joint components. The surrounding muscle and tendons also can be involved. In the early stages of OA, the cartilage becomes swollen and loses elasticity, which results in the formation of tiny cracks within cartilage tissue that hinder joint function and leave the cartilage vulnerable to further damage. The fragmentation of the cartilage surface can lead to remodeling of the bone and invasion by blood vessels. Inflammation also commonly occurs in the synovium, causing pain and swelling, and can exacerbate cartilage deterioration. Osteoarthritis is not a systemic disease and only occurs in those joints with deterioration, most commonly affecting the joints of the spine, knee, hand, foot, and hip.

Rheumatoid Arthritis

Rheumatoid arthritis is a chronic, systemic, inflammatory autoimmune disorder affecting the synovium and leading to joint damage and bone destruction. The disease begins in the small joints, such as the hands and feet, and extends to larger joints. In RA, the immune system attacks the tissues that line joints, including cartilage. The inflamed synovium proliferates across the joint and becomes heavily infiltrated with inflammatory cells. The invading synovium also produces enzymes that decrease cartilage integrity and stimulate bone erosion. Additionally, the surrounding soft tissue becomes inflamed, and new blood vessel growth occurs. Together with the invasion of cartilage and bone into the joint surface, this leads to deformity and progressive physical disability. Intestinal inflammation, abnormal gut microflora, and lipid abnormalities, including insulin resistance correlated to inflammation, also are associated with RA.

Epidemiology

Osteoarthritis is a much more common disease than is rheumatoid arthritis. The number of people affected by arthritis is large with a wide-ranging impact on society. Approximately one in three people with arthritis (31 percent) between the ages of 18 and 64 report work limitations due to arthritis, and arthritis is strongly associated with major depression (CDC 2016). Worldwide, approximately 9.6 percent of men and 18 percent of women have OA, and about 0.3 percent to 1 percent of people have RA (WHO 2016). Rheumatoid arthritis has a relatively lower prevalence in poorer countries (WHO 2016). Both OA and RA are more prevalent in women; it has been noted that 24.3 percent of women and 18.3 percent of men in the United States have been diagnosed with arthritis; the prevalence increases with age and is higher among women than men in every age group (CDC 2016).

Although premature mortality is quite low in people with arthritic diseases, the morbidity associated with the disease can be very high, varying greatly among individuals. Joint stiffness and pain are the most prominent symptoms, and arthritis often causes reduced mobility and a lower level of physical activity that result in some degree of physical disability (CDC 2016). This morbidity related to arthritis also comes as an economic cost to both the individual and to society. Arthritis is among the most common reasons for working days lost, amounting to a huge economic impact worldwide. In 2003, the total cost attributed to arthritis and other rheumatic conditions in the United States was $128 billion, up from $86.2 billion in 1997 (CDC 2016).

Symptoms and Diagnosis

General signs and symptoms of arthritis include swelling in one or more joints, stiffness around joints that lasts for at least an hour in the morning, constant or recurring pain or tenderness in a joint, difficulty in moving joints, and warmth or redness around joint (CDC 2016). A general physician or rheumatologist often will review a patient's medical history and order lab tests, including blood and urine tests and imaging tests such as x-rays or MRIs, to make a diagnosis (CDC 2016). Both OA and RA can be classified according to severity using criteria set out by the American College of Rheumatology. Osteoarthritis can manifest in different ways, but it is usually diagnosed when health care providers note a loss of cartilage within synovial joints, associated with loss of bone mass and the thickening of the joint capsule. (The joint capsule is the thin, fluid-filled sac that surrounds the joint and that contains lubricating fluid.) Rheumatoid arthritis usually is diagnosed when patients have arthritis of at least one joint area and achieve a certain "score" that is based on the American College of Rheumatology's criteria. These criteria include location and number of involved joints; symptom duration; severity of RA symptoms, such as swelling or deformity; and positive blood results for serum rheumatoid factor.

Causes and Risk Factors

Osteoarthritis sometimes is brought about by another disease or condition. This includes trauma or repetitive use, infectious diseases, or other inflammatory diseases, such as gout. Gout is a complex form of arthritis that occurs when either the kidney does not excrete enough uric acid or the body produces too much, and consequently, uric acid crystals can accumulate in joints. The accumulation of crystals results in inflammation, swelling, and severe attacks of pain. Obesity is another common contributor to OA because excess adipose tissue increases systemic inflammation and can put added stress on damaged joints, particularly the knees and hips.

Rheumatoid arthritis appears to be caused by the interaction among many genetic and environmental factors. Genetic susceptibility can be seen in twin and family studies that have shown an increase in the risk of developing RA among relatives. Certain shared alleles, called "rheumatoid epitopes," could help predict disease severity and outcome. Rheumatoid arthritis seems to peak in the fifth decade of life, and socioeconomic status seems to affect the outcome of—rather than cause of—the disease; lower socioeconomic status is linked with a worse prognosis. Smoking and dietary choices also are likely to affect the risk of developing RA and also the outcome of the disease. People in geographic zones that eat a Mediterranean diet—including a lifelong consumption of fish, olive oil, and cooked vegetables—have lower rates of RA occurrence and severity.

Treatments

Arthritis treatment recommendations vary greatly from lifestyle changes to prescription medicine therapies and depend on type and severity of arthritis and the individual. Because arthritis has no cure, the goals of treatment are to reduce pain, limit joint damage, maximize function, and maintain or improve the quality of life. Treatment usually consists of a combination of medication and nonpharmacologic therapies, such as physical therapy, occupational therapy, patient education, and weight loss (for people who are overweight).

There are many medications on the market to help in the management of arthritis, including analgesics, nonsteroidal anti-inflammatory drugs (NSAIDs), disease-modifying antirheumatic drugs (DMARDs), biologic response modifiers, and corticosteroids (CDC 2016). These medications aim to reduce pain and decrease inflammation, often by slowing or blocking the immune system—which can leave the patient susceptible to other health problems (CDC 2016). Other suggested practices include exercise, proper nutrition, rest and relaxation, surgery (in some cases), and heat/cold therapies (CDC 2016).

Nutrition

People with arthritis are at risk for nutritional deficiencies. One reason could be that inflammation is associated with the production of cytokines, the activators of immune cells that increase resting metabolic rate and protein breakdown. Medications also can cause conditions that are associated with decreased appetite, such as peptic ulcers or gastritis. People with arthritis who experience significant disability frequently have difficulty shopping for groceries and preparing nutritious meals. For people with arthritis, a proper diet means eating a variety of foods that balance caloric intake and physical activity; choosing a diet with plenty of vegetables and fruits; and choosing foods low in synthetic trans fats, added sugars, and alcohol. Following a healthy diet nurtures a healthy weight and improves overall health, which might be important in managing arthritis and its symptoms. Additionally, foods with anti-inflammatory properties might help reduce the inflammation associated with both OA and RA.

Some of the dietary components and eating patterns that have been investigated as possible factors in the management of OA and RA include omega-3 fatty acids and gamma linolenic acid. Omega-3 fatty acids play a role in modifying the inflammation process and the regulation of pain, decreasing cytokine activity and cartilage breakdown. It has also been suggested that omega-3 levels are inversely correlated with cardiovascular disease, which is seen in many patients with RA; are associated with lower risk of developing the disease; and can work alongside other medications, such as NSAIDs, to decrease inflammation (Stamp et al. 2005). Omega-3 fatty acids can be found in oily fish (e.g., salmon, tuna, mackerel), some vegetables (including soybeans, tofu, kale, collard greens, and winter squash), walnuts, flaxseed, and pecans. Gamma linolenic acid (GLA) is a fatty acid precursor to anti-inflammatory compounds made by the body. Gamma linolenic acid is found in evening primrose oil, borage oil, and black currant oil supplements, though caution should be used with supplements because they are not well regulated.

Eating foods rich in antioxidants could decrease the oxidation that leads to increased cell and tissue damage in inflammatory arthritis. Antioxidants such as vitamin C, vitamin E, selenium, carotene, lycopene, and flavonoids slow the process of oxidation and remove free radicals. Colorful vegetables and fruits are rich in antioxidants: leafy greens (including spinach and kale), beets, blueberries, and cranberries. Beans, nuts, green tea, red wine, dark chocolate, and certain spices such as cinnamon, ginger, and turmeric also are rich in antioxidants. Vitamin D also could exert anti-inflammatory effects. Probiotic foods and high-quality supplements could help to address the intestinal inflammation present with RA.

Glucosamine and glucosamine chondroitin supplements are often used or suggested for people with osteoarthritis, but, as the Arthritis Foundation reports, "most studies assessing their effectiveness show modest to no improvement compared with placebo in either pain relief or joint damage" (Hess 2015).

Specialty and Controversial Diets

Some research suggests that vegetarian and vegan diets could improve clinical symptoms of arthritis as could many low-fat diets that aim to reduce animal product consumption. Another beneficial eating plan may be the Mediterranean diet.

Little research supports the notion that elimination diets, fasting, and "miracle" food diets are safe and effective ways to reduce inflammation. There is little scientific evidence to show that cutting out a specific food, or relying on one as a cure, are effective treatment options. Fasting, although associated with reduced inflammation in the short term, can lead to dehydration and serious nutritional deficiencies and is not recommended as a viable long-term treatment option.

Barbara A. Brehm and Micaela A. Young

See also: Arthritis; Diet and Nutrition; Gout; Inflammation; Juvenile Arthritis; Osteoarthritis; Reactive Arthritis; Rheumatoid Arthritis; Vitamin D

Further Reading

Brehm, B. A. (2015). *Nutrition: Science, Issues, and Applications,* Santa Barbara, CA: ABC-CLIO.

Centers for Disease Control and Prevention (CDC). (2016). Arthritis. Retrieved from http://www.cdc.gov/arthritis/index.htm.

Hess, A. (2015). Chondroitin sulfate and glucosamine supplements in osteoarthritis. Arthritis Foundation. Retrieved from http://www.arthritis.org/living-with-arthritis/treatments/natural/supplements-herbs/glucosamine-chondroitin-osteoarthritis.php.

Lorig, K., & Fries, J. F. (2006). *The Arthritis Helpbook: A Tested Self-Management Program for Coping with Arthritis and Fibromyalgia,* 6th ed. New York: Da Capo Press.

National Center for Complementary and Alternative Medicine (NCCAM). (2013). Rheumatoid arthritis and complementary approaches. Retrieved from http://nccam.nih.gov/health/RA/getthefacts.htm.

Nelson, J., & Zeratsky, K. (2013, March 16). Does diet have a role in rheumatoid arthritis? Retrieved from http://www.mayoclinic.com/health/diet-and-rheumatoid-arthritis/MY02387.

Stamp, L., James, M., & Cleland, L. (2005). Diet and rheumatoid arthritis: A review of the literature. *Seminars in Arthritis and Rheumatism, 35,* 77–94.

World Health Organization (WHO). (2016). Chronic rheumatic conditions. Retrieved from http://www.who.int/chp/topics/rheumatic/en/.

ASTHMA

Asthma is a chronic medical condition that causes inflammation, narrowing, and increased mucus in the airways, the part of the body that brings air into and out of the lungs. This tightening of the airways can result in shortness of breath, tightness in the chest, coughing, and wheezing. The degree to which asthma affects the lives of those with the condition varies. For some, it can be a minor nuisance, while for others, it can greatly affect their everyday lives and potentially lead to an asthma attack, which can be life-threatening. The majority of those with asthma develop the condition during childhood. It is estimated that more than 25 million people in the United States have asthma.

There are two different types of asthma: extrinsic and intrinsic. In *extrinsic asthma*, the airways begin to narrow because of an allergic reaction to an allergen such as pollen, dust, mold, or animal fur. It is the most common form of asthma, and individuals with atopy, a condition that causes hypersensitivity to allergens, are especially susceptible to the condition. In *intrinsic asthma*, the airways will also begin to tighten, but the reaction is not caused by allergens. Typical triggers of intrinsic asthma include cold air, exercise, and smoke.

While the specific cause of asthma is not known, there are several factors that are believed to contribute to the development of the condition. One cause is atopy, which can be inherited or acquired due to environmental factors such as an overly hygienic environment, which can affect how a child's immune system develops. The hypersensitivity to allergens caused by atopy can make individuals with the condition very susceptible to developing asthma. In addition, asthma can be inherited if a parent has the condition. Children can develop asthma as a result of certain kinds of respiratory infections or through exposure to allergens while their immune system is still developing.

Regardless of underlying cause and immediate trigger, the symptoms of asthma include inflammation and sensitivity of the airways. When the airways become irritated, they begin to narrow and fill with mucus, which limits air flow to the lungs. As the airways continue to narrow, a variety of symptoms may occur, such as difficulty breathing, tightness in the chest, and coughing. The severity of asthma symptoms varies and can be lessened with the use of medication.

If asthma symptoms worsen, it can lead to an asthma attack. During an asthma attack, the airways will continue to narrow and fill with mucus. Symptoms include heavy coughing; chest pain; rapid, short breathing; and tightening in the neck and chest muscles. While mild asthma attacks may dissipate within a few minutes, severe attacks require immediate medical attention. If an individual suffering from a severe asthma attack does not receive medical care, congestion in the airways may lead to oxygen deprivation and, potentially, death.

In order to diagnose asthma, a health care professional will begin by examining the patient's medical and family history. The doctor will then conduct a physical exam to assess the patient's breathing and more closely observe any signs of asthma, such coughing and swollen nasal passages. In order to determine the condition of the patient's lungs, the doctor will perform a lung function test known as a spirometry. This test measures how much air the patient can breathe in and out of the lungs, as well as how fast he or she can blow air out. The doctor may also give the patient medicine and perform the test again to see if the results improve. If the patient has an easier time breathing after receiving the medication and if he or she has a medical history of symptoms associated with asthma, the doctor may diagnose asthma. For children with asthma symptoms, lung function tests are difficult to perform if the child is under the age of five, which is when most children develop asthma. As a result, when diagnosing young children, doctors rely mostly on the child's medial history as well as a physical examination to determine whether or not the child has asthma.

There is no known cure for asthma, but the condition can be effectively controlled in several different ways. Asthma symptoms can be combated with quick-relief medications such as inhaled short-acting beta2-agonists, which relax smooth muscle and dilate bronchial passageways. In order to reduce the inflammation of the airways and prevent asthma symptoms from occurring, long-term control medications are required. Long-term asthma medications usually take the form of inhaled corticosteroids, which are administered through an inhaler into the lungs. If taken on a regular schedule, inhaled corticosteroids can greatly reduce the swelling of the airways and make asthma symptoms more manageable. While inhaled corticosteroids are generally safe, they can cause side effects such as thrush. For individuals with severe asthma, a corticosteroid pill or liquid may be required. In addition to taking medication, avoiding triggers of asthma symptoms can make it easier to control the condition.

The Greek physician Hippocrates is believed to be the first medical practitioner to describe asthma, around 450 BCE. The term comes from the Greek word for "panting." The condition is also believed to have been present in ancient Egypt. In 1864, Dr. Henry Hyde Salter found animal hair to be a trigger for asthma symptoms, and in the early 1900s, Italian physician Bernardino Ramazzini made a connection between asthma and poor working conditions. During the late 1800s and up until the early 1900s, inhaling asthma medications in the form of smoke was one of the preferred methods of treatment. In 1901, Jokici Takamine, a Japanese scientist, developed the first bronchodilator, a medication that dilates portions of the airways to make breathing easier, which served as one of the first effective treatments for asthma. In the 1960s, researchers learned that asthma is an inflammation of the airways and that individuals with the condition tend to have weaker immune systems, making them more susceptible to allergens. In 1972, inhaled corticosteroids were introduced and remain one of the most effective medications for controlling asthma long-term.

Today, approximately 235 million people around the world have asthma, and it is the most common noncommunicable disease among children. While cases of asthma tend to be more prevalent in developed nations, individuals in developing nations who have the condition are more likely to die from complications resulting from asthma. In the United States, the rates of asthma as well as asthma-related hospitalization and death are higher among African Americans than for any other racial group.

Renee Dubie

See also: Allergies; Asthma, Children and Youth; Immune System Disorders; Inflammation; Respiratory Diseases

Further Reading

Adams, Francis. (2006). *The Asthma Sourcebook*, 3rd ed. New York: McGraw-Hill.

American Academy of Allergy Asthma & Immunology. (2015). Asthma overview. Retrieved from https://www.aaaai.org/conditions-and-treatments/asthma.

Centers for Disease Control and Prevention. (2015). Asthma. Retrieved from http://www.cdc.gov/asthma/default.htm.

Fanta, C. H., Cristiano, M., & Haver, K. E., with Waring, N. (2003). *The Harvard Medical School Guide to Taking Control of Asthma: A Comprehensive Prevention and Treatment Plan for You and Your Family.* New York: Free Press.

Pescatore, F. (2008). *The Allergy and Asthma Cure: A Complete 8-Step Nutritional Program.* Hoboken, NJ: John Wiley & Sons.

ASTHMA, CHILDREN AND YOUTH

Bronchial asthma is the most commonly diagnosed chronic (long-lasting) disease in children throughout the United States. An estimated 6.8 million children are affected by bronchial asthma nationwide (Bloom et al. 2013). In New York City, 22.2 percent of children have received an asthma diagnosis, accounting for 38,000 school-aged children affected by the disease (NYC Youth Risk Behavior Survey 2009). Among these New York City children, those living in high risk-neighborhoods report higher rates of asthma, with East and Central Harlem at 30 percent, the South Bronx at 28.5 percent, and North and Central Brooklyn at 27.2 percent. Low income, poor housing conditions, adverse environmental factors, and low health literacy contribute to the disproportionately high rates. While this disease cannot be cured, it can be effectively kept under control with good medical treatment, increased health education to improve self-management skills, and avoidance or reduction of exposure to environmental triggers. Inadequate asthma management and treatment can have devastating consequences, including permanent lung damage and death.

Because bronchial asthma is a lifelong diagnosis, physicians are often reluctant to declare this diagnosis in children under six months of age without the presence of a strong family history and/or close and constant monitoring of symptoms to substantiate the diagnosis. Absence of symptoms for long periods of time is not an indication of the absence of the disease; rather, it signifies that the disease is under control and that there have been no immediate exposures to an individual's environmental triggers. Contrary to popular myths, asthma does not simply go away, nor can it be outgrown.

Asthma is a disease of the lungs, characterized by continuous swelling and mucus buildup inside the airways coupled with a squeezing of the muscles on the outside of these airways. Swelling, mucus buildup, and muscle constriction lead to an asthma attack, making it difficult for the individual to breath.

The impact of asthma varies greatly among individuals, with some only exhibiting mild symptoms and others being severely incapacitated by the disease. Asthma severity has been classified into four categories based on the number of daytime

Table 3   Asthma Severity Classifications

	Daytime Symptoms	Nighttime Symptoms	Need for Rescue Medication
Mild intermittent	2 days or fewer per week	2 times per month or fewer	2 days or fewer per week
Mild persistent	More than 2 days per week	3–4 times per month	More than 2 days per week but not daily
Moderate persistent	Everyday	More than once per week but not nightly	Everyday
Severe persistent	Symptoms throughout the day	Every night	Several times a day

Source: National Heart, Blood and Lung Institute. (2007). Guidelines for the Diagnosis and Management of Asthma (EPR-3). Washington, DC: National Institutes of Health.

symptoms and the number of nighttime symptoms present as well as the need for use of reliever (rescue) medications during a 30-day period (see Table 3).

Treatment regimens are determined by the need to control the most severe symptoms. For example, a child with daytime symptoms two days per week, consistent with "mild intermittent" asthma, and with nighttime symptoms every night, consistent with a severe persistent classification, would be classified for treatment as the most severe or "severe persistent" overall asthma in order to attain the best possible clinical outcomes. Seasonal asthma symptoms would be categorized as "mild intermittent" because individuals are most commonly affected by pollen during the spring season and/or by ragweed and other tree allergens during the fall season.

The exact cause of bronchial asthma is still not fully understood; however, environmental and genetic factors have been associated with its development. Although not always the case, a previous family history of asthma increases the likelihood that a child will develop the disease. While there have been many advances in the overall understanding and treatment of asthma, research indicates (Akinbami & Schoendorf 2002; Malveau 2009; NYC Youth Risk Behavior Survey 2009) that asthma prevalence rates have remained consistently high. Hospitalization rates have also remained high, although recent improvements have been noted. The East Harlem community has the highest rates of asthma-related hospitalizations in all of New York City. This is particularly significant because the lowest hospitalization rates have been reported just one city block away on the Upper East Side. Socioeconomic (financial) status has been cited as one of the most plausible explanations for such a disparity.

Well-controlled asthma can help increase the number of symptom-free days, reduce the number of missed school days for the child and work days for the parent, increase physical activity, and allow child to sleep well during the night. Most significantly it will decrease emergency room visits and hospitalizations due to asthma and potentially save a life.

Good asthma education provides asthmatics with the tools necessary to effectively manage symptoms and environmental triggers. The National Heart Lung and Blood Institute (NHLBI) of the National Institutes of Health (2007) and the Centers for Disease Control and Prevention (CDC 2011) list common asthma symptoms as coughing with or without phlegm production, shortness of breath, wheezing (whistling sound when breathing), tightness of the chest, and constant fatigue. Individual asthma symptoms may vary; therefore, early identification of asthma symptoms for each individual is essential.

As with asthma symptoms, individuals are sensitive to different environmental triggers that may bring on an asthma attack. It is also important to adequately identify asthma triggers in order to remove or reduce exposure to these elements. These triggers are elements in our environment that are harmless to most people. Some commonly known indoor triggers include dust; dust mites (microscopic insects that irritate the airways); mold; roaches and mice allergens; pet dander; exposure to harsh, strong-smelling chemicals, including cleaning detergents and personal products; and wood smoke, smoking in the home, and cooking odors. Outdoor exposures include pollen, pollution, car exhaust, and exposure to secondhand smoke. Allergies, colds, flu, and other respiratory and sinus infections can also trigger an asthma attack.

Adherence to prescribed treatment regimens is essential to the proper control and management of asthma. There are two main types of asthma medications. Inhaled corticosteroid (long-term controller) medications are used to reduce swelling and to decrease mucus buildup inside the airways. This medication is taken every day whether symptoms are present or not. Bronchodilator medications are also known as reliever or rescue medications because they are life-saving, quick-acting relievers to release the squeezing of the muscles around the airways. Bronchodilator reliever medications are to be taken as prescribed by the physician and/or half an hour prior to exercise or exposure to a known environmental trigger. Prednisone will be prescribed to treat severe asthma attack episodes. It is given as emergency care, usually for a short period of time. This medication should not be taken frequently or as a substitute for regular treatment.

Aside from medications, physicians often provide several tools so that their patients can monitor and self-manage their asthma. The first is called an asthma action plan. This is a form containing the names and dosages of prescribed medications, a list of possible symptoms, and lung function scores determined by a peak flow meter, a small plastic tubular breathing apparatus that measures how well the lungs are working. Through health education, the physician or other clinical personnel instructs the patient/parent on how to obtain the child's personal best score using the peak flow meter. This is used as a baseline measure to determine levels of asthma control.

Levels of asthma control are defined using the colors of the traffic light. The green zone indicates that the child is experiencing no symptoms and/or limitations to normal daily activities and that the child is doing well. A child diagnosed with mild, moderate, or severe persistent asthma will need to take preventive controller medication to reduce the risk of having an asthma attack. The yellow zone indicates the presence of mild symptoms usually associated with some limitations to daily activities. It is an indication that the child's asthma is getting worse. Symptoms seen at this time can include some wheezing, tightness in the chest, shortness of breath, and inability to sleep through the night. Treatment at this time would include the use of the preventive controller medication plus the prescribed dosage of a reliever medication to alleviate the symptoms. Patients are asked to slow down their activities in order to allow the medications to take effect. The red zone indicates a medical alert and dangerous signs that should not be ignored. A child in the "red" will exhibit severe symptoms, which may include, but are not limited to, severe shortness of breath, blue lips and/or fingernails, and an inability to engage in any of the normal activities. Prescribed reliever medications may not be working and symptoms may be getting worse. Immediate medical attention must be sought in these cases. If a regular primary care physician is unavailable, the child should be taken to the emergency room for immediate care.

Another tool for school-aged children is the medication administration form (MAF), provided to school nurses and personnel as a prescription and authorization for children to receive reliever medications while in school. These forms are completed each year or when there are any changes to the treatment plan. Spacers, plastic tubes to facilitate use of medications, are also prescribed. Additional treatment strategies and enhanced asthma education curriculums continue to emerge.

Significant efforts to reduce the impact of asthma in underserved communities are currently under way. The New York City Department of Health and Mental Hygiene (NYC DOHMH), the NHLBI, the CDC, and other government entities are developing multiple programs to address the prevalence and hospitalization rates. The East Harlem Asthma Center of Excellence is one such effort. It is an initiative of former Mayor Michael Bloomberg in conjunction with the Go-Green East Harlem Initiative of Manhattan Borough President Scott Stringer. It started in 2007 with building a state-of-the art facility and inaugurated in 2010 in collaboration with the NYC DOHMH. The center provides education, information, support, and referrals to asthma counseling and medical care. Other milestones for asthma care and management include continuous efforts by the Communities in Action Asthma Initiatives by the Environmental Protection Agency and, most recently, CDC's renewed commitment to asthma control through the $25.4 million approved by Congress for the National Asthma Control Program, delineating the continued need to address, through programming and services, the multiple factors negatively affecting children in the United States today (CDC 2011).

Betty Perez-Rivera

See also: Allergies; Asthma; Immune System Disorders; Inflammation; Respiratory Diseases

Further Reading
Akinbami, L. J., & Schoendorf, K. C. (2002). Trends in childhood asthma: Prevalence, health care utilization, and mortality. *Pediatrics, 110,* 2, 315–322.

Bloom, B. L., Jones, I., & Freeman, G. (2013). Summary health statistics for U.S. children: National Health Interview Survey 2012. *Vital and Health Statistics*, *10*, 258.

Centers for Disease Control and Prevention. (2011). *Vital Signs: Asthma in the US, Growing Every Year*. Atlanta, Georgia.

Cloutier, M. M., Wakefield, D. B., Hall, C. B., & Bailit, H. L. (2002). Childhood asthma in an urban community: Prevalence, care system, and treatment. *Chest*, *122*, 1571–1579.

Gelfand, E. W. (2009). Pediatric asthma. *Proceedings of the American Thoracic Society*, *6*, 278–282.

Gold, D. R., & Wright, R. (2005). Population disparities in asthma. *Annual Review of Public Health*, *26*, 89–113.

Halterman, J. S., Szilagyi, P. G., Yoos, L., Conn, K. M., Kaczorowski, J. M., Holzhauer, R. J., Lauver, S. C., Neely, T. L., Callahan, P. M., & McConnochie, K. M. (2004). Benefits of a school-based asthma treatment program in the absence of secondhand smoke exposure results of a randomized clinical trial. *Archives of Pediatric and Adolescent Medicine*, *158*, 460–467.

Mackay, D., Haws, S., Ayres, J. G., Fischbacher, C., & Pell, J. P. (2010). Smoke-free legislation and hospitalizations for childhood asthma. *The New England Journal of Medicine*, *36*(12), 1139–1145.

Malveaux, F. J. (2009). The state of childhood asthma: Introduction. *Pediatrics*, *123*, S129–S130.

National Heart, Blood and Lung Institute (2007). *Guidelines for the Diagnosis and Management of Asthma* (EPR-3). Washington, DC: National Institutes of Health.

NYC Health. (2009). NYC Youth Risk Behavior Survey. Retrieved from https://www1.nyc.gov/site/doh/data/data-sets/nyc-youth-risk-behavior-survey.page.

Nicholas, S. W., Jean-Louis, B., Ortiz, B., Northridge, M., Shoemaker, K., Vaughan, R., Rome, M., Canada, G., & Hutchinson, V. (2005). Addressing the childhood asthma crisis in Harlem—The Harlem children's zone asthma initiative. *American Journal of Public Health*, *95*(2), 245–249.

Silverman, R. A., Stevenson, L., & Hastings, H. M. (2003). Age-related seasonal patterns of emergency department visits for acute asthma in an urban environment. *Annals of Emergency Medicine*, *42*(4), 577–587.

Stewart, M., McGhan, S., Watt, S., Anderson, S., Masuda, J. R., Letourneau, N., & Sharpe, H. M. (2010). Health professionals' preparation for supporting children and parents affected by asthma and allergies. *Journal of Asthma and Allergy Educators*, *1*(6), 223–231.

Strachan, D. P., & Sanders, C. H. (1989). Damp housing and childhood asthma; respiratory effects of indoor air temperature and relative humidity. *Journal of Epidemiology and Community Health*, *42*, 7–14.

ATHEROSCLEROSIS

Overview

Atherosclerosis a slow, progressive disease that occurs when plaque builds up inside the arteries, or the blood vessels carrying oxygen and nutrients from the heart to the rest of the body. Made of cholesterol and other fatty substances, plaque thickens and stiffens the arteries, which can restrict blood flow. If the plaques burst, they can create blood clots. Narrowed or blocked arteries can affect any part of the body and can lead to other diseases. Coronary artery disease is the result of blocked arteries to the heart; carotid artery disease refers to the block arteries to the brain; peripheral arterial disease occurs if arteries to the arms and legs are blocked; chronic kidney disease can occur if plaque builds up in the arteries leading to the kidneys.

The cause is not known, but atherosclerosis starts when the layer of cells lining the blood vessels is damaged, most likely due to high blood pressure, smoking, or high cholesterol; the damage leads to the formation of plaque. Millions of people in the United States may have atherosclerosis, but symptoms are not evident until it becomes severe. Depending on where an artery is affected, symptoms can appear as chest or leg pain, shortness of breath, numbness, infection, dizziness, confusion, weakness, loss of appetite, changes in skin color or toenails, hair loss, and swelling of hands or feet. Sometimes referred to as hardening of the arteries, the disease may begin in childhood and may not pose a danger until age 60 or older; some hardening of the arteries is a normal part of aging. Healthful lifestyle changes, medications, and surgical procedures are recommended treatments.

Symptoms

The symptoms of atherosclerosis depend on which arteries are affected. If plaque builds up in the carotid arteries, which supply blood to the brain, symptoms may include sudden weakness; dizziness; trouble walking; loss of balance or coordination; unexplained falls; paralysis or numbness of the face, arms, or legs; confusion; trouble speaking or understanding; vision or breathing problems; loss of consciousness; and a sudden and severe headache. If plaque affects the coronary arteries providing blood to the heart, symptoms may include angina (chest pain), shortness of breath, arrhythmias, sleep problems, fatigue, feeling faint, lack of energy, vomiting, extreme anxiety, and coughing.

If the blood supply affects in the renal arteries, chronic kidney disease can result. Symptoms may not appear until they worsen and cause a loss of kidney function, which can cause fatigue, changes in urination, loss of appetite, nausea, swelling in the hands or feet, itching or numbness, and difficulty concentrating. When peripheral arteries, usually the legs, become blocked, the most common symptom is leg pain, often described as heaviness, cramping, or dullness in the muscles; other symptoms may include hair loss on legs or feet, erectile dysfunction, numbness or weakness in the legs, changes in skin color or toenail thickness, and occasionally, infections.

Causes and Risk Factors

Although the precise cause of atherosclerosis is unknown, atherosclerosis may start in childhood and develop more quickly with aging. It begins with damage to the inner cell layer of the arteries, which allows plaque to build up. Factors that cause damage include smoking and other use of tobacco, high blood cholesterol and triglycerides, diabetes or high blood sugar due to insulin resistance, and inflammation from diseases or infections. Additional risk factors that increase the likelihood of developing atherosclerosis include aging, obesity, family history of early heart disease, lack of exercise, and an unhealthy diet. Other possible risk factors may include high levels of the C-reactive protein in the blood (which is a sign of inflammation), sleep apnea, stress, and heavy alcohol consumption.

Diagnosis

A physical exam may suggest signs of damaged arteries such as a weak or absent pulse below a narrowed artery, decreased blood pressure in an affected limb, whooshing sounds over an artery, signs of an aneurysm in the abdomen or behind the knee, or poor wound healing in the area of restricted blood flow. Other diagnostic tools include blood tests for levels of cholesterol and other fats or proteins; an electrocardiogram that measures the heart's electrical activity; a chest x-ray to look for heart failure; an ankle/brachial index test that can detect signs of peripheral arterial disease; echocardiography for information about the size and shape of the heart, how well it is working, and areas of poor blood flow; an ultrasound to check for changes in blood pressure in arteries where blood flow may be blocked; cardiac CT scan for early symptoms of coronary heart disease; cardiac stress testing; and angiography to see if plaque is blocking the arteries.

Treatments

The focus of treatments is to relieve symptoms, reduce risk factors for the buildup of plaque and formation of blood clots, widen or bypass blocked arteries, and prevent diseases caused by atherosclerosis. Recommended treatment includes making healthy lifestyle changes such as eating a heart-healthy diet of a variety of fresh fruits and vegetables, whole grains, lean meats, and good fats; getting regular physical exercise; maintaining a healthy body weight; avoiding tobacco products; and managing stress with relaxation techniques such as meditation, walking, or yoga, as well as talking to a mental health care provider or loved ones.

Medications may be prescribed to lower cholesterol, blood pressure, or blood sugar; prevent blood clots; and prevent inflammation. If necessary, surgical procedures include angioplasty to open blocked or narrowed coronary arteries, bypass surgery to allow blood to flow around a blocked or narrowed artery, and endarterectomy to remove plaque buildup from the carotid arteries in the neck.

Prevention

It is possible to prevent atherosclerosis by reducing many risk factors with the same lifestyle changes that help treat it: a heart-healthy diet, exercising regularly, a healthy body weight, no tobacco products, and using coping techniques to manage stress.

Prognosis and Outcomes

The effects of atherosclerosis cannot be reversed, but lifestyle changes and medications can prevent it from worsening. Although atherosclerosis leads to coronary artery disease, the main cause of death in the United States, people with the disease are living longer with better quality of life with the help of healthy lifestyle, an appropriate diet, and medications to lower LDL (bad) cholesterol.

Ray Marks

See also: Angina; Angiogram; Arrhythmias/Dysrhythmias; Coronary Heart Disease; Gangrene; Heart Diseases; High Blood Pressure; Kidney Diseases

Further Reading

American Heart Association. (2014). Atherosclerosis. Retrieved from http://www.heart.org /HEARTORG/Conditions/Cholesterol/WhyCholesterolMatters/Atherosclerosis_UCM _305564_Article.jsp.

Mayo Clinic. (2014). Arteriosclerosis/atherosclerosis. Retrieved from http://www.mayoclinic .org/diseases-conditions/arteriosclerosis-atherosclerosis/basics/definition/con -20026972.

Medical News Today. (2015). Atherosclerosis: Causes, symptoms and treatments. Retrieved from http://www.medicalnewstoday.com/articles/247837.php.

National Heart, Lung, and Blood Institute. (2015, September 22). What is atherosclerosis? Retrieved from http://www.nhlbi.nih.gov/health/health-topics/topics/atherosclerosis/.

ATRIAL FIBRILLATION

The term *atrial fibrillation* or *flutter* describes a type of very irregular heartbeat, which is usually too rapid. It is a type of arrhythmia and is caused by a disorder in the internal electrical system of the heart that regulates the rate and rhythm of the heartbeat. It can affect both men and women, and the risk for this condition increases with age and is common in people over 60 years of age. It is also called *auricular fibrillation*.

If atrial fibrillation is not diagnosed, treated, controlled, and monitored, it can be dangerous and can lead to chest pain, heart attack, heart failure, and stroke. It occurs when the two upper chambers of the heart, or atria, beat rapidly and irregularly or chaotically because the electrical signals to these two chambers are disorganized.

The main problem in atrial fibrillation is that the blood can pool in the atria and is not pumped completely to the two heart chambers below, called ventricles. The four chambers thus do not work in a coordinated way, and if this is not controlled or treated properly, it sometimes requires emergency treatment and can lead to complications.

Symptoms of Atrial Fibrillation

Symptoms may be chronic or may come and go or only occur on occasion and can include:

Chest pain
Confusion
Decreased blood pressure
Dizziness or light-headedness
Fainting
Fatigue
Feeling tired
Palpitations
Poor exercise tolerance
Shortness of breath
Weakness

In the occasional type of atrial fibrillation, symptoms may come and go and can last for a few minutes to a few hours, and can then stop on their own.

In the chronic type of atrial fibrillation, the heart rhythm is always abnormal.

In some people, atrial fibrillation causes no symptoms.

Causes of Atrial Fibrillation

In addition to age, some causes or risk factors for atrial fibrillation include:

- Alcohol abuse (especially binge drinking)
- Congestive heart failure
- Coronary artery disease
- Family history
- Heart disease caused by high cholesterol
- Heart surgery
- Heart valve disease
- History of a heart attack
- High blood pressure, especially if not well controlled
- Hypertrophic cardiomyopathy
- Lung disease
- Medications
- Overactive thyroid gland (hyperthyroidism)
- Pericarditis
- Sleep apnea

Diagnosis

A medical practitioner can use a physical examination—including a pulse check, a blood pressure check, and an electrocardiogram test—to examine the electrical waves of the heart. Other tests include exercise stress tests, ultrasound tests, tests to examine the state of the blood vessels, and angiograms.

Treatments

Medications to try to alter the hearts' electrical system and promote a normal heart rhythm may be used depending on the severity of the problem.

Procedures to restore normal rhythm—for example, using a pace maker or electrical shock treatment—or surgical and catheter procedures can also be implemented.

To prevent atrial fibrillation and its consequences, avoidance of binge drinking and frequent checkups or self-screening of one's pulse twice a year are important. A normal pulse is between 60 and 100 beats per minute and is strong and regular.

Treating the cause of atrial fibrillation often normalizes the heartbeat. If a person has a pulse that is irregular or too fast or too slow, however, or if the person has one or more symptoms of atrial fibrillation—such as chest pain, palpitations, shortness of breath, bleeding, or falling—he or she should see a health care provider. And, in the case of chest pain and serious shortness of breath, emergency medical care should be sought immediately.

Lifestyle changes that can improve overall heart health—such as eating heart-healthy foods, using less salt, increasing physical activity levels, and giving up smoking and caffeinated drinks—are other recommended strategies.

Clinical trials for atrial fibrillation can be explored at www.clinicaltrials.gov.

Ray Marks

See also: Angina; Angiogram; Arrhythmias/Dysrhythmias; Coronary Heart Disease; Heart Diseases; Heart Valve Disorders; High Blood Pressure; Kidney Diseases; Lung Diseases; Thyroid Disease

Further Reading

Mayo Clinic. (2015). Atrial fibrillation. Retrieved from http://www.mayoclinic.com/health/atrial-fibrillation/DS00291.

National Heart Lung and Blood Institute. (2001). What is atrial fibrillation? Retrieved from http://www.nhlbi.nih.gov/health/health-topics/topics/af/.

Shea, J. B., & Sears, S. F. (2008). Cardiology patient page. A patient's guide to living with atrial fibrillation. *Circulation, 117,* e340–e343.

U.S. National Library of Medicine, National Institutes of Health. (2011). Atrial fibrillation. Interactive tutorial. Patient Education Institute. Retrieved from http://www.nlm.nih.gov/medlineplus/tutorials/atrialfibrillation/htm/index.htm.

Women's Heart Foundation. (2011). Pulse check. Retrieved from http://www.womensheart.org/content/Stroke/pulse_check.asp.

ATROPHIC VAGINITIS

Overview

Atrophic vaginitis occurs in women who have low levels of estrogen, the hormone that keeps the vagina lubricated. When estrogen levels drop, vaginal tissue shrinks and thins, leading to dryness and inflammation. This most often takes place in women beginning in perimenopause and during menopause; up to 40 percent of postmenopausal women experience this condition, which is also known as vaginal or urogenital atrophy. Symptoms range from vaginal soreness, itching, burning, and discharge to painful intercourse and urinary tract infections; changes in the vagina can also increase the risk of vaginal infections. Mild symptoms can be managed with the application of nonprescription lubricants or moisturizing cream; hormone therapy may be prescribed for some women.

Symptoms

Atrophic vaginitis can affect the genital and urinary tracts. In addition to vaginal dryness, genital symptoms may include burning, discharge, inflammation, irritation, lesions, soreness, tenderness, and itching. Vaginal dryness increases the risk for uncomfortable or painful sexual intercourse, tears or sores in the vaginal walls, and the likelihood of developing yeast or bacterial infections. Symptoms affecting the urinary tract may include infection, blood in urine, and stress incontinence, which is an involuntary loss of small amounts of urine usually associated with movement.

Causes and Risk Factors

Atrophic vaginitis is caused by a decrease in estrogen, which occurs naturally after menopause. Other factors that can also reduce estrogen levels include medications or hormone therapy for breast cancer, endometriosis, uterine fibroids, or infertility; surgical removal of the ovaries; radiation therapy in the pelvic area; chemotherapy; postpartum or while breastfeeding; major depression or stress; and intense exercise.

Soaps, detergents, lotions, perfumes, and douches can irritate the vagina; tight clothing and synthetic materials may worsen symptoms. The immune disorder Sjögren's syndrome, as well as allergy and cold medications and certain antidepressants, tampons, condoms, douching, and smoking tobacco, may worsen vaginal dryness. Risk factors that may contribute to developing atrophic vaginitis include smoking tobacco, which reduces blood circulation; not having given birth vaginally; and no sexual activity, which increases the flow of blood to the vagina and maintains elasticity in the tissues.

Diagnosis

Diagnosis of atrophic vaginitis is based on a pelvic exam; blood and urine tests, which can indicate estrogen levels; and tests that measure the acid balance in the vaginal fluids and the presence of cells and bacteria that are common with the condition.

Treatments

Treatments focus on relieving vaginal dryness and other symptoms. Nonprescription topical lubricants and vaginal moisturizing creams can alleviate dryness, and water-soluble vaginal lubricants lessen pain or discomfort during intercourse.

Prescription topical estrogen, available in a variety of forms, is the most common treatment; it delivers estrogen only to the vaginal area to improve natural elasticity and moisture.

Severe symptoms may be treated with estrogen replacement therapy, often called hormone replacement therapy, which is effective in treating the condition. Long-term studies suggest that these types of treatment may increase the risks for stroke, breast cancer, heart attacks, or endometrial cancer.

Prevention

In addition to using nonprescription lubricants or moisturizing creams before symptoms become severe, women who stay sexually active increase vaginal blood circulation that stimulates natural moisture. Wearing cotton underwear and loose-fitting clothing can improve air circulation in the genital area, creating an environment that is not conducive for the growth of bacteria.

Prognosis and Outcomes

Atrophic vaginitis is not an inevitable result of reduced levels of estrogen. Correct diagnosis and appropriate treatment choices usually relieve symptoms of atrophic vaginitis. While hormone replacement therapy is effective, individuals must weigh its risks and benefits against their personal or family medical histories.

Future

Because even small amounts of estrogen may increase the risk of breast and endometrial cancers, scientists are working to create other types of treatments for atrophic vaginitis and its symptoms.

Ray Marks

See also: Sjögren's Syndrome; Vaginal Diseases; Women's Health

Further Reading
HealthLine. (2015). Postmenopausal atrophic vaginitis. Retrieved from http://www.healthline
.com/health/atrophic-vaginitis#Overview1.
Mayo Clinic. (2013, April 23). Vaginal atrophy. Retrieved from http://www.mayoclinic.org
/diseases-conditions/vaginal-atrophy/basics/definition/CON-20025768.
MedicineNet.com. (2015, February 23). Vaginal dryness and vaginal atrophy. Retrieved from
http://www.medicinenet.com/vaginal_dryness_and_vaginal_atrophy/article
.htm#what_causes_vaginal_dryness_and_vaginal_atrophy.
Medical News Today. (2014, September 11). What is atrophic vaginitis (vaginal trophy)?
What causes atrophic vaginitis? Retrieved from http://www.medicalnewstoday.com
/articles/189406.php.
MedlinePlus. (2013, November 10). Vaginal dryness. Retrieved from https://www.nlm.nih
.gov/medlineplus/ency/article/000892.htm.

ATTENTION DEFICIT HYPERACTIVITY DISORDER (ADHD)

Attention deficit hyperactivity disorder, commonly referred to as ADHD, is a chronic neurobehavioral condition that affects children and youth and often continues into adulthood. Children with ADHD can have difficulty sustaining attention and controlling impulsive behaviors and, in some cases, may have extreme levels of activity. ADHD is one of the most common behavioral disorders among school-aged children. Studies indicate rates of diagnosis among young people, ranging from 1 to 13 percent of youth in North America.

Signs and symptoms of ADHD can appear in children before the age of seven and can persist into adulthood. ADHD can be difficult to diagnosis because most healthy children have aspects and qualities of the disorder at some point in their development. However, these qualities become an area of concern when they inhibit an individual's ability to accomplish developmental tasks, such as forming relationships in school or in their family life, and achieving academic success.

Because the prevalence of ADHD is so high, much attention has been focused on research to discover the causes that will better inform treatment. Presently, ADHD is being treated through a combination of drug and behavioral therapy. The outcomes of treatment plans are good, and children often grow into successful adults who are able to manage the symptoms of ADHD.

History

Despite breakthroughs in research and an expansion in definitions, ADHD is not a new condition. In 1798, Sir Alexander Crichton published a book in which he described a "mental restlessness" that had similar symptoms to what we now know as ADHD. ADHD was previously referred to as attention deficit disorder (ADD). However, ADHD has become the preferred term because this most accurately describes the primary conditions discovered through research: inattention and hyperactive-impulsive behavior. The cause is still unknown, but recent studies have been focusing on genetic influences.

The signs and symptoms of ADHD commonly appear in many school-aged children, but for a child with ADHD, these behaviors are persistent and disruptive to their daily life. Signs and symptoms of ADHD include that the youth or child:

- May not appear to be listening
- Frequently day dreams
- Has a hard time paying attention
- Is easily distracted from school work or play
- Has a poor memory
- Acts and speaks on impulse
- Is in constant motion and has a hard time sitting still
- Is often seen fidgeting
- Is unable to play quietly

The Mayo Clinic suggests the emotional and social outcomes of this disorder can affect a child's self-esteem, ability to develop and maintain healthy relationships, and performance in school (2011). ADHD interferes with a child's learning process because he or she has difficulty paying attention and relating to peers and adults. ADHD is not a learning disability, but rather impedes a child's ability to learn.

Most children with ADHD also have at least one other developmental, behavioral, or psychiatric disorder. This may include oppositional defiant disorder, conduct disorder, depression, anxiety disorders, learning disabilities, or Tourette syndrome. ADHD doesn't cause any other psychological or developmental problems but often exists alongside another. The symptoms of these disorders make diagnosis of ADHD more difficult.

ADHD behaviors can appear differently in boys and girls. Girls tend not to be diagnosed as frequently because they tend to be quietly inattentive. Girls who have trouble paying attention may daydream more frequently, making it harder for adults to observe problematic behavior. And boys tend to be primarily hyperactive and less compliant with teachers and other adults. Boys' inattentive behaviors are often expressed through play or fidgeting.

Types

The Centers for Disease Control and Prevention (CDC) distinguishes between three different types of ADHD (2016):

Predominantly inattentive presentation: It is hard for the individual to organize or finish a task, to pay attention to details, or to follow instructions or conversations. The person is easily distracted or forgets details of daily routines.

Predominantly hyperactive-impulsive presentation: The person fidgets and talks a lot. It is hard to sit still for long (e.g., for a meal or while doing homework). Smaller children may run, jump, or climb constantly. The individual feels restless and has trouble with impulsivity. Someone who is impulsive may interrupt others a lot, grab things from people, or speak at inappropriate times. It is hard for the person to wait their turn or listen to directions. A person with impulsiveness may have more accidents and injuries than others.

Combined presentation: Symptoms of the above may change over time as well.

The type of ADHD is determined by which symptoms are strongest in the individual. It is not uncommon for a child to have a combination of types, although the *Diagnostic and Statistical Manual of Mental Disorders (DSM-5)* and most other research, groups hyperactive and impulsive symptoms together. For the purposes of distinguishing behaviors associated with each type, the preceding list indicates three types.

Diagnosis

Because the cause of ADHD is unknown, there is no specific test for diagnosis. If a child is suspected of having ADHD, an evaluation will be completed by a doctor or health care professional. This evaluation may include questionnaires completed by parents, teachers, and sometimes the child; psychological evaluation of the child and family; and complete developmental, mental, nutritional, physical, and psychosocial examinations.

Children are often diagnosed prior to the age of seven and as early as the age of two or three. Because many of the signs and symptoms are regular aspects of maturation, in order to be diagnosed, consistent inattentive or hyperactive-impulsive behavior must be observed for a minimum of six months.

The *DSM-5* also indicates that six or more of the signs and symptoms within the inattentive or hyperactive-impulsive categories must be present, must have caused impairment in the child's daily life, and must affect the child's relationships in more than one setting (i.e., school or family relationships). When a child is diagnosed with ADHD, he or she is often given a specific diagnosis based on the types reviewed earlier.

Deciding if a child has ADHD can be complicated by the fact that mental health issues and intellectual problems such as anxiety and depression have some of the same or similar symptoms. Comorbidity of ADHD is common, and doctors will often test for other illnesses and disorders. Another complication in diagnosis exists when assessing very young children, developmental problems—such as language delays—can be mistaken for ADHD. In these circumstances, evaluations are conducted by or in consultation with a specialist, such as a psychologist, psychiatrist, speech pathologist, or developmental pediatrician.

Treatment

ADHD cannot be cured, but through individual treatment plans and methods, ADHD can be successfully managed. There is no single solution that works for all children and youth; research indicates success is found through utilizing a variety of approaches.

Treatment has focused on managing the symptoms of ADHD so that children and youth can engage in tasks of daily living in the best possible way. Approaches have varied from drug treatment to cognitive behavioral therapy to supporting youth in developing healthy self-esteem, decreasing negative thoughts, and enhancing their problem-solving skills.

Medication may be an option to mitigate the behavior problems that led to conflict in peer, academic, and familial settings. Medication can affect children differently— one child may respond well to a certain type while another child does not. Currently, stimulant and nonstimulant medications are commonly prescribed to treat ADHD. The most common stimulant medications prescribed are methylphenidate, dextro-amphetamine-amphetamine, and dextroamphetamine. These stimulant medications boost and balance neutrotransmitters. They also improve the core signs and symptoms of inattention, impulsivity, and hyperactivity. These dramatic results are time limited, and the right dose for each individual child must be determined to work best.

Counseling is another form of treatment that assists children manage the behavioral symptoms and effect the disorder has on their self-esteem. Counseling can exist in a number of different forms, from behavioral therapy that teachers and parents can learn to deal with difficult behavior to behavioral strategies that support children in learning coping techniques. Behavior therapy for ADHD focuses on creating clear, direct, instructions and reward systems.

Because of the high prevalence of ADHD and its impact on a child's academic functioning, many educational settings have adopted policies to assist in a comprehensive treatment plan for children with ADHD in schools.

Expected Outcomes

With the treatment available, ADHD can be managed well in childhood and adolescence. Side effects from taking stimulants might include loss of appetite and difficulty maintaining the same height and weight growth rate; however, children taking stimulants for ADHD will likely reach their full growth potential by adulthood.

Most children with ADHD will continue to display symptoms into adulthood, but by this time, they will likely have developed coping strategies and techniques to manage/hide the symptoms. The symptoms associated with ADHD frequently decrease with age.

Research is currently under way to learn more about genetics, brain imaging, behavioral research, and their relationship to the causes of the ADHD. Expected changes in treatment will likely come out of this research as scientists seek to understand the different ways people respond to medication and how ADHD can be treated in younger children, with minimal side effects from drugs.

Andrea D'Souza

See also: Family Health; Mental Disorders; Social Health

Further Reading

Center for Disease Control and Prevention. (2016). Facts about ADHD. Retrieved from http://www.cdc.gov/ncbddd/adhd/facts.html

Hallowell, E. M., & Ratey, J. J. (2011). *Driven to Distraction: Recognizing and Coping with Attention Deficit Disorder,* rev. ed. New York: Anchor.

Mayo Clinic. (2011). Attention-deficit/hyperactivity disorder. Retrieved from http://www.mayoclinic.com/health/adhd/DS00275.

National Institute of Mental Health. (2008). Attention deficit hyperactivity disorder (ADHD). Retrieved from http://www.nimh.nih.gov/health/publications/attention-deficit-hyperactivity-disorder/what-efforts-are-under-way-to-improve-treatment.shtml.

Wender, P. H. (2000). *ADHD: Attention-Deficit Hyperactivity Disorder in Children and Adults.* Oxford: Oxford University Press.

AUTISM

Overview

Autism results from a neurological disorder that prevents the normal progression of brain development in the areas of social interaction and communication. Also referred to as autism spectrum disorder (ASD), it exists along a spectrum of neurodevelopmental disorders that affect how people communicate and interact with others. The range and intensity of disability varies, but all people with autism face challenges with learning, communication, and social skills.

Autism can affect any gender, race, culture, or socioeconomic status. In the United States, it's estimated that about 1 out of every 88 children is born with autism. There is no definitive cause or cure for this chronic disorder, which usually becomes evident in the first three years of life. Treatment has focused on behavior management, medication, and educating parents and school personnel. Depending on the symptoms, individualized approaches and treatment can help people with autism develop the tools and skills needed to lead healthy and productive lives.

History

Autism was recognized as early as 1867 by Henry Maudsley, a psychiatrist who observed very young children with marked deviation delays and distortions in development. During that time period, children with serious developmental delays or differences were categorized as having psychoses. In 1943, psychiatrist Leo Kanner outlined a clearer description of the childhood disorder we know today as autism.

Kanner described a group of children who had delayed or deviant language development, who preferred to be alone, and who could not anticipate being picked up by caregivers. They also displayed repetitive behavior and poor eye contact and showed fear of change and a preference for pictures and nonliving objects. Kanner predicted that the disorder would be more common than previously acknowledged and that many children had been misdiagnosed with mental retardation and schizophrenia.

Prior to 1980, children with such pervasive developmental disorders were generally diagnosed with schizophrenia. Historically, autistic disorder was called early infantile autism, childhood autism, or Kanner's autism. It is now known as autism spectrum disorder (ASD), which reflects the wide array of symptoms and severity. No two people are identical in their combination or degree of symptoms.

Symptoms

Children with autism respond to their environments differently from other children, and they process information in unique ways. Symptoms are usually noticed in a child before 18 months. Children can be observed to have difficulties with pretend play, social interaction, and verbal and nonverbal communication activities. Regressive autism occurs when a child appears to reach normal developmental milestones but suddenly regresses before the age of one or two, losing previously acquired language and social skills.

Other symptoms of autism may include resistance to change, odd repetitive motions, preference for being alone, aversion to cuddling, avoiding eye contact, inappropriate attachments to objects, hyperactivity or underactivity, and overactive or underactive sensory responsiveness.

Causes and Risk Factors

No single cause is known, but abnormalities in brain structure or function appear to be generally accepted as a cause. Genetics and environmental factors are also thought to contribute; no reliable evidence-based study has linked ASD and vaccines. The disorders can affect any child, but some factors have been studied for increased risk: boys (about four times more likely than girls), family history, preterm babies, and children born to older parents, as well as those with fragile X syndrome, tuberous sclerosis, Tourette syndrome, and Rett syndrome.

Diagnosis

A diagnosis is based on abnormal functioning in at least one of the following before the age of three: sustained impairment in comprehending and responding to social cues; unusual language development and usage; and restricted, stereotypical, or self-stimulatory behavior patterns such as hand flapping, tapping ears, or rocking.

Treatments

Early intervention treatment, from birth to age three, has been shown to greatly improve development and help children learn valuable skills. Interventions focus on reducing autistic behaviors that prevent children from performing in school, developing meaningful relationships, and learning skills that lead to healthy independent lives as adults. Behavioral interventions are used to treat self-injurious and self-stimulatory behavior (rocking) and to increase verbal and nonverbal communication and self-care.

Some people may be treated with medication, but no one specific drug is effective in treating the symptoms of autism. For some children, medication can help decrease behaviors such as self-injury or aggression. The drug risperidone is approved to treat irritability in children with autism who are between 5 and 16 years old; it is the only FDA-approved drug for the treatment of specific autism symptoms. Medication has been shown to be most effective in combination with behavioral interventions. Some dietary treatments have been developed, but many of these are not supported by scientific evidence.

Prevention

Although it is not possible to prevent the development of autism, it can be treated so that children can improve their social and communication skills.

Prognosis and Outcomes

Autism is a lifelong disorder, but some autism symptoms improve with treatment and age. Some children may grow up to lead normal or near-normal lives. Some adults with autism remain severely handicapped and cannot live independently. The prognosis for dependent living is improved if a child has a supportive environment that meets his or her complex needs. The quality of life for adults living with autism is affected significantly over time; ongoing support systems are necessary for their educational, medical, social, recreational, family, and employment needs.

Future

Researchers are studying biological factors unrelated to genetics that could be involved in the causes of autism, including problems with brain connections, metabolism, and the immune system. The U.S. Centers of Excellence in Autism Research conduct investigations into the causes, diagnosis, early detection, prevention, and treatment of autism.

Andrea D'Souza

See also: Environment; Genetics and Genomics; Mental Disorders; Neurological Diseases; Schizophrenia; School Wellness Programs; Social Health; Vaccines

Further Reading

Autism Society. (2014). About autism. Retrieved from http://www.autism-society.org/what-is/.

Centers for Disease Control and Prevention. (2015). Autism spectrum disorder (ASD). Retrieved from http://www.cdc.gov/ncbddd/autism/screening.html.

Eunice Kennedy Shriver National Institute of Child Health and Human Development. (2014, January 16). Autism spectrum disorder (ASD): Overview. Retrieved from http://www.nichd.nih.gov/health/topics/autism/Pages/default.aspx.

Landy, S. (2015). Autism: Symptoms, causes, assessment, and treatment. Retrieved from http://www.autism.net/images/pdf/AUTISM.pdf.

Mayo Clinic. (2015). Autism. Retrieved from http://www.mayoclinic.com/health/autism/DS00348.

Melillo, R. (2013). *Autism: The Scientific Truth about Preventing, Diagnosing, and Treating Autism Spectrum Disorders—And What Parents Can Do Now.* New York: The Penguin Group.

AUTOIMMUNE DISEASE

An autoimmune disease is a condition in which the immune system, which normally protects the body from infection and illness, attacks and destroys healthy body tissue. That is, the immune system is unable to recognize one or more entities of the body and produces autoantibodies that attack its own cells, tissues, and/or organs in error. As a result, inflammation and damage to the body occur, leading to autoimmune disorders. Autoimmune diseases have been found in almost every organ in the human body. According to the National Institutes of Health, there are more than 80 known types of autoimmune diseases.

Autoimmune diseases are common and affect more than 23.5 million people in the United States. Autoimmune diseases can affect individuals of any age and sex, but certain groups of people are more at risk such as women of childbearing age, people with a family history of autoimmune diseases, people exposed to specific environmental conditions (sunlight and viral and bacterial infections), and people of certain races/ethnicities. For example, Hispanic and African American people are more prone to lupus, and Type I diabetes is most common among White people. Autoimmune diseases are one of the leading causes of disability and death in the United States. Some autoimmune diseases are more rare than others.

The cause of autoimmune diseases remains unknown; however, in some cases, autoimmune diseases can be inherited (such as lupus and multiple sclerosis). There are other types of autoimmune diseases (such as rheumatic fever) that are triggered by a virus or infection with bacteria. In this case, antibodies and T-cells attack normal cells because they resemble the infecting microorganism. There are two general types of autoimmune disorders: (1) those that are systemic autoimmune diseases damaging many organs and (2) those that are localized, affecting a single organ or tissue. There are some instances in which the immune system does not attack a particular tissue or organ, but rather, antibodies reacts to substances (phospholipids), which are normal components of platelets and cell membranes, leading to blood clots in blood vessels.

While symptoms of autoimmune disorders vary, there are some common symptoms, including feeling tired, dizzy, and feverish. In fact, because many symptoms of autoimmune disorders are similar to each other and to other types of ailments, it is often difficult for doctors to diagnose an autoimmune disease. Diagnosis is thus a long and stressful process. There are laboratory tests, however, that can be performed to diagnose an autoimmune disorder such as the autoantibody test, the antinuclear antibody test, and other tests for inflammation.

Definitive cures for autoimmune diseases are not available, but there are treatments to autoimmune diseases, which depend on the particular disease, the severity of the disease, and the symptoms. People who suffer from pain can take over-the-counter pain medication. Others might need prescriptions for pain, depression, anxiety, fatigue, and sleep problems. Some might need surgery. Other treatments include replacing certain vital substances the body can no longer produce. For instance, with the case of diabetes, people need to take insulin injections to regulate blood sugar. Some people need to take drugs to suppress their immune system activity, controlling the disease process and organ functioning. Some people use alternative treatments that include acupuncture, herbal products, and hypnosis, but there is a need for more studies to confirm effectiveness of alternative treatments.

Many autoimmune disorders are chronic, affecting the quality of life of those who have them. Nonetheless, many diseases can be managed by treatment (mentioned earlier) or by practicing certain behaviors conducive to health. For instance, individuals with autoimmune diseases can eat well-balanced meals, including fruits and vegetables, whole grains, and lean sources of protein; they should avoid foods with trans fats, salt, added sugar, and cholesterol. Regular physical activity and getting sufficient sleep are also important. Last, finding ways to reduce anxiety and stress can reduce having a flare-up, the worsening of symptoms.

Dena Simmons

See also: Celiac Disease; Dermatitis; Diabetes, Type 1; Felty Syndrome; Hashimoto's Disease; Immune System Disorders; Inflammation; Lupus; Multiple Sclerosis; Rheumatic Fever; Rheumatoid Arthritis

Further Reading

Autoimmune Disease Research Center. (2015). Autoimmune disease. Retrieved from http://autoimmune.pathology.jhmi.edu/faqs.cfm.
Lab Tests Online. (2015). Autoimmune disease. Retrieved from http://labtestsonline.org/understanding/conditions/autoimmune/.
MedlinePlus. (2015). Autoimmune disease. Retrieved from http://www.nlm.nih.gov/medlineplus/ency/article/000816.htm.
Whitacre, C. (2001). Sex differences in autoimmune disease. *Nature Immunology*, 2, 777–780.
Women's Health. (2015). Autoimmune disease. Retrieved from http://www.womenshealth.gov/publications/our-publications/fact-sheet/autoimmune-diseases.cfm#a.

AUTONOMIC NERVOUS SYSTEM DISORDERS

Overview

As part of the body's nervous system, the autonomic nervous system controls involuntary actions, meaning it operates without any conscious effort by an individual. Involuntary actions include breathing and the heart beating, digestion, and body temperature. The autonomic nerves supply the circulatory and digestive systems, as well as the lungs, liver, bladder, eyes, genitals, and other major organs; they control the processes of blood pressure, metabolism, water balance, sexual response, and others.

When the autonomic nervous system, which consists of the sympathetic and parasympathetic divisions, undergoes damage, a variety of health conditions can arise, affecting one area of the body or entire systems within it. Although some disorders may be temporary, prolonged conditions can result in life-threatening consequences.

Symptoms

Damage to the autonomic nervous system may result in dizziness caused by the sudden drop in blood pressure; difficulty breathing, swallowing, or digesting; and abnormal sweating that affects body temperature regulation. The eyes, bladder, and heart can be affected, and men may experience erectile dysfunction.

Causes

Diabetes, alcoholism, Parkinson's disease, and other chronic health conditions can negatively affect the autonomic nervous system, as can cancer and chemotherapy, infections, nerve injuries, and inherited and autoimmune disorders. Autonomic nervous system disorders may also occur in the absence of any other underlying problem.

Diagnosis

During a physical examination, a doctor will perform blood pressure tests, as well as heart rate, breathing, and sweat tests. Tests for underlying illnesses are conducted, if necessary.

Treatments

Once identified, the underlying illness or other cause will be treated. Otherwise, treatments—including medications and lifestyle and dietary changes—alleviate symptoms associated with low blood pressure; sweating; and urinary, gastrointestinal, and sexual function problems.

Prognosis and Outcomes

Some types of autonomic nervous system disorders may worsen over time, while others may improve, especially if the underlying cause can be treated. Some types have no cure, so treatment is aimed at preventing excess disability and managing symptoms through medications, the use of devices, or personal lifestyle adaptations.

Ray Marks

See also: Alcoholism; Autoimmune Disease; Diabetes, Nerve/Neurological Diseases; Parkinson's Disease

Further Reading

Mayo Clinic. (2015). Autonomic neuropathy. Retrieved from http://www.mayoclinic.org/diseases-conditions/autonomic-neuropathy/basics/definition/CON-20029053.

Merck Manual. (2011). Overview of the autonomic nervous system. Retrieved from http://www.merckmanuals.com/home/brain-spinal-cord-and-nerve-disorders/autonomic-nervous-system-disorders/overview-of-the-autonomic-nervous-system.

National Institute of Neurological Disorders and Stroke. (2013). NINDS dysautonomia information page. Retrieved from http://www.ninds.nih.gov/disorders/dysautonomia/dysautonomia.htm.

B

BACK PAIN

Back pain is pain experienced in the posterior region of the thorax. Usually caused by injury, it is sometimes a symptom of another chronic condition or illness. Pain originating in another area of the body may sometimes be displaced and experienced as back pain. Back pain can have a profound impact on motion and general well-being due to the back's centrality to overall body movement.

The most common back injuries are sprains, strains, spasms, and tears of muscles and ligaments in the lumbar region, or lower back. These injuries result from excessive tissue stress, such as from unaccustomed heavy lifting or rapid movement, and tissue weakness, which can result from poor posture, excess body weight, and sedentary habits, or it can be secondary to another injury or condition. Incidence of such injuries increases with age, and they are very common during pregnancy, when the weight of the growing fetus and expanding abdomen stress the lumbar region. Lumbar pain is also called lumbago.

Bone, cartilage, and nerve injuries are rarer and more dangerous than connective tissue and muscle injuries. They can permanently impair movement and sensation. Such injuries may result from accidents or violence or be caused by progressive degenerative conditions, such as osteoporosis, arthritis, and multiple sclerosis. Shoulder blade, pelvis, and rib injuries may cause significant back pain. Spinal bone injuries increase the risk of cartilage and nerve damage. Cartilage injuries include herniated disks, where inflamed or displaced cartilage presses directly on the spinal cord. Nerve injuries can cause paralysis.

Internal organ injuries and some illnesses may include back pain as a symptom. The kidneys and their attached adrenal glands are located in the lumbar region. Kidney damage or urinary infection may cause pain in this area. Lung damage or disease may cause thoracic back pain. Nerves in the female reproductive system can be closely associated with the lower back, and it is common for reproductive disorders, such as ovarian cysts, as well as normal reproductive events, such as menstruation and childbirth, to include severe, displaced lumbar pain.

The spinal cord and vertebral column allow almost all movement of and communication throughout the body. The spine, pectoral girdle, rib cage, and pelvic girdle are the primary support systems for motion. Severe back pain can render large regions of the body inoperative, especially because such pain usually feels worse during movement. This is a self-perpetuating problem because avoiding motion further weakens back and abdominal muscles and decreases bone density, which contributes to more and greater injury and pain.

Back pain is a subjective condition diagnosed by the patient's self-report. Specific causes are diagnosed through patient history and tests, which may include x-rays, other imaging technology, and tests for internal organ function and certain diseases.

Treatment depends on the cause of the pain and its manifestation. Acute back pain is defined as sudden pain that lasts less than 12 weeks. Chronic back pain lasts longer than three months, whereas recurrent back pain appears to end but reappears later, following a consistent pattern. Progressive back pain is chronic pain that grows worse over time. Pain may occur only during specific motions or activities or be constant. Treatment includes pain relief and addressing the underlying cause. Short-term relief options include painkilling drugs, anti-inflammatories, manual techniques (such as heat application, acupuncture, chiropractic, massage, and certain yoga poses), and postural supports (such as back braces). Long-term relief strategies include posture- and strength-enhancement techniques, such as tailored exercise and weight loss programs, and ergonomic support during sleep and sitting. Resting for longer than two days is not recommended for pain control because it may increase muscle weakness and degeneration.

Back pain due to serious injury requires repair or treatment of the injury and may include surgery. Treatment of pain from underlying disease processes and chronic conditions includes interventions to address the underlying condition. The details of individual treatments are strongly dependent on the cause of back pain in the individual patient.

Around 80 percent of people experience acute or chronic back pain at some point in their lives. Women are at higher risk than men, and black women are at highest risk. Risk factors for back pain include age greater than 30; overweight condition; sedentary lifestyle; pregnancy; activities that involve heavy lifting, sudden twisting motions, or poor posture; smoking; breathing disorders such as emphysema; injury to the torso, shoulders, or pelvis; and arthritis, cancer, osteoporosis, or diseases and disorders affecting the kidneys, adrenal glands, or female reproductive tract.

Angela Libal

See also: Arthritis; Kidney Diseases; Multiple Sclerosis; Osteoporosis; Urinary Tract Infections

Further Reading

National Institute of Arthritis and Musculoskeletal and Skin Diseases. (2015). What is back pain? Retrieved from http://www.niams.nih.gov/Health_Info/Back_Pain/back_pain_ff.asp.

National Institute of Neurological Disorders and Stroke. (2015). NINDS back pain information page. Retrieved from http://www.ninds.nih.gov/disorders/backpain/backpain.htm.

Sarno, J. E. (1986). *Mind Over Back Pain*. New York: Berkley-Penguin.

Sarno, J. E. (2004). *Healing Back Pain: The Mind-Body Connection*, audio CD. New York: Mac-Millan Audio.

U.S. Department of Health and Human Services, Office of Disease Prevention and Health Promotion. (2015). The basics: Types of back pain. Retrieved from http://healthfinder.gov/HealthTopics/Category/everyday-healthy-living/safety/prevent-back-pain#the-basics_2.

BASAL CELL CARCINOMA

Basal cell carcinoma (BCC) is a common form of skin cancer. It is the most common type of skin cancer in the United States, where an estimated 2.8 million people are diagnosed with BCC every year. BCC is a slow-growing cancer. It usually appears on the neck and face or on other parts of the body that are most often exposed to the sun, and it generally looks like a waxy bump or reddish growth on the skin.

A slow-growing cancer, BCC begins in the outermost layer of skin, the epidermis. This cancer starts to grow as a mutation within the basal cells, the type of cells that generate new skin cells to replace older skin cells as they die. The abnormal basal cells will reproduce more rapidly than usual and continue growing instead of dying off like a normal basal cell. Eventually, the collection of abnormal basal cells can grow together to form a cancerous lesion or tumor. It is thought that cumulatively high exposure to ultraviolet radiation from the sun or a tanning lamp is the main cause of mutated basal cells; however, chronic inflammatory skin disorders, tattoos, or complications from burns or scars are also among possible risk factors.

Although BCC commonly appears as a raised bump or growth, it can also look like a flat, scaly patch of discolored skin or, in rare incidences, a shiny, white scar. Persistent, nonhealing sores may also be early forms of BCC. Complications of its occurrence can include reoccurring BCC or higher risk for other forms of cancer. Although BCC can be disfiguring, death from this disease is extremely rare. In some cases, untreated BCC will spread beyond the skin to the liver, lungs, or other organs and can eventually lead to death. Because this happens so rarely, there is very little study on the subject; only 400 documented cases of secondary cancerous growth from BCC have been reported since the late 1800s. BCC can affect anyone, but those at higher risk include people with a fair complexion and light-colored eyes, families with a history of skin cancer, and people who live in a sunny environment or at a higher altitude. Most BCC occurs in adults 50 and older, and research has shown that men have a higher rate of BCC than women.

To diagnose BCC, a medical practitioner will conduct a physical exam to evaluate unusual skin growths or discolorations. If a portion of the skin looks suspicious, a sample will be removed for a skin biopsy, which means it will be sent to a laboratory for testing. The size, shape, location, and severity of the BCC, combined with a patient's overall health, will determine course of treatment for the cancer. Some common treatment methods include scraping the top skin and then searing the remaining tumor with an electric needle, surgically removing the tumor and some surrounding tissue, freezing the tumor with liquid nitrogen to kill the cells, or removing the cancer cells one layer at a time until only healthy skin remains (called Mohs surgery). Of these, Mohs surgery has the highest success rate in treating BCC—some 98 percent of BCC tumors are fully removed with this surgery. Radiation is also a treatment option and presents with a 90 percent success rate; laser surgery, which has a cure rate of between 70 percent and 90 percent, is another treatment option. If BCC is in its early stages, medicated ointment or cream may be the only treatment needed.

While unnamed, there is evidence that skin cancer was identified as a disease in early Egypt and Greece. Tumors were cauterized, or burned off, in a similar fashion as the liquid nitrogen or electric needles used to treat BCC in modern times. By the mid-1800s, there was record of treating skin cancer with a caustic paste made of arsenic and herbs, and by the start of the 20th century, BCC itself had been identified as a specific type of cancer. In 1936, Dr. Frederic E. Mohs perfected his technique of horizontally removing each layer of abnormal skin cells, a surgery now routinely used to treat BCC.

Since Dr. Mohs's surgical developments, more has been learned about BCC and how to prevent it. Little had been done, however, to combat advanced BCC until the 21st century. In 2012, a new chemotherapy drug was introduced to fight advanced BCC. Called vismodegib (sold as Erivedge), it is an oral medication approved for use only when surgery or radiation is not a viable option.

Tamar Burris

See also: Melanoma; Skin Cancer; Squamous Cell Carcinoa

Further Reading

Goldsmith, C. (2011). *Skin Cancer*. Minneapolis, MN: Twenty-First Century Books.

Mayo Clinic. (2015). Basal cell carcinoma. Retrieved from http://www.mayoclinic.org/diseases-conditions/basal-cell-carcinoma/basics/definition/con-20028996.

Memorial Sloan Kettering Cancer Center. (2015). About basal cell carcinoma. Retrieved from https://www.mskcc.org/cancer-care/types/basal-cell-carcinoma/about-basal-cell-carcinoma.

Neville, J. A., et al. (2007). Management of nonmelanoma skin cancer in 2007. *Nature Reviews Clinical Oncology, 4*, 462–469.

Rubin, A. I., et al. (2005, November 24). Basal-cell carcinoma. *New England Journal of Medicine, 353*, 2262–2269.

Tung, R. (2009). Nonmelanoma skin cancer. Cleveland Clinic. Retrieved from http://www.clevelandclinicmeded.com/medicalpubs/diseasemanagement/dermatology/nonmelanoma-skin-cancer/.

BEHCET'S SYNDROME

Overview and Facts

Behcet's disease is a chronic disease that affects multiple systems of the body, including the spinal and freely moving joints of the body and the blood, digestive, and nervous systems. The eyes, genital organs, mouth, and skin can also be involved. The disease occurs worldwide, but it is more common in Asian and eastern Mediterranean countries and less common in the United States. Individuals of all ages can develop Behcet's disease, but it mainly affects individuals in their twenties or thirties, though it can affect people as young as four years of age or as old as 70.

History

In 1937, Hulushi Behcet, a Turkish dermatologist and scientist, described a syndrome characterized by a set of three symptoms: mouth sores, genital ulcers, and uveitis, a disease of the eye. Since Behcet's description, there have been many additional articles regarding the illness, with clinical descriptions involving almost the entire system.

Causes

The underlying problem in this condition is thought to involve inflammation of the blood vessels or vasculitis, and the arteries and veins of any organ can be affected. The precise cause is not clear though. However, both genetic and environmental factors, such as microbes and bacteria and viruses, have been suggested to cause a defect either at birth that can be hereditary or one occurring later on in the immune system that then leads to the development of the disease. These bacteria or viruses may cause the immune system to attack the blood vessels, but Behcet's disease is not contagious and does not spread from one person to another.

Symptoms

The symptoms of Behcet's disease differ from one person to the next. Some individuals may experience only mild symptoms, such as sores in the mouth, while others may experience more severe problems, such as vision loss. In extreme cases, arteries can become inflamed and cause a stroke if the oxygen supply to the brain is affected. If the veins are affected, they can develop blood clots. If these loosen, they can cause lung blockage and destruction.

The five most common symptoms of Behcet's disease are:

- Mouth sores
- Genital sores
- Other skin sores
- Swelling of parts of the eye
- Pain, swelling, warmth, tenderness, and stiffness of the joints

The most frequent symptom of the disease, though, is the involvement of the musculoskeletal system. This includes arthritis or inflammation of the joints and joint pain. Muscles, ligaments, and bone may all be involved as well. Except for a small number of cases, individuals with these arthritic symptoms experience periodic flare-ups that can stop on their own, and this usually does not produce deformity or joint destruction. The disease commonly affects one of the larger joints such as the knee, wrist, ankle, or elbow. There may also be thinning of the bone, or bone death, as well as inflammation of the sacroiliac and other spinal joints or eye problems that can lead to impaired vision and bone destruction. There may also be an exaggerated skin reaction to scratches.

Less common symptoms include:

- Inflammation of the brain and spinal cord
- Blood clots
- Central nervous system problems
- Bowel problems
- Depression
- Ear problems
- Chest problems

Diagnostic Tests

Although laboratory tests exist, the diagnosis is usually confirmed through a clinical examination and by meeting internationally agreed-upon criteria. This may take a long time because the symptoms do not always occur together.

A special skin test called a pathergy test may be helpful. Other tests include skin biopsy, lumbar puncture, MRI of the brain, and bowel tests.

Treatment

The treatment is based on the type of problem that is identified and its severity, and it is aimed at preventing complications. This may involve pain medications, rest if pain is excessive, and anti-inflammatory medications and steroids plus moderate exercise.

Practitioners who treat this condition include rheumatologists, neurologists, gastroenterologists, ophthalmologists, and immunologists.

See your doctor if you notice any reoccurring symptoms related to the mouth, skin, genitals, eyes, joints, or digestive and blood systems or experience headaches, disorientation, fever, or poor balance.

Summary

Behcet's disease is a rare chronic multisystem disease that comes and goes and can disappear spontaneously, similar to other autoimmune diseases. It may last for a few weeks, with intervals of months or years between attacks. Behcet's disease is produced by the body's immune system, which is over-reactive. This produces unpredictable episodes of inflammation that affect many body parts, especially the small blood vessels. Symptoms may occur wherever there is a blood supply and can mostly be suppressed by the correct treatment.

Ray Marks

See also: Arthritis; Environment; Eye Diseases; Genetics and Genomics; Immune System Disorders; Inflammation; Musculoskeletal Disorders

Further Reading

American Behcet's Disease Association. (2014). Behcet's disease. Retrieved from http://www .behcets.com/site/c.8oIJJRPsGcISF/b.9196317/k.904C/Behcets_Disease.htm.

Johns Hopkins Vasculitis Center. (2015). Behcet's disease. Retrieved from http://www.hopkinsvasculitis.org/types-vasculitis/behcets-disease/.

Mayo Clinic. (2011). Behcet's disease. Retrieved from http://www.mayoclinic.org/diseases-conditions/behcets-disease/basics/definition/con-20027549.

National Institute of Arthritis and Musculoskeletal and Skin Diseases. (2015, August). Questions and answers about Behcet's disease. Retrieved from http://www.niams.nih.gov/Health_Info/Behcets_Disease/default.asp.

National Institute of Neurological Disorders and Stroke. (2012, February 6). NINDS Behcet's disease information page. Retrieved from http://www.ninds.nih.gov/disorders/behcet/behcet.htm.

BELL'S PALSY

Also known as idiopathic peripheral facial palsy and cranial mononeuropathy, Bell's palsy is a condition in which muscles of the face become paralyzed, usually on one side, as a result of damage or dysfunction of the nerve that supplies the face muscles, called the facial nerve. As a result, the affected muscles may feel stiff, and half of the face can start to droop and become distorted. It may be hard for the affected individual to smile and to close the affected eye.

The condition can affect anyone. It can start round about age 15, but most cases occur over the age of 50. It can occur in newborn babies and affects males and females and all races to the same extent.

In many cases, the condition does not become chronic and disappears in a short period of time. However, in about 10 percent of cases, the condition may reappear, either on the same side or sometimes on the opposite side of the face. A small percentage also continue to experience the problems for life.

In rare cases, both sides of the face may be affected. In general, the symptoms vary from person to person and can range from mild weakness to total paralysis.

Historical View

Bell's palsy is named after a Scottish anatomist, Charles Bell (1774–1842), who was the first to describe the condition after studying the nerve and the supply of the facial muscles by the facial nerve 200 years ago.

Types of Symptoms

The symptoms and signs of this condition may occur suddenly in the form of:

A rapid development of mild weakness or the total paralysis of one side of the face.
It may not be possible to make facial expressions easily or close the affected eye.
There may be pain around the jaw or in and around the ear on the affected side.
There may be increased sensitivity to sound on the affected side.
Other problems include headaches, twitching of the muscles, decreased taste perception, facial tingling, drooling, numbness on the affected side of the face, impaired speech, difficulty eating or drinking, and changes in the amount of saliva or tears that can be produced.

Causes and Risk Factors

The most common cause of Bell's palsy is thought to be the herpes simplex virus, but other viruses have also been thought to cause this condition, such as the chickenpox virus called herpes zoster, the virus called Epstein-Barr, and the virus called cytomegalovirus.

These viruses may affect the facial nerve on one side and cause it to swell or become inflamed. The nerve passes through a very narrow opening behind the ear, and if swollen, the transmission along the facial nerve from the brain to the face muscles can be disrupted. All structures and areas of the face as well as the fluids produced in the mouth and eye that are controlled by the facial nerve can be affected. Those at highest risk are:

Commonly pregnant, especially in the last three months of pregnancy, or the first week of birth
Older people
Those with diabetes
Those who have an upper respiratory infection, such as the flu
People who experience brain tumors, stroke, and Lyme disease
Those that have immune system health problems such as HIV/AIDS
Those with tumors, high blood pressure, chronic middle-ear infections, and facial injury or trauma to the skull

There may be a family history of Bell's palsy in those with repeated attacks, suggesting genetics may be involved. Alternately, trauma, stress, and factors in the environment may trigger the reoccurrence of the problem.

Major complications may include:

- A chronic loss of taste sensation
- Chronic facial spasm
- Corneal infections of the eye
- Incomplete regeneration of the facial nerve
- Irreversible damage to the facial nerve
- Misdirected regrowth of facial nerve fibers, resulting in involuntary contraction of certain muscles when others are moving (synkinesis)—for example, when the person smiles, the eye on the affected side may close
- Partial or complete blindness of the eye that won't close, due to excessive dryness and scratching of the cornea, the clear protective covering of the eye

Diagnostic Tools

Diagnosis is usually arrived at by excluding other possibilities.
Tests may include:

Clinical, physical, and neurological examinations
Blood tests
Nerve conduction tests
Electromyography
Imaging scans such as MRI, x-rays, or CT scans

Treatments

Corticosteroids or antiviral drugs or vitamin therapy to restore nerve function may be of help, but most people recover within 10 days.

If the eye is affected, protecting the eye may be important until the condition resolves. Special eye protectors, glasses or goggles to protect eyes may help, as may ointments and tear-like eye drops that keep eye moist.

Physical therapy, including exercise and electrical muscle stimulation, can be helpful for retraining the muscles in long-standing cases. Some forms of physical therapy may be helpful for reducing pain on the affected side.

Mouth care and dental care may be required, including eating soft foods to prevent swallowing problems and frequent brushing and flossing.

In extreme cases, decompression of the nerve or cosmetic or reconstructive surgery may be carried out.

Prevention

If you notice any weakness or changes in your face muscles, neck pain, or pain behind the ear, you should see a doctor. The doctor can determine if this is due to Bell's palsy or something more serious such as a stroke, which may produce similar problems.

Ray Marks

See also: Diabetes; Ear Diseases; High Blood Pressure; Immune System Disorders; Lyme Disease; Neurological Diseases; Stroke

Further Reading

Mayo Clinic. (2015). Bell's palsy. Retrieved from http://www.mayoclinic.com/health/bells -palsy/DS00168.

MedicineNet.com. (2011). Bell's palsy symptoms. Retrieved from http://www.medicinenet .com/script/main/art.asp?articlekey=156337.

MedlinePlus. (2014, May 20). Bell's palsy. Retrieved from https://www.nlm.nih.gov/medline plus/ency/article/000773.htm.

National Institute of Neurological Disorders and Stroke. (2015, April 16). Bell's palsy fact sheet. Retrieved from http://www.ninds.nih.gov/disorders/bells/bells.htm.

Parker, J. N., & Parker, P. M. (2003). *Bell's Palsy: A Medical Dictionary, Bibliography, and Annotated Research Guide to Internet References*. San Diego, CA: ICON Health Publications.

BILE DUCT CANCER

The bile duct is a four- to five-inch long, tube-like structure that connects the liver to the intestine and transports bile from the liver to the intestine. The top half of the bile duct is associated with the liver, while the bottom half of the bile duct is associated the pancreas.

Bile duct cancer, also known as cholangiocarcinomas, involves tumors that occur in the bile duct. They are uncommon tumors but are serious problems that do occur at the rate of approximately 4,000 new cases each year in the United States.

The condition usually develops in people older than 65 years old and is more common in Israel and Japan and in American Indians than in the general U.S. population. In England and Wales, there are approximately 2.8 cases per 100,000 females and two cases per 100,000 males.

Bile duct cancer begins when normal cells in the bile duct change and grow uncontrollably, forming a mass called a tumor. A tumor can be benign (noncancerous) or malignant (cancerous, meaning it can spread to other parts of the body).

Cancer can occur in any part of the bile duct. To be able to treat bile duct cancer, doctors look at the exact location of the tumor:

Extrahepatic. The part of the bile duct that lies outside the liver is called extrahepatic. It is in this part of the bile duct where cancer usually begins. A common site for bile duct cancer is at the point where the right and left hepatic ducts join.

The two major types of bile duct tumors that are found are:

- *Distal bile duct tumors:* tumors affecting the bottom half of the bile duct
- *Klatskin's or Perihilar or Hilar tumors:* Tumors affecting the upper part of the bile duct

Intrahepatic. About 5 to 10 percent of bile duct cancers are intrahepatic, or occur inside the liver.

Patients with intrahepatic bile duct cancer diagnoses usually have a poor prognosis, and the tumor metastasizes early. This tumor has been associated with thorium dioxide, ulcerative colitis, and sclerosing cholangitis; surgery is the only chance for successful. They can sometimes be confused with cancers that start in the liver cells, which are called *hepatocellular carcinomas*.

Bile duct cancers can occur as a primary or main condition or as a secondary condition due to the spread of cancers from another source in the body. Primary tumors are most common and occur 95 percent of the time; they are slow-growing and usually do not spread or metastasize quickly.

Not all bile duct tumors are cancerous, however. Bile duct hamartomas and bile duct adenomas are benign or non-cancerous tumors.

Symptoms, Causes, and Risk Factors

Symptoms of bile duct cancer include abnormal liver tests, abdominal pain, anorexia, chills, diarrhea, fever, itching, jaundice (yellowness of the skin), poor appetite, weakness and fatigue, and weight loss.

Causes and risk factors include a family history of congenital fibrosis or cysts, parasitic infestations, gallstones, primary sclerosing cholangitis (psc), ulcerative colitis, toxic materials, chronic typhoid infections, chronic biliary infections, and biliary cirrhosis.

Prevention

Early detection using abdominal ultrasound or abdominal computerized tomography scan is indicated if a person is jaundiced.

If you have signs of jaundice or other symptoms, contact your physician or medical provider.

Other diagnostic tests include:

- CT scan-directed biopsy
- Cytology

Blood tests that may be done include:

- Liver function tests (especially alkaline phosphatase or bilirubin levels)

Cholangiography via a transhepatic or endoscopic approach may be required to define the biliary anatomy and extent of the lesion.

Magnetic resonance cholangiography is a noninvasive alternative available in an increasing number of centers.

A percutaneous transhepatic cholangiogram (PTCA) may be required.

Ray Marks

See also: Abdominal Diseases; Eating Disorders; Liver Diseases; Ulcerative Colitis

Further Reading

American Cancer Society. (2014, November 1). What is bile duct cancer? Retrieved from http://www.cancer.org/Cancer/BileDuctCancer/DetailedGuide/bile-duct-cancer-what -is-bile-duct-cancer.

CancerNet. (2015). Bile duct cancer. Retrieved from http://www.cancer.net/cancer-types/bile -duct-cancer.

Center for Pancreatic and Biliary Diseases. (2012). Bile duct cancer. Retrieved from http:// www.surgery.usc.edu/divisions/tumor/pancreasdiseases/web%20pages/BILIARY%20 SYSTEM/cholangiocarcinoma.html.

Cholangiocarcinoma Foundation. (2015). Overview—A silent disease. Retrieved from http:// cholangiocarcinoma.org/the-disease/defined/.

Mayo Clinic. (2013, April 3). Bile duct cancer. Retrieved from http://www.mayoclinic.org /bile-duct-cancer/.

National Cancer Institute. (2015). Bile duct cancer treatment. Retrieved from http://www .cancer.gov/types/liver/patient/bile-duct-treatment-pdq.

BILIARY CIRRHOSIS

Overview

Biliary cirrhosis is a rare form of liver cirrhosis caused by disease or defects of the bile ducts. Symptoms usually include cholestasis (accumulation of bile in the liver). There are two types of biliary cirrhosis:

- Primary biliary cirrhosis
- Secondary biliary cirrhosis

In 1851, the clinical picture of progressive obstructive jaundice that was not due to mechanical obstruction of the large bile ducts was observed. Later, in 1950, Ahrens and coworkers termed this disease *primary biliary cirrhosis* according to

Pyrsopoulos and Reddy (2009). It is also known as chronic nonsuppurative destructive cholangitis.

Primary Biliary Cirrhosis

Primary biliary cirrhosis is a chronic or long-standing health condition that involves the progressive inflammation and destruction of the small and medium-sized bile ducts of the liver, which are tubules that form a type of "plumbing system" for the liver. This form of irritation and swelling blocks the normal flow of bile, a fluid essential for the proper digestion of fats from the liver into the small intestine. As it spreads, it causes damage to the cells of the liver, and this plus the toxicity that emerges from the bile trapped in the liver cells leads to irreversible scarring or cirrhosis of the areas of destruction if the condition is not resolved. The scarring makes it impossible for the liver to carry out its specific functions. The condition most commonly affects middle-aged women between 30 and 60 years of age. It is considered an uncommon disease but is not rare; having a family history of the condition raises the risk for developing this condition.

Secondary Biliary Cirrhosis

Secondary biliary cirrhosis results from prolonged bile duct obstruction or narrowing or closure of the bile duct for other reasons, such as a tumor.
Clinical Stages of the disease include:

Preclinical—absence of symptoms (for 2 to 10 years)
Asymptomatic—absence of symptoms, abnormal liver tests (2 to 20 years)
Symptomatic—symptoms, abnormal liver tests (3 to 11 years)
Advanced stages—symptoms, complications, abnormal liver tests (0 to 2 years)

The prolonged inflammation of the bile ducts eventually causes a loss of liver function.

Symptoms

More than 50 percent of cases may have no symptoms at time of diagnosis. The symptoms that do occur usually develop gradually and may involve:

Abdominal pain
Digestive problems
Enlarged liver
Fatigue
Fatty deposits under skin
Fatty stools
Hyperpigmentation
Itching
Jaundice
Malignancy
Metabolic Bone Disease
Soft yellow spots on eyelids

Vitamin deficiencies
Xanthomas or cholesterol deposits

Causes and Risk Factors

The precise cause is not known.

There may be a predisposition as a result of genetics, autoimmunity, or infection that may induce primary biliary cirrhosis.

Environmental factors such as exposure to chemicals found in cigarette smoke may be involved.

The disease may be associated with exogenous estrogens and several autoimmune diseases including:

Celiac disease
Hypothyroidism
Raynaud's phenomenon
Scleroderma
Sicca or dry eyes or mouth syndrome

Possible Complications

Brain damage
Bleeding and bruising
Cognitive impairment if toxins that cannot be removed from blood by liver accumulate in the brain
Edema or swelling of the feet and abdomen (ascites)
Enlarged veins
Fluid and electrolyte imbalance
Insulin resistance and Type 2 diabetes
Liver cancer
Malabsorption of fats and fat-soluble vitamins
Malnutrition
Osteomalacia or soft bones
Osteoporosis or weak bones
Rheumatoid arthritis
Risk of infection
Sensitivity to medications

Diagnostic Tools

Tests may involve:

Blood tests
Liver biopsy
Liver dysfunction tests
Liver disease tests
Magnetic resonance imaging
Serum autoantibody testing
Ultrasound imaging

Treatments

Treatments aimed at relieving symptoms and pain may be used.
Liver transplants may be successful if done early enough.

Prevention

Medication and use of vitamin replacements, plus calcium supplements, and drugs to treat itching can reduce the symptom and possibly slow the progression of the disease. However, if the disease is not adequately treated, most patients will require a liver transplant to prevent death.

About 25 percent of patients with this condition will experience liver damage. If you have a first-degree relative such as a parent with this condition, your doctor can screen for this disease or monitor your health over time.

Treating the disease complications, as well as any underlying disease, and starting treatment early may help to minimize progressive disability and improve the outcome of the condition. Social support and being educated about the disease and leading a healthy lifestyle, eating nutritious meals, and avoiding alcohol and other substances may also be beneficial.

Ray Marks

See also: Autoimmune Disease; Biliary Diseases; Celiac Disease; Genetics and Genomics; Hypothyroidism; Liver Diseases; Raynaud's Phenomenon

Further Reading

Dickerson, J. L. (2006). *The First Year: Cirrhosis: An Essential Guide for the Newly Diagnosed.* Boston, MA: Da Capo Press.

Kumagi, T., & Heathcote, E. J. (2008). Primary biliary cirrhosis. *Orphanet Journal of Rare Diseases,* 3(1). doi:10.1186/1750-1172-3-1.

Massachusetts General Hospital. (2015). Biliary cirrhosis/bile duct cancer. Retrieved from http://www.massgeneral.org/conditions/condition.aspx?id=63.

Mayo Clinic. (2014, November 22). Primary biliary cirrhosis. Retrieved from http://www.mayoclinic.org/diseases-conditions/primary-biliary-cirrhosis/basics/symptoms/con-20029377.

National Institute of Diabetes and Digestive and Kidney Diseases. (2014, March). Primary biliary cirrhosis. Retrieved from http://www.digestive.niddk.nih.gov/ddiseases/pubs/primarybiliarycirrhosis/.

Pyrsopoulos, N. T., & Reddy, K. R. (2009). Primary biliary cirrhosis. Retrieved from http://emedicine.medscape.com/article/171117-overview.

BILIARY DISEASES

Overview

The biliary system is the organ and duct system that creates, transports, stores, and releases bile into the duodenum, or first part of the small intestine, to aid digestion.

It consists of the gall bladder, the bile ducts in and outside the liver, the hepatic duct, the common bile duct, and the cystic duct.

Biliary tract disorder is an abnormality of function, structure, or both of the organs, ducts, and other structures that participate in the secretion, storage, and delivery of bile into the duodenum.

Biliary diseases can affect the gall bladder and small bile ducts in the liver or any part of the biliary tract involved in the production and transportation of bile, a greenish-yellow fluid that is secreted by the liver and used to remove wastes and break down fat during digestion. Biliary diseases are common chronic health conditions. Their disease presentation is not uniform, however, and biliary diseases can present with no symptoms or with varying signs and symptoms. These diseases can affect as many as 20 percent of the population at any point in time and usually involve gallstones that block the biliary tract and possibly the pancreas. There may also be a tumor in the biliary tract or pressure on the biliary tract from a tumor of the pancreas that causes a biliary tract disorder. If untreated, gallstones or blockages can lead to serious complications.

Types of biliary disorders mentioned in various sources include:

- Gallbladder disorders:
  - Gallstones
  - Gall bladder cancer
  - Gall bladder inflammation or cholangitis
  - Primary sclerosing cholangitis
- Bile duct disorders:
  - Cholecystitis—bile duct inflammation
  - Bile duct cancer
  - Fascioliasis
- Jaundice
- Biliary colic

Primary biliary cirrhosis is a chronic disease in which there is destruction of the small bile ducts to the liver as a result of progressive inflammation. The bile ducts serve as channels that link the liver and gall bladder. Bile ducts carry bile, which contains substances required for digestion and fat absorption. If the bile ducts are progressively scarred and damaged by inflammation, and if bile collects in the liver, this leads to cirrhosis, where there is widespread scarring of the liver.

Symptoms

Right upper abdominal pain
Jaundice
Jaundice and abdominal pain
Nausea and vomiting
Hyperpigmentation
Pruritis or itching or the need to scratch
Fatigue

Weight loss
Fatty food intolerance
Malignancy
Metabolic bone disease

Causes and Risk Factors

Causes and risk factors include gallstones, infection, hereditary history, female gender, age more than 40 years, family history, obesity, history of five or more pregnancies, rapid weight loss, sickle cell or other hemolytic disorders, or diabetes.

Diagnostic Tools

Diagnostic tools may include:

Clinical, physical, and medical examination
Blood tests
Endoscopic retrograde cholangiopancreatography, which allows access to the bile ducts and pancreas ducts. Also allows for therapy such as removing stones from the bile ducts or pancreas ducts.
Imaging-ultrasound, CAT scans, x-rays
Hepatobiliary scintigraphy

Treatments

Treatments will be medical management by a physician, as well as possibly endoscopic management (the physician using a flexible tube with a light and camera to examine the digestive system on a screen), surgery, and/or diet.

Ray Marks

See also: Autoimmune Disease; Liver Diseases

Further Reading

American College of Gastroenterology. (2013, July). Biliary tract disorders, gallbladder disorders, and gallstone pancreatitis. Retrieved from http://patients.gi.org/topics/biliary-tract-disorders-gallbladder-disorders-and-gallstone-pancreatitis/.
American Liver Foundation. (2014, January 14). Primary sclerosing cholangitis (PSC). Retrieved from http://www.liverfoundation.org/abouttheliver/info/psc/.
Cleveland Clinic. (2010, August). Gallbladder and biliary tract disease. Retrieved from http://www.clevelandclinicmeded.com/medicalpubs/diseasemanagement/hepatology/gallbladder-biliary-tract-disease/.
CDEM Self Study Module. (2010). Abdominal pain: Biliary tract disease. Retrieved from http://www.cdemcurriculum.org/ssm/gi/biliary/biliary.php.
Johns Hopkins Medicine. (2015). Gastrointestinal, liver and pancreatic diseases and conditions. Retrieved from http://www.hopkinsmedicine.org/gastroenterology_hepatology/diseases_conditions/.

Mayo Clinic. (2013, July 5). Gallstones. Retrieved from http://www.mayoclinic.org/diseases
-conditions/gallstones/basics/definition/con-20020461.
National Library of Medicine Genetics Home Reference. (2015, October 26). Retrieved from
http://ghr.nlm.nih.gov/condition/primary-sclerosing-cholangitis.

BIPOLAR DISORDER

Bipolar disorder, often called manic depression or manic depressive disorder, is associated with mood swings that range from depression to mania or from very low moods to inflated, excessively excited type of moods. This means, at times, those affected by the condition may lose interest in their activities or feel hopeless, and at other times, they may feel full of energy or euphoria.

It is one of several medical conditions that are categorized as depressive disorders. In addition to manic depression and manic depressive disorder, it is also called manic depressive illness, bipolar mood disorder, and bipolar affective disorder.

Depressive disorders affect the way an individual's brain functions, and in bipolar disorder, there may be mood shifts that occur several times a day or periodically at intervals over several months. Sometimes, both types of symptoms occur at the same time. This is called a mixed bipolar disorder state.

Usually, a bipolar disorder lasts for a long time and can require treatment and careful management in order not to disrupt a person's life. Sometimes, it is not readily easy to spot and may go untreated for many years. Although some individuals with this condition may experience psychotic symptoms, such as hallucinations or delusions, others may have behavioral problems, relationship problems, or school- or work-related problems. Bipolar disorder is a treatable condition, however, and with correct treatment, people with this condition can lead full, active, productive lives.

The condition often develops in a person's late teens or early adult years. The majority of cases start before age 25. Some may develop the symptoms in childhood or late adulthood, however.

Signs and Symptoms

As noted in the National Institute of Mental Health website (2016), there are four types of bipolar disorder:

1. Bipolar I disorder: This is the most severe type, where mood swings cause significant difficulty and periods of mania can put the person at risk for injury if severe.
2. Bipolar II disorder: This is less severe than bipolar disorder I and is usually accompanied by an elevated mood, irritability, and some functional changes. Instead of full-blown mania, the person has hypomania, which is less severe. Periods of depression usually last longer than periods of hypomania in this type.
3. Cyclothymia: This is a mild form of bipolar disorder. Here, the highs and lows are not as severe as in other two types.
4. Bipolar disorder not otherwise specified.

These different forms have been classified to show that the disorder can present differently in different individuals. In general, young people with bipolar disorder may experience very rapid mood changes and other symptoms such as irritability and high levels of anxiety. In a mixed episode of bipolar disorder, a person can experience the symptoms of mania, or an excessively high mood, and major depression, or an excessively low mood, nearly every day for at least one week.

If an individual has a specific type of bipolar disorder, the treatment can be targeted toward this type of problem, rather than treating the problem in a generic way.

Symptoms of Mania (Highs)

Mood changes
    A long period of feeling happy or euphoric
    Extremely irritable mood, feeling jumpy or agitated
Behavioral changes
    Talking rapidly
    Jumping from one idea to the next
    Easily distracted
    Increased energy
    Restless
    Talking a lot
    Decreased need for sleep
    Having unrealistic belief in one's abilities
Behaving impulsively
Taking on too many projects
    Aggressive behavior
    Reckless behavior and lack of control, such as binge eating, drinking, and/or drug use; poor judgment; sex with many partners; spending sprees

Symptoms of Depression

Mood changes
    A long period of feeling low
    Loss of interest in previously pleasurable activities
    Anger, worry, and anxiety
    Feelings of guilt or worthlessness
    Loss of self-esteem
Behavioral changes
    Feeling tired
Having problems concentrating
Memory problems
    Being restless or irritable
Changing one's eating, sleeping behaviors
    Suicidal or death-related thoughts
    Pulling away from friends or activities previously enjoyed

Causes

Causes may include genetics; biochemical differences in the person; biological-brain changes; life changes-such as childbirth (which can trigger a manic episode); neurotransmitters and chemical imbalances; hormone imbalances; environment stress, abuse, significant loss; medications such as antidepressants or steroids; periods of sleeplessness; and recreational drug use.

Common coexisting problems include substance abuse, anxiety disorders, thyroid diseases, migraine headaches, diabetes, and obesity.

Diagnosis

A diagnosis should be done by a psychiatrist or doctor, with a psychiatric or psychological assessment and review of medical history. Brain imaging studies may be used to understand process of disease.

Treatment

Although bipolar disorder cannot be cured, it can be treated. Medications may include lithium, anticonvulsant medications such as valproic acid, mood stabilizers, antipsychotics, and sleep medications. Treatment may include cognitive behavioral therapy, family-focused therapy, interpersonal therapy, psychoeducation, and electroconvulsive therapy if medications don't work. If the condition is severe, hospitalization may be necessary.

Bipolar disorder is not a sign of weakness. It is a medical condition that requires treatment. Early treatment is preferable, especially for mixed episodes of bipolar disorders, and is usually undertaken with a team of medical professionals, and in the case of teens, family members. Maintaining the treatment after that is also very important. Lifestyle changes, such as reducing stress, eating well, and getting enough sleep and exercise, as well as joining a support group, can help an individual with this condition to manage his or her life more effectively.

Where to Go for Help

Mental health specialists
Community mental health centers
Hospital psychiatry departments
Family services, social agencies
Medical practitioners
Peer support groups
Private clinics

If someone is in crisis or has the warning signs of harming him- or herself, call the doctor or health care provider. Or call 911 or go to a hospital emergency room. Call toll-free, the 24-hour hotline of the National Suicide Prevention Lifeline at 1-800-273-TALK (or 1-800-273-8255).

Ray Marks

See also: Anxiety; Depression; Environment; Genetics and Genomics; Mental Disorders; Psychotic Disorders; Social Health

Further Reading

Jamison, K. R. (2009). *An Unquiet Mind*. New York: Vintage Books.

Mayo Clinic. (2015) Bipolar disorder. Retrieved from http://www.mayoclinic.com/health
/bipolar-disorder/ds00356.

Miklowitz, D. J. (2011). *The Bipolar Disorder Survival Guide: What You and Your Family Need
to Know*, 2nd ed. New York: Guilford Press

Mondimore, F. M. (2006). *Bipolar Disorder: A Guide for Patients and Families,* 2nd ed. Baltimore: Johns Hopkins University Press.

National Institutes of Mental Health. (2016). Bipolar disorder. Retrieved from https://www
.nimh.nih.gov/health/topics/bipolar-disorder/index.shtml.

PubMed Health. (2015). Bipolar disorder. Retrieved from http://www.ncbi.nlm.nih.gov
/pubmedhealth/PMH0001924/.

Teens Health. (2015). Bipolar disorder. The Nemours Foundation. Retrieved from http://
kidshealth.org/teen/your_mind/mental_health/bipolar.html.

WebMD. (2014). Slideshow: Understanding bipolar disorder. Retrieved from http://www
.webmd.com/bipolar-disorder/ss/slideshow-bipolar-disorder-overview.

BLACK LUNG DISEASE

Overview

Black lung disease is a common term used to describe any lung disease that develops as a result of inhaling coal dust. This name comes from the fact that those with the disease have lungs that look black instead of pink. It is also called anthracosis or coal workers' pneumoconiosis.

There are two forms of the condition: a simple form, known as coal workers' pneumoconiosis (CWP), and a complicated form known as progressive massive fibrosis (PMF). About 15 percent of simple cases develop PMF.

The disease in its simplest form is due to the inhalation and accumulation of coal dust into the lungs, but there may be no symptoms or noticeable effects of this on quality of life or only very mild symptoms, such as a cough and mucus production, in response to the inhalation of coal dust, but this may be more a matter of dust-induced bronchitis. As the condition progresses and becomes more complex, a more persistent cough and shortness of breath develop, along with sputum and moderate to severe airway obstruction, and quality of life starts to decrease.

Because pneumoconiosis is a reaction to accumulated dust in the lungs, it may appear and get worse during exposure to any dust or even after exposure has ceased.

The severity of pneumoconiosis depends on the type of coal mine and the dust conditions in the work environment. Once PMF starts to occur, it seems to continue aggressively, even if the dust exposure is reduced. It may lead to chronic obstructive lung disease.

Although it is preventable, it is estimated that 1,500 former coal miners die each year from black lung, especially in isolated rural communities.

The risk of having black lung disease is directly related to the amount of dust inhaled over the years, and the disease typically affects workers over age 50 or older workers.

In the last 10 years, cases of black lung among minors have doubled in the United States.

Causes and Symptoms

When a minor repeatedly breathes in fine coal dust particles when he or she is in the mine, these cannot be destroyed within the lungs or removed from them, so they build up. Eventually, this buildup becomes denser and can cause scarring in the lungs, thus making them less able to supply oxygen to the blood.

The primary symptom of the disease is shortness of breath, which often gradually gets worse as the disease progresses. In severe cases, the patient may develop cor pulmonale, an enlargement and strain of the right side of the heart caused by chronic lung disease. This may eventually cause right-sided heart failure.

Some patients also develop emphysema, which is associated with damage of the tiny air sacs in the lungs, and this can lead to shortness of breath and lung and heart failure. Others may develop the severe type of black lung disease called progressive massive fibrosis.

Diagnostic Tools

Pneumoconiosis is diagnosed through an occupational history and chest x-rays. Lung function tests may be used to determine how badly the lungs are damaged. Bronchoscopy may be undertaken to examine related damage to the bronchi or smaller airways.

Occupational history is very important to the diagnosis of CWP—if a person has not been exposed to coal dust, he or she cannot have CWP. The occupational history should include not only recent and past full-time employment, but also summer jobs, student jobs, military history, and short-term jobs.

The diagnosis of CWP has legal public health implications because some states require that all cases be reported.

Treatments

There is no treatment or cure for this condition, although it is possible to treat complications such as lung infections and cor pulmonale. Further exposure to coal dust should cease altogether.

Prevention

This disease will not occur of the person does not inhale coal dust. This could mean an affected person may have to quit her or his job.

The only way to prevent black lung disease is to avoid long-term exposure to coal dust. Coal mines may help prevent the condition by lowering coal dust levels and providing protective clothes to coal miners.

Ray Marks

See also: COPD (Chronic Obstructive Pulmonary Disease); Cor Pulmonale; Emphysema; Lung Cancer; Lung Diseases; Pneumonia

Further Reading

MedlinePlus. (2013, May 30). Coal worker's pneumoconiosis. Retrieved from https://www.nlm.nih.gov/medlineplus/ency/article/000130.htm

Merck Manual. (2015). Coal workers' pneumoconiosis. Retrieved from http://www.merckmanuals.com/home/lung-and-airway-disorders/environmental-lung-diseases/coal-workers-pneumoconiosis

Pneumoconiosis. (2015) Coal workers pneumoconiosis. Retrieved from http://www.pneumoconiosis.org.uk/coal-workers-pneumoconiosis

United Mine Workers of America. (2015). Black lung. Retrieved from http://www.umwa.org/?q=content/black-lung

BLADDER CANCER

Overview

Bladder cancer is a form of cancer that develops in the lining of the bladder, a hollow organ in the lower part of the abdomen that stores and releases urine. It commonly affects older adults, but it can occur at any age, and those who smoke and men are more likely to develop it. It is the sixth most common cancer in the United States. Its most usual form is transitional cell carcinoma, which begins in the cells of the bladder's innermost layer of tissue.

Superficial bladder cancer is confined to the lining, while invasive cancer spreads to nearby organs and lymph nodes, occasionally forming a secondary tumor. The disease is categorized in stages: Stage 0 refers to abnormal cells found in tissue lining the inside of the bladder that may become cancer and spread to nearby tissue. Stage I is a cancer that has formed and spread to the tissue layer underneath the inner lining. Stage II has spread to the inner or outer half of the bladder muscle wall. Stage III has spread from the bladder to the surrounding fatty layer of tissue and possibly to the reproductive organs. Stage IV has spread from the bladder to the wall of the abdomen or pelvis or to one or more lymph nodes or other body parts, including the rectum, ureters, bones, liver, lungs, the prostate in men, or the uterus and vagina in women.

Symptoms

Bladder cancer is usually first visible as blood in the urine. Other common symptoms include an urgency to urinate, including without producing urine; more frequent or painful urination; and the need to strain to empty the bladder. Additional symptoms are abdominal, pelvic, lower back, or bone pain; fatigue; loss of appetite; leg swelling; incontinence; and weight loss.

Causes and Risk Factors

The cause of bladder cancer is unknown, but changes in the DNA of bladder cells may be one factor. Exposure to environmental chemicals, such as paints and dyes, cigarette smoke, and other agents that irritate the bladder lining can lead to cell changes. Other bladder irritants include long-term catheters, radiation treatment, or the tropical parasite that causes the infection schistosomiasis.

Smoking may cause nearly half of all bladder cancers in men and women. Other risk factors for the disease include age (older), gender (male), race (Caucasian), eating a high-fat meat diet, and having a long-term bladder infection.

Diagnosis

In addition to a physical exam, a series of tests and procedures are available to diagnose bladder cancer: CT scan (also called CAT scan), a computerized x-ray that produces cross-sectional images of the body; urine tests to check for red and white blood cells, sugar, protein, and abnormal cells; cystoscopy, a thin, lighted tube (cystoscope) inserted through the urethra into the bladder for viewing; biopsy, which removes cells or tissues for examination by a pathologist; and intravenous pyelogram (IVP), a set of x-rays of the kidneys, ureters, and bladder that look for the presence of cancer cells.

Treatments

Treatment depends on the stage of the cancer, the severity of symptoms, and overall health. Standard treatment options are surgery, radiation therapy, chemotherapy, and biologic therapy, which makes use of the body's the immune system to fight the disease or provide protection from potential treatment side effects.

Chemoprevention, or drugs used to inhibit the development changes in cells, and photodynamic therapy, or medications that make cancer cells vulnerable to lasers, are among the new types of treatments being tested in clinical trials to determine safety and effectiveness.

Prognosis and Outcomes

In addition to a person's age and general state of health, a prognosis depends on the stage of the cancer, as well as whether it is superficial or invasive and if it has spread. Early bladder cancer can be cured, although it may reappear elsewhere in the body. Those who give up smoking improve their prognosis.

Ray Marks

See also: Urethral Cancer; Urethral Disorders; Urinary Incontinence

Further Reading

Dartmouth-Hitchcock. (2013, April 13). Bladder cancer. Retrieved from http://www .dartmouth-hitchcock.org/medical-information/health_encyclopedia/uh1360.

Mayo Clinic. (2011). Bladder cancer. Retrieved from http://www.mayoclinic.com/health /bladder-cancer/DS00177.

MedicineNet. (2011). Bladder cancer. Retrieved from http://www.medicinenet.com/bladder _cancer/article.htm.

MedlinePlus. (2011). Bladder cancer. U.S. National Library of Medicine. National Institutes of Health. Retrieved from http://www.nlm.nih.gov/medlineplus/bladdercancer.html.

National Cancer Institute. (2011). Bladder cancer. Retrieved from http://www.cancer.gov /cancertopics/types/bladder.

BLADDER DISEASES

Overview

Located in the pelvis, the bladder is a hollow muscular organ that stores and expels urine. Beginning the process of urination, nerves signal the brain with an urge to empty the bladder once it fills to capacity. A variety of diseases can affect the bladder, ranging from types of incontinence, or urine leakage, to cancer. Other common diseases include cystitis, a bacterial infection that occurs most often in women; interstitial cystitis, also known as painful bladder syndrome, that is a chronic pelvic pain often worsened by increased urine in the bladder; overactive bladder, or the sudden urge to urinate that is difficult to stop that is often experienced by older adults with cognitive or physical disorders; and urinary retention, or the inability to empty the bladder, usually seen in men as they age, that is characterized by weak urine stream, a delay in starting to urinate, and a sense that the bladder remains full.

Causes of bladder diseases include nerves impaired by damage or disease, muscle weakness, infections, bladder or kidney stones, tumors, injuries, inflammation, diseases, and physical abnormalities. Symptoms vary, but they commonly include irritation, pain, frequent or increased urgency to urinate, and abnormal colors or odors of urine. Bladder diseases, which can affect children and adults, can be treated depending on their nature with medications, exercises, and occasionally surgery.

Symptoms

The symptoms of many bladder diseases are common, including pelvic pain or discomfort, burning or painful urination, frequent or increased urgency to urinate, difficulty urinating, excessive urination at night, excessive amounts of urine, urine leakage or involuntary urination, bloody or cloudy urine, and urine that smells foul or otherwise abnormal. Bladder infections that spread to the kidneys can cause back or abdominal pain, as well as fever; urine buildup due to urinary retention may damage the bladder, and backflows into the kidneys can also cause serious damage. Bladder infections, cancer, and injury occasionally lead to life-threatening and serious symptoms that require immediate medical attention; these include a change in consciousness level or mental status; fever higher than 101°F; inability to produce urine; severe pain in the abdomen, pelvis, or back; severe nausea and vomiting; and uncontrolled or heavy bleeding.

Causes and Risk Factors

Because the nerves signal the brain when to empty the bladder, the nervous system is vital to normal bladder function. Symptoms of bladder diseases are commonly caused by nerve damage, which can result due to vaginal childbirth; brain or spine infections or injuries; diabetes; stroke; multiple sclerosis; and poisoning from heavy metals. Some children have congenital nerve disorders that can prevent the release of urine.

Other causes of bladder symptoms include infections and associated inflammation; trauma, or injury, to the bladder and nearby organs; weak muscles in the pelvis and around the urethra; medication side effects; benign bladder or nearby tumors; kidney or bladder stones; muscle tightness on the pelvic floor; diverticulae, or outpouchings, of the bladder or urethra; in men, benign prostatic hyperplasia, or an enlarged prostate that usually occurs with age, and urethral stricture or narrowing; and in women, cystocele, or when the bladder bulges into the vagina, as well as hormones and pressure on the bladder during pregnancy.

Diagnosis

In addition to a physical exam and a medical history, bladder diseases are diagnosed with urinalysis, or urine lab tests for infection, traces of blood, or other abnormal substances; cystoscopy to examine inside the lining of the bladder and urethra; and ureteroscopy, which provides a look inside the ureters and kidneys. Imaging tests—including x-rays, ultrasounds, MRIs, and CT scans—can also detect bladder and kidney stones, infections, tumors, injuries, and cysts. Specific tests for an overactive bladder may include a focused neurological exam and urodynamic tests that measure urine left in the bladder following urination, urine flow volume and speed, and bladder pressure. Urinary retention may be diagnosed with the same tools as well as electromyography, or sensors that measure the electrical activity of the bladder and sphincter muscles and nerves. Because no one test can diagnose interstitial cystitis, it is diagnosed by the presence of bladder pain along with frequency and urgency of urination and by ruling out other diseases with similar symptoms with urinalysis, urine culture, cystoscopy, biopsy of the bladder wall and urethra, and distention of the bladder.

Treatments

Treatment depends on the type of bladder infection and its cause. Medications are commonly prescribed for bacterial and interstitial cystitis, overactive bladder, and urinary retention. Other forms of treatment for urinary retention include bladder drainage, urethral dilation and stents, and surgery. Treatments for overactive bladder and interstitial cystitis may include behavioral interventions, including Kegel exercises to strengthen the pelvic floor; limiting fluids; and bladder training, or a gradual delay in time between feeling the urge and urinating. Nerve stimulation and bladder distention may improve also symptoms of interstitial cystitis. Usually, surgery is considered after implementing other treatments.

Prevention

While they are not entirely preventable, risk factors for some bladder diseases can be reduced, including restricting nighttime fluids and keeping well hydrated during the day; avoiding caffeinated and alcoholic beverages; maintaining a healthy body weight; practicing Kegel exercises; urinating regularly to empty the bladder fully; and following good hygiene practices, particularly to prevent bacteria from entering the urethra and bladder. Treating and managing the symptoms of underlying disorders and illnesses, such as an enlarged prostate or constipation causing urinary retention or diabetes causing overactive bladder, may help prevent the development of bladder diseases.

Prognosis and Outcomes

The prognoses for cystitis and overactive bladder are generally good as long as symptoms are treated promptly and treatment protocols are followed. Treatment results vary among individuals with interstitial cystitis; dietary changes may help control symptoms for some people, but others may respond only to extensive treatment or surgery. Prevention of urinary retention is based on treatment of its underlying cause.

Jean Kaplan Teichroew

See also: Bladder Cancer; Diverticular Disease; Kidney Diseases; Urinary Incontinence; Urinary Tract Infections

Further Reading

Healthgrades. (2013, August 23). Bladder symptoms. Retrieved from http://www.health grades.com/symptoms/bladder-symptoms.

Healthline. (2015). Urologic diseases: Overview. Retrieved from http://www.healthline.com /health/renal-and-urological-disorders.

Mayo Clinic. (2014, September 26). Overactive bladder. Retrieved by http://www.mayoclinic .org/diseases-conditions/overactive-bladder/basics/risk-factors/con-20027632.

MedlinePlus. (2015, September 15). Bladder diseases. Retrieved from https://www.nlm.nih .gov/medlineplus/bladderdiseases.html.

National Institute of Diabetes and Digestive and Kidney Diseases. (2014, January 22). Urinary tract and how it works. Retrieved from http://www.niddk.nih.gov/health-information/health-topics/Anatomy/urinary-tract-how-it-works/Pages/anatomy.aspx.

BLEEDING DISORDERS

Description

Bleeding disorders are an acquired or inherited tendency to bleed excessively. Bleeding disorders occur when your body does not form a blood clot to stop bleeding. In cases of injury, bleeding may be very heavy and last for a long time or for periods of time longer than normal. Bleeding disorders are also termed coagulopathy, abnormal bleeding, and clotting disorders.

Bleeding problems can range from mild to severe.

Symptoms

- Bleeding into joints
- Excessive bruising
- Easy bleeding
- Heavy bleeding
- Heavy menstrual bleeding
- Nosebleeds

In severe cases, complications include:

Bleeding into the brain, or severe bleeding as a result of injury or problems in the gastrointestinal tract
Scarring of the joints or joint disease
Vision loss from bleeding into the eye
Chronic anemia or low red cell count from blood loss
Neurological or psychiatric problems
Death

Which problems occur depends on the specific bleeding disorder, and how severe it is.

Causes and Risk Factors

Bleeding disorders occur if an individual does not have enough platelets or clotting factors in her or his blood. So these clotting factors, which involve as many as 20 different plasma proteins or coagulation factors, do not work in the way they were designed to form a substance along with other chemicals, called fibrin, because they are low or are missing.

Sometimes, this occurs in response to certain medications. Bleeding disorders can also be due to diseases such as liver disease or deficiencies in vitamin K; immune system–related diseases, such as allergic reactions to medications or infections, such as HIV; and cancers such as leukemia, which is a blood cancer.

They can also be inherited such as hemophilia and von Willebrand's disease; they can occur in families and following surgery, dental visits, or trauma.

Other causes are bone marrow problems, kidney failure, disseminated intravascular coagulation, pregnancy-associated eclampsia or toxicity, organ transplant rejection, and antibodies that can destroy clotting factors.

The condition can also start on its own or because the veins or arteries of the body are injured or have structural problems and the blood clotting mechanism is deficient.

Diagnosis

Diagnosis is through laboratory tests, including:

- History and physical examination
  - Blood cell counts
  - Bleeding time
  - Partial thromboplastin time
  - Platelet aggregation test
  - Prothrombin time

Treatment Approaches

Treating the underlying disease, disorder, or condition may improve bleeding. Treatment may include:

- Medications, to help prevent the normal breakdown of blood clots after they have formed
- Clotting factor replacement to replace a specific clotting factor
- Corticosteroids, such as prednisone, to suppress the immune system in people who have developed antibodies that inhibit specific clotting factors (acquired hemophilia)
- Desmopressin acetate (DDAVP) to temporarily increase factor VIII clotting activity
- Immune therapies to suppress the immune system in people with acquired hemophilia
- Plasma transfusions to supplement all the clotting factors; transfusion of fresh frozen plasma may be used after a bleeding episode or before certain procedures to control bleeding
- Platelet transfusions to increase the number of platelets in the bloodstream
- Vitamin supplementation for bleeding disorders caused by vitamin K deficiency

People who have bleeding disorders should try:

- Avoiding injury or contact sports
- Having regular checkups with their health care provider
- Informing their dentist that they have a bleeding disorder
- Protecting their joints through regular exercise and maintaining a healthy weight
- Receiving immunizations for hepatitis A and B
- Seeking prompt treatment when bleeding occurs
- Seeking help from counselors or support groups

Prognosis or Outcome

Outcome depends on the extent of the disorder. Uncontrolled internal or external bleeding can lead to serious, life-threatening complications, such as anemia, dangerous blood loss, shock, and damage to vital internal organs such as the brain.

It is usually possible however, to stop the excess bleeding and treat the underlying disease, if this is the cause.

Those who experience any unusual bleeding or excessive bruising after a minor injury, bleeding gums, nosebleeds, or heavy menstrual bleeding should contact their medical provider or call 911.

Prevention depends on the type of problem.

Ray Marks

See also: Anemia; Hemophilia; Neurological Diseases; Uterine Cancer; Uterine Diseases

Further Reading

American Association for Clinical Chemistry. (2012). Lab Tests Online. Retrieved from http://labtestsonline.org/understanding/conditions/bleeding-disorders.

American Society of Hematology. (2015). Bleeding disorders. Retrieved from http://www.hematology.org/Patients/Blood-Disorders/5219.aspx.

Centers for Disease Control and Prevention. (2015, October 2). Blood disorders. Retrieved from http://www.cdc.gov/ncbddd/blooddisorders/index.html.

Jones, P. (2002). *Living with Haemophilia*, 5th ed. New York: Oxford University Press.

National Hemophilia Foundation. (2015). Types of bleeding disorders. https://www.hemophilia.org/Bleeding-Disorders.

National Heart, Lung, and Blood Institute. (2015). Blood disorders. Retrieved from http://www.nhlbi.nih.gov/health/resources/blood.

World Federation of Hemophilia. (2012, May). What are bleeding disorders? Retrieved from http://www.wfh.org/en/page.aspx?pid=1282.

BLOOD CANCERS

Overview

Blood cancer, sometimes called hematologic cancer, is the term for a group of cancers that affect normal cell production or function in the blood, bone marrow, and lymph nodes. The diseased blood cells rapidly multiply and cause life-threatening damage to the immune and circulatory systems. They can affect anyone of any age; it is estimated that more than 100,000 people in the United States receive a diagnosis of blood, bone marrow, and lymph node cancers, resulting in more than 50,000 deaths. Leukemia is the most common cancer and the leading cause of cancer death in children and teens.

The main forms of blood cancer are leukemia, lymphoma, and multiple myeloma. Leukemia, which can be acute or chronic, begins in the bone marrow. It is caused by a rapid production of abnormal white blood cells that impair the ability of the bone marrow to produce red blood cells and platelets. The acute form is characterized by a large number of abnormal white blood cells that fight infection; the chronic form is the slow development of too many normally functioning white blood cells.

Lymphoma, primarily Hodgkin lymphoma and non-Hodgkin lymphoma, describes the blood cancers that develop in the lymphatic system, which drains excess fluids from the body and produces immune cells. Lymphocytes are the white blood cells that fight infection, but abnormal lymphocytes that become lymphoma cells eventually impair the immune system and its ability to fight infections. Myeloma begins in the bone marrow when plasma cells begin to grow uncontrollably, compromising the immune system and damaging the production and function of white and red blood cells leading to bone disease, organ damage, anemia, and other illnesses; multiple myeloma is the most common type.

Because leukemia and myeloma affect the bone marrow, symptoms can include easy bruising, anemia, bleeding problems, and frequent infections. Enlarged lymph nodes are a typical symptom of lymphoma. What precisely causes these cancers is not known, but general risk factors that increase the chances of developing blood cancer include aging; exposure to certain chemicals, radiation, or types of chemotherapy; family or personal history of blood cancer, certain blood disorders, or genetic disorders; certain viral infections; and a compromised immune system. Treatments include chemotherapy, radiation, and stem cell transplantation.

Symptoms

Symptoms of leukemia depend on the type and stage of the disease, but typically they include fever, chills, night sweats, and flu-like symptoms; weakness and fatigue; swollen or bleeding gums; headache; enlarged liver or spleen; swollen tonsils; bone pain; pale skin; tiny red spots on the skin; and unexplained weight loss. Symptoms of lymphoma, which affects the lymphatic system, include swollen lymph nodes in the neck, armpits, or groin; fever; weakness and fatigue; unexplained weight loss; sweating; difficulty breathing; chest pain; and a rash or itchy skin. Symptoms of myeloma, occurring in the bone marrow, include the excessive calcium in the blood; anemia; kidney failure; thirst; changes in urination; dehydration; constipation; increased susceptibility to infection; osteoporosis or bone pain, swelling, or fracture; high protein levels in the blood or urine; weakness; confusion; and unexplained weight loss.

Causes and Risk Factors

The causes of leukemia, lymphoma, and myeloma are unknown. For many people, there are no obvious reasons for developing blood cancer. But risk factors that increase the chance of developing leukemia include exposure to high levels of radiation, repeated or prolonged exposure to benzene and certain other chemicals, having had chemotherapy, Down syndrome and some genetic disorders, being Caucasian, age (younger than 15 and older than 50), and a strong family history. Risk factors for developing lymphoma include older age, being male or Caucasian, having an autoimmune disease, infection with Epstein-Barr or HIV/AIDS viruses, a diet high in meats and fat, and exposure to some pesticides. Age is the most significant risk factor for developing myeloma, particularly over the age of 67; others include being African American, male, or obese; exposure to radiation, pesticides, fertilizers, or Agent Orange; and work in petroleum-related industries.

Diagnosis

A physical exam can indicate symptoms typical of blood cancers, and a medical history helps identify other risk factors. Diagnostic tools and procedures for blood cancers typically include blood and urine tests and bone marrow aspiration and biopsies. Imaging tests may include x-rays, CT, MRI, and PET scans.

Treatments

Treatment for blood cancer is required by a hematologist-oncologist, a specialist in the diagnosis and treatment of blood cell cancers. Depending on the specific form of cancer, its progression, and an individual's overall health, treatments vary, but they commonly include stem cell transplantation, which places healthy blood-forming cells into the body; chemotherapy, or medications to stop the growth of cancer cells; targeted therapy, or the use of drugs or other substances that precisely identify and attack cancer cells; immunotherapy, which uses the body's immune system to attack cancer cells; and radiation therapy to destroy cancer cells or relieve pain or discomfort.

Prevention

Because so few of the known risk factors for leukemia, lymphoma, or myeloma can be changed, it is not possible to prevent the diseases.

Prognosis and Outcomes

The prognosis for those with blood cancer has improved after decades of research that brought about significant improvements in treatments, which has resulted in higher remission and survival rates. Many are alive today and may have active cancer or may be in remission from blood cancer. After treatment, many people with leukemia live many years with good quality of life. Lymphoma, once fatal, is now one of the most curable forms of cancer due to research; those with slow-growing non-Hodgkin lymphoma can live for many years with treatment. Research has also improved the prognosis and survival rates for myeloma.

Ray Marks

See also: Autoimmune Disease; Bone Cancer; Bone Diseases; Cancer; Leukemia; Lymphoma; Multiple Myeloma

Further Reading

American Cancer Society. (2015). Leukemia. Retrieved from http://www.cancer.org/cancer
/leukemia/index.

American Cancer Society. (2015). Lymphoma. Retrieved from http://www.cancer.org/cancer
/lymphoma/index.

American Cancer Society. (2015). Multiple myeloma. Retrieved from http://www.cancer.org
/cancer/multiplemyeloma/index.

American Society of Hematology. (2015). Blood cancers. Retrieved from http://www
.hematology.org/Patients/Blood-Disorders/Blood-Cancers/5229.aspx.

Leukemia and Lymphoma Society. (2015). Types of blood cancer. Retrieved from http://www
.lls.org/disease-information.

BLOOD DISORDERS

Blood, which is made up of cells such as red blood cells (carry oxygen), white blood cells (fight infection), and platelets (help blood to clot), and fluid, called plasma, can be subject to different types of disorders. Blood disorders are also termed *hematological diseases.*

These disorders are considered to represent a serious public health problem and include:

- Bleeding disorders, including hemophilia due to disorders in substances responsible for clotting
- Platelet disorders
- Anemia, one of the more common blood disorders due to decreased number of red blood cells, of which there are up to 400 types
- Increased number of red blood cells or white cells called polycythemia, which thickens blood and can cause shortness of breath, headaches, dizziness, and confusion.

Some other blood related health problems include:

Deep vein thrombosis—clot in a deep vein

Hemochromatosis—too much iron in body

Idiopathic thrombocytopenic purpura—a bleeding disorder due to low number of blood platelets

Lymphoma—form of cancer in which white blood cells become malignant

Leukemia—form of cancer in which white blood cells become malignant

Malaria—red blood cell infection

Multiple myeloma—blood cancer in which plasma cell within the white blood cells multiply and cause organ damage

Pulmonary embolism—sudden blockage in a lung artery

Sickle cell disease—an inherited disorder in which the body produces sickle-shaped red blood cells that can block blood flow

Thalassemia—inherited blood disorders; common hereditary blood disorder

Thrombocythemia and thrombocytosis—condition in which there are too many blood platelets

Thrombocytopenia—fewer than normal numbers of blood platelets

These blood disorders affect millions of people in the United States each year, including people of all ages regardless of race, sex, and socioeconomic status. Many Americans and others across the globe thus live with one of these conditions and its complications, which may include pain. Many blood disorders are life-threatening as well. Others are chronic, but do not affect longevity, such as acute leukemia.

Symptoms

These are often vague and nonspecific. There may however be evidence of fatigue, dizziness, shortness of breath, loss of concentration, noise in the ear, fast heartbeat and weakness in the presence of anemia.

There may fever and infection if there are low numbers of white blood cells or bleeding problems that affect the blood cells or blood clotting mechanism that lead to easy bruising or bleeding or red spots on the lower extremities. There may be nose bleeds, bleeding of mouth and gums, and blood in urine or stools with a low platelet count. There may also be abnormal blood clots that lead to warm, painful areas in the legs or sudden shortness of breath, chest pain, or both.

Other symptoms include swelling of the joints, internal bleeding, tightness of the joints.

Causes and Risk Factors

Causes can include inherited disorders; secondary manifestations due to another illness or primary disorder; or secondarily due to chemotherapy or radiation treatments. The overuse of recreational drugs, chemical exposure, pregnancy complications, viral infections, can often cause or influence blood disorders. Risk factors include high dose radiation treatments, chemical exposure, or toxic exposure in foods, drinks, or other consumable items.

Diagnosis

A hematologist uses physical examinations, a review of the patient's history and laboratory tests to make a diagnosis of a blood disorder, including blood smears, blood tests, bone marrow examination, hemoglobin counts, and total blood counts.

Inherited blood diseases are usually diagnosed in childhood, but the diagnosis may not be made if the symptoms are mild.

Treatment

Treatments and prognosis for blood diseases vary, depending on the blood condition and its severity. They can include simple observation, antibiotics, anticoagulation therapy, growth factor supplementation, iron supplementation, steroids, immune modulating therapies, transfusions, chemotherapy, plasma infusions, bone marrow transplantation, and chemically engineered blood products that can be added to deficient blood.

Prognosis

With proper preventive actions and early intervention, many of these disorders and their complications can, to a large extent, be eliminated. The Centers for Disease Control and Prevention (CDC) is working toward developing a comprehensive public health agenda to promote and improve the health of people with blood disorders. Optimum diet, ample rest, and a supportive environment are recommended.

Exercising, if indicated, may be helpful. Good dental care and following the physician's recommendations are highly recommended as well.

Ray Marks

See also: Anemia; Bleeding Disorders; Deep Vein Thrombosis; Hemochromatosis; Leukemia; Lymphoma; Multiple Myeloma; Platelet Disorders; Sickle-Cell Disease; Thrombophlebitis

Further Reading

Centers for Disease Control and Prevention. (2011). Blood disorders. http://www.cdc.gov/ncbddd/blooddisorders/index.html.

Cleveland Clinic. (2011). Blood disorders. Retrieved from http://my.clevelandclinic.org/disorders/diseases/blood_disorders/can_overview.aspx.

Merck Manuel Home Health Book. (2011). Diagnosis of blood disorders. Retrieved from http://www.merckmanuals.com/home/blood_disorders/symptoms_and_diagnosis_of_blood_disorders/diagnosis_of_blood_disorders.html.

Merck Manuel Home Health Book. (2011). Symptoms of blood disorders. Retrieved from http://www.merckmanuals.com/home/blood_disorders/symptoms_and_diagnosis_of_blood_disorders/symptoms_of_blood_disorders.html?qt=&sc=&alt=.

National Heart and Lung Institute. People Science Health. (2011). Blood diseases and resources information. Available at: http://www.nhlbi.nih.gov/health/public/blood/index.htm.

Nemours Foundation. (2011). Blood. Retrieved from http://kidshealth.org/parent/general/body_basics/blood.html.

BLOOD PRESSURE

Overview

The heart is a muscle that pumps blood into the arteries of the body. Blood pressure (BP) is the force or pressure of the circulating blood in the blood vessels. Blood pressure changes all the time. It decreases when a person is at rest or sleeping, and rises when a person is active. Blood pressure is also affected by emotions, as when someone is excited, nervous, or scared.

Measuring Blood Pressure

Blood pressure is recorded in millimeters of mercury. It is written as mmHg. There are always two numbers given when measuring blood pressure: one is systolic pressure and the other is diastolic pressure. For each heartbeat, there is a peak of pressure in the arteries. This is systolic pressure. Diastolic pressure is the minimum amount of pressure in the arteries when the heart relaxes between contractions. A typical normal blood pressure measurement is 120 mmHg systolic and 80 mmHg diastolic pressure. It is written as 120/80 mmHg, or verbally, it is stated as one-twenty over eighty. The measure of blood pressure, along with temperature, respiratory rate, and pulse, is considered a vital sign, an essential physiological measurement of a basic bodily function. At the doctor's office, a physician will place a sphygmomanometer around the bicep of the patient and use a stethoscope to measure blood pressure. A sphygmomanometer uses an inflatable cuff that restricts blood flow. It measures when blood flow is starting and stopping. The cuff is inflated until the blood flow to the artery to the arm is stopped. A doctor slowly releases the pressure, and listens with a stethoscope to determine when blood flow restarts. This is the systolic blood pressure. As the pressure is released, the sound of the beating of the heart fades away until it disappears. This is the diastolic pressure.

History

More than 2,000 years ago, the Egyptians were the first to discover that blood circulated the body (Booth 1977). It was not until Stephen Hales (1677–1761), a British veterinarian, that blood pressure was defined. In volume II of the *Statical Essays*, Hales described how he inserted a pipe into the artery of a horse and noticed how the blood rose. He concluded that pressure in the body was pushing the blood. In France, Jean Poiseuille (1799–1869) then created the mercury manometer to measure blood pressure. This instrument enabled Poiseuille to prove that pressure was maintained in large and small arteries of animals. He also showed that arterial pressure controlled venous pressure, or pressure in the veins. Due to his discovery of measuring blood pressure with mercury, that mmHg is still recorded today. According to the National Library of Medicine, Nikolai Korotkoff (1874–1920) from Russia was the first scientist to measure diastolic pressure by listening to sounds in the arteries when pressure was applied (National Library of Medicine 1987). Despite these advances in measurement, it was not until the 1950s that the dangers of high and low blood pressure were understood.

Types

There are several different types of blood pressure. According to the Centers for Disease Control and Prevention, high blood pressure, also called hypertension, is measured as systolic > 140 mmHg or diastolic > 90 mmHg (CDC 2016). Hypertension puts stress on the heart and creates tissue growth inside the arteries, which is also called atherosclerosis. This makes the arteries harden or become more resistant to blood flow, hence requiring more pressure. High blood pressure usually has no warning signs or symptoms, so many people do not realize that they have it. Eating too much sodium is a major contributor to high blood pressure. Smoking,

Table 4   Stages of High Blood Pressure in Adults

Stages	Systolic (Top Number)	Diastolic (Bottom Number)
Normal blood pressure	Below 120	Below 80
Prehypertension	120–139	80–89
High blood pressure, stage 1	140–159	90–99
High blood pressure, stage 2	160 or higher	100 or higher

The ranges in the table are blood pressure guides for adults who do not have any short-term serious illnesses. People with diabetes or chronic kidney disease should keep their blood pressure below 130/80 mmHg.
Source: Adapted from National Heart, Lung, and Blood Institute. (2015, September 10). Description of high blood pressure. http://www.nhlbi.nih.gov/health/health-topics/topics/hbp.

obesity, inactivity, stress, excessive alcohol use, old age, and kidney disease, as well as some thyroid disorders, can increase risks for developing hypertension. People with family members who have high blood pressure as well as African Americans tend to have higher risks as well. Left untreated, hypertension can lead to angina, heart disease, stroke, heart failure, renal failure, and eye damage.

Hypotension, on the other hand, is defined as having low blood pressure, or pressure that is lower than 90 (systolic) and 60 mmHg (diastolic). Hypotension is a medical concern if dizziness and fainting are prevalent and if the person has heart disease. According to the National Lung and Blood Institute, symptoms and signs of hypotension include dizziness, fainting, cold skin, tiredness, or nausea (NLBI 2010).

Table 4 shows the different types of blood pressure.

Symptoms

High blood pressure or hypertension generally has no symptoms, although severe hypertension may exhibit headaches, nausea, or other symptoms. With low blood pressure, people may experience dizziness or fatigue.

Treatment

A cardiologist may recommend modifications to lifestyle, medications, and dietary changes (such as reduced sodium intake) to treat hypertension.

Medications that may be prescribed for hypertension include:

Diuretics, sometimes called water pills, which help kidneys remove some salt from the body; blood vessels don't have to hold as much fluid and your blood pressure goes down

Beta-blockers, which make the heart beat at a slower rate and with less force

Angiotensin-converting enzyme inhibitors (also called ACE inhibitors), which relax the blood vessels and lower blood pressure

Angiotensin II receptor blockers (also called ARBs), which work approximately the same way as angiotensin-converting enzyme inhibitors

Calcium channel blockers, which relax blood vessels by stopping calcium from entering cells (MedlinePlus 2015)

Other medications may be prescribed.

The treatment of hypotension depends on the underlying cause. A cardiologist will check the results of an ECG, or electrocardiogram, to make sure a patient's heart rate and rhythm are normal. Next, a blood sample will be drawn to test for anemia, or iron deficiency, and blood sugar levels. An increase of sodium and water intake may be recommended. Medications prescribed may include fludrocortisone to increase blood volume or midodrine to stop feelings of dizziness when standing up.

Megan Aronson

See also: Angina; Atherosclerosis; Kidney Failure; Heart Diseases Hypertension; Hypotension; Stroke

Further Reading

American Heart Association. (2015). About high blood pressure. Retrieved from http://www.heart.org/HEARTORG/Conditions/HighBloodPressure/AboutHighBloodPressure/About-High-Blood-Pressure_UCM_002050_Article.jsp.

Booth, J. (1977, Nov.). A short history of blood pressure measurement. *Proceedings of the Royal Society of Medicine*, 70(11), 793–799.

Centers for Disease Control and Prevention (CDC). (2016). High blood pressure. Retrieved from https://www.cdc.gov/bloodpressure/.

Chang, L. (2010). An overview of blood pressure treatment. *WedMD.com*. Retrieved November 22, 2011, from http://www.webmd.com/hypertension-high-blood-pressure/guide/hypertension-treatment-overview.

MedlinePlus. (2015). High blood pressure. Retrieved from https://www.nlm.nih.gov/medlineplus/ency/article/000468.htm.

National Library of Medicine. (1987). *A Century of American Physiology: Based on an Exhibit Commemorating the Centennial of the American Physiological Society as the National Library of Medicine.* National Institute of Health. Bethesda, Maryland: National Library of Medicine. Retrieved on November 15, 2011, from http://www.nlm.nih.gov/hmd/pdf/century.pdf.

National Heart, Lung, and Blood Institute. (2010). What is hypotension? Retrieved from http://www.nhlbi.nih.gov/health/health-topics/topics/hyp/.

Sheps, S. G. (2002). *Mayo Clinic on High Blood Pressure*. Rochester, MN: Mayo Clinic.

BODY MASS INDEX (BMI)

Body mass index (BMI) is a method used for indicating the weight status of adults. It is a measure that reflects a ratio between the weight of an individual divided by the square of their height. For adults over age 20, the BMI is used often used to calculate the extent of his or her body fat. According to the National Institutes of Health, a BMI that is lower than 18.5 is considered to be underweight. A normal

BMI is from 18.5 to 24.9. A BMI of 25–29.9 is considered to represent overweight status; and a BMI of 30.0 and above is considered a state of obesity.

Using the standard mathematical formula listed for calculating one's BMI, the National Institutes of Health provides an online BMI calculator that can compute one's BMI after he or she enters his or her height in feet and inches along with his or her weight in pounds. There are limits to using the BMI as the measure may overestimate body fat in athletes or underestimate body fat in an individual who has lost muscle.

For children and teens, BMI is calculated based on gender and age-specific charts, and the thresholds for weight status are based on percentiles derived from comparison with other children of the same gender and age. Underweight for children means that the individual is less than the 5th percentile. A healthy weight is greater or equal to the 5th percentile but is less than the 85th percentile. Overweight is greater or equal to the 85th percentile, but is less than the 95th percentile. Obesity is categorized as being greater than or equal to the 95th percentile.

This means if your weight is at the 50th percentile, you are close to the average weight of an individual young person of the same age and gender as yourself. You will be classified as overweight if your body weight falls between the 85th and 95th percentile for your age and gender and as obese if you exceed the 95th percentile.

BMI and Health

The BMI ranges are based on the effect body weight has on disease and death, although they change in young people due to growth and are not always totally accurate in muscular people or smaller or older people who have lost muscle. As BMI increases, the risk for some diseases generally increase as well. Some of these conditions include:

Breathing problems
Cardiovascular disease
Gallstones
High blood pressure
Osteoarthritis
Some forms of cancer
Type 2 diabetes

It is important to understand, however, that BMI is only one component of an individual's health and health care providers can help an individual interpret his or her BMI as it relates to the overall health of the individual. The best way to determine the BMI is to have a health professional do it. That way you will know the measure is accurate, and you can discuss the result with the doctor, who can give you sound advice if you need it. If you need to control your weight, your doctor can help you to do this safely because being underweight is also very unhealthy. There are very good resources for helping you to control your weight at www.nhlbi.nih .gov/health/public/heart/obesity/lose_wt/control.htm, and losing a small amount of weight if you are overweight will lower your risk of developing a health condition.

Some of these include setting the right goals, following a healthy eating plan, watching portion sizes, being physically active, and reducing sedentary time.

Ray Marks

Further Reading

Centers for Disease Control and Prevention (CDC). (2015). Body mass index (BMI). Retrieved from http://www.cdc.gov/healthyweight/assessing/bmi/index.html.

Kids Health. (2016). Body mass index (BMI). Retrieved from http://kidshealth.org/en/parents/bmi-charts.html.

National Institutes of Health. (n.d.) Calculate your body mass index. Available at http://www.nhlbi.nih.gov/health/educational/lose_wt/BMI/bmicalc.htm.

National Heart, Lung and Blood Institute. (2011). Body mass index tables. Available at http://www.nhlbi.nih.gov/health/educational/lose_wt/BMI/bmi_tbl.htm.

National Heart, Lung and Blood Institute. (2015). Aim for a healthy body weight. Retrieved from www.nhlbi.nih.gov/health/public/heart/obesity/lose_wt/control.htm.

BONE CANCER

Description

Bone cancer, also called sarcoma, usually occurs when cancer from another body site such as the breast or lung spreads to the bone. This form is called metastatic cancer. On rare occasions, however, cancer can start in the bone, and this is called primary bone cancer. Malignant cancer of the bone is due to a cancerous tumor of the bone that destroys normal bone tissue. Bone tumors can also be benign or inactive, and these are more common than malignant tumors. Both may grow and compress healthy bone tissue, but benign tumors do not destroy bone tissue. Another type of bone cancer is called multiple myeloma, and it is the most common type of bone cancer.

The three types of sarcomas or primary bone cancers are:

- Osteosarcomas, which arise in new tissue in growing bones, usually between ages 10 and 25, are most commonly found in the knee and upper arm.
- Chondrosarcomas, which arise in cartilage that lines the joints, usually occur after age 50; they can occur in the pelvis, upper leg, and shoulder. If they contains cancerous bone cells, the tumor condition is termed osteosarcoma.
- Ewing's sarcomas, which arise in the nerve tissues of the bone marrow of young people, or in their soft tissues such as muscle, fat, blood vessels, or other supporting tissues, often appear after treatment of another health condition with radiation or chemotherapy and commonly occur in or along the spine or in the middle part of the bones of the pelvis, legs and arms, or ribs.

Most often, bone cancer affects the bones of the arms and legs, but it can occur in any bone.

Signs and Symptoms

Pain is the most common symptom, but there may be other symptoms, depending on the cancer type and location.

Other signs and symptoms include:

Anemia
Swelling and tenderness near affected bone area
Fatigue, fever, weight loss
Stiffness
Unintended weight loss
Lump on the bone palpable through the skin

Pathological fractures may also occur due to weakened bones, and this is more common in the lower than upper part of the body.

The symptoms of bone cancer tend to develop slowly and the rate depends on the type, location, and size of the tumor.

Causes

Most bone cancers occur in people with identifiable risk factors, including high doses of radiation therapy for cancer; exposure to petroleum products, benzene, herbicides, and insecticides; treatment with certain anticancer drugs; heredity; Paget's disease of the bone, and other bone diseases.

Diagnosis

X-rays may show destruction of the bone.

CT scans, MRI, and radionuclide bone scans or a skeletal examination may be done to pinpoint which bones are affected.

Tissue or needle biopsies may also be used.

Tests to Determine the Extent (Stage) of the Bone Cancer

Once a doctor diagnoses bone cancer, he or she may seek to determine the extent (stage) of the cancer. The cancer's stage guides the treatment options.

Stages of bone cancer include:

Stage I. At this stage, bone cancer is limited to the bone and hasn't spread to other areas of the body. It is considered low grade and not aggressive.
Stage II. This stage of bone cancer is limited to the bone and hasn't spread to other areas of the body. Here, the bone cancer is high grade and considered aggressive.
Stage III. At this stage, bone cancer occurs in two or more places on the same bone. The bone cancer is high grade and considered aggressive.
Stage IV. This stage of bone cancer indicates that cancer has spread beyond the bone to other areas of the body, such as the brain, liver, or lungs.

Treatment

Treatment for cancer that has spread to the bones depends on where the cancer started and the extent to which it has spread, as well as the patient's age and general health.

For metastatic cancer, management of the cancer and the symptoms produced by the bone tumor are important. Surgery is the most common form of treatment. Other forms of treatment include:

Amputation
Biphosphonates to reduce bone pain and slow down bone damage
Chemotherapy
Cytotoxic drugs
Hormone therapy
Immunotherapy
Pain medications
Radiation therapy

With modern surgical techniques, 90 percent of cases will not need amputation.

Prognosis or Outcome

The outcome is affected by age, size of tumor, grade and stage of tumor, duration of symptoms, and location of tumor.

Ray Marks

See also: Anemia; Cancer; Environment; Multiple Myeloma; Osteoporosis

Further Reading

American Cancer Society. (2015). Bone cancer. Retrieved from http://www.cancer.org/cancer/bonecancer/detailedguide/index.

Hasan, H. (2009). *Bone Cancer: Current and Emerging Trends in Detection and Treatment.* New York, NY: Rosen Publishing.

Mayo Clinic. (2015, March 17). Bone cancer. Retrieved from http://www.mayoclinic.org/diseases-conditions/bone-cancer/home/ovc-20126418

National Cancer Institute. (2015). Bone cancer. Retrieved from http://www.cancer.gov/types/bone/bone-fact-sheet.

University of Maryland Medical Center. (2014, May 26). Bone cancer. Retrieved from http://www.umm.edu/altmed/articles/bone-cancer-000023.htm.

BONE DISEASES

Description

Bones are an essential component of the body, providing for both structure and mobility. Over the childhood and teenage years, new bone is constantly being added to the old, which is partially removed and replaced. After approximately age 20, new bone is no longer added at a rate that is greater than the bone removal rate. This can become a health problem if the bones are not adequately built up in the teenage years and during childhood. A bone disease is any disease that affects the bone.

Among the different types of bone related problems that exist, the following are the most common:

- Bone cancer or bone tumors
- Bone infection
- Osteoporosis, due to low bone density—the most common bone disease
- Osteogenesis imperfect—a genetic disease
- Osteonecrosis—bone death
- Osteomalacia
- Osteopetrosis—present at birth is a disease that results from impaired bone remodeling leading to dense bone
- Paget's disease of the bone—a metabolic disease that causes bones to become fragile and deformed, as well as larger
- Proteus syndrome—atypical growth of bones
- Rickets—abnormal bone formation in children
- Skeletal fluorosis—an arthritic bone disease

A bone disease can make the bone very weak and brittle and liable to fracture. Weak bones can you put you at risk for infections, skin conditions, and heart conditions.

Signs and Symptoms

Each bone disorder or condition has its own unique symptoms. The most common symptoms and signs are:
Bone deformities, bone pain and tenderness, fractures, joint pain, and nerve damage

More rarely there may be:
Hearing loss, loss of appetite, or vomiting

Causes

Bone diseases may result due to age, excess alcohol usage, blood disorders, and deficiencies in calcium and vitamin D intake, as well as developmental defects, excessive exposure to fluoride, exercise deficiencies, genetic factors, infectious diseases, and malnutrition. Other causes include the presence of other health conditions—for example, chronic kidney disease and neurological disorders—and problems with the rate of bone growth or bone building. Smoking and excess steroid usage are other causes.

Diagnosis

Bone diseases are diagnosed using alkaline phosphatase blood tests, bone density scans, bone biopsies, x-rays, and blood tests. Blood tests can check levels of calcium, phosphorus, and parathyroid hormone, plus vitamin D.

Treatment

Treatment depends on age, overall, health, and the nature of the condition.

Bone and tissue transplantation, bone building medications, bone cancer treatments, casts, crutches, surgery, traction, braces, and exercise are some of the common treatments.

Prevention

Adequate diet, avoiding tobacco, exercising, following one's treatment plan, genetic testing, the use of nutrition supplements, and regular oral health care are recommended.

Prognosis

Prognosis depends on the cause and seriousness of the condition.

Ray Marks

See also: Bone Cancer; Legg-Calve-Perthes Disease; Osteoporosis; Paget's Disease of the Bone; Rickets

Further Reading

American Kidney Fund. (2015). Bone disease. Retrieved from http://www.kidneyfund.org/kidney-disease/kidney-failure/bone-disease/.

Mayo Clinic. (2014, December 13). Osteoporosis. Retrieved from http://www.mayoclinic.org/diseases-conditions/osteoporosis/basics/definition/con-20019924.

Mayo Clinic. (2013, February 13). Paget's disease of bone. Retrieved from http://www.mayoclinic.org/diseases-conditions/pagets-disease-of-bone/basics/definition/con-20020138.

National Institute of Arthritis and Musculoskeletal and Skin Diseases. (2015). Bone basics. Retrieved from http://www.niams.nih.gov/Health_Info/Bone/Bone_Basics/.

National Institute of Arthritis and Musculoskeletal and Skin Diseases. (2015). Osteogenesis imperfecta. Retrieved from http://www.niams.nih.gov/Health_Info/Bone/Osteogenesis_Imperfecta/.

BOWEL INCONTINENCE

Overview

Bowel incontinence refers to the inability to control the passage of small amount of stool, liquid or solid, or control flatus (passing gas). It is also termed uncontrollable passage of feces, loss of bowel control, and fecal incontinence.

Bowel incontinence is a chronic health condition that may affect more than 5 million Americans, where an individual over the age of four years loses voluntary control over bowel movements. This may be very disabling due to the involuntary presence of stools, the occasional leakage of a small amount of the stool, or the complete loss of bowel control.

Most commonly, people over 65 years of age are affected, and women are affected more than men.

There are numerous potential causes, and many patients have more than one reason to cause loss of bowel control. Complications may include emotional distress, skin irritations, stigma, and reduced quality of life, especially if untreated.

Symptoms

People are sometimes reluctant to discuss their lack of bowel control because of the social stigma attached to it. Their initial complaint might be *pruritis ani,* breakdown of the skin in the buttock area, and ulcers of the skin.

Causes

- Bowel surgery
- Certain medications, such as antibiotics or Neurontin
- Chemotherapy
- Chronic constipation causing muscles involved in bowel functions to stretch/ weaken
- Chronic laxative use
- Conditions associated with chronic diarrhea or constipation
- Decreased awareness of sensation in the bowel area
- Dementia
- Diabetes
- Emotional problems
- Gynecological, prostate, or rectal surgery
- Injury to muscles in rectal area due to childbirth
- Improper diet
- Multiple sclerosis
- Nerve or muscle damage from trauma, tumors, or radiation
- Physical disability
- Severe diarrhea
- Severe hemorrhoids or rectal prolapse
- Spinal cord damage
- Stress
- Stroke

Diagnostic Tools

After a medical history for diagnosis of the cause of the incontinence, the following tools and techniques might be used: anal electromyography, barium enema, blood tests, endoscopy, MRIi or x-ray defecography, nerve tests, physical exam, rectal or pelvic ultrasound, stool culture and testing, tests of anal sphincter tone (anal manometry), and/or x-rays using a special dye (a balloon sphincterogram).

Treatments

The treatment is to regulate bowel movements, decrease frequency, and increase stool consistency.

Appropriate treatment can help or eliminate the problem for most people and include:

- The prevention of constipation leading to impaction of the fecal mass
- Removal of impacted material from the rectal area
- Dietary changes and medications
- Bowel retraining, surgery, the use of an external pouch or colostomy bag
- Biofeedback
- Sacral nerve stimulation
- Kegel exercises
- Skin care
- Social support
- Using absorbent undergarments

Prognosis

Unfortunately, many times the cause of incontinence is childbirth anal surgery. It may be years until the symptoms of incontinence arise.

The frequency of fecal incontinence increases with age. Once it occurs, the patient may be able to control the symptoms with diet, medication, and exercise. Many patients may initially benefit from surgery, but that benefit gradually decreases over the years and incontinence may recur.

Whatever the cause, although fecal incontinence can be embarrassing, the Mayo Clinic suggests not shying away from talking to a doctor. According to the Cleveland Clinic website, no matter how serious the problem appears to be, this condition can be significantly improved and, in most cases, it may be cured.

Prevention

By knowing one's own limitations, understanding the health condition, and preparing ahead of time to meet all eventualities, the affected individual can control his or her situation reasonably successfully.

Patricia A. McGarry-Strizak

See also: Stress; Wellness

Further Reading

Cleveland Clinic. (2012). Bowel incontinence. Retrieved from http://my.clevelandclinic.org /disorders/bowel_incontinence/hic_bowel_incontinence.aspx.

Mayo Clinic. (2012). Fetal incontinence. Retrieved from http://www.mayoclinic.com/health /fecal-incontinence/DS00477/METHOD=print.

MedlinePlus. (2014). Bowel incontinence. United States National Library of Medicine. National Institutes of Health. Retrieved from http://www.nlm.nih.gov/medlineplus/ency /article/003135.htm.

BRADYCARDIA

Bradycardia is the medical term for a slow heart rate. The normal resting heart rate range for a healthy adult is between 60 and 100 beats per minute. In a person with bradycardia, the heart beats fewer than 60 times per minute due to some type of blockage or slowing of the natural electrical signals in the heart. In the United States, the condition is more prevalent in men—some 15 percent of all men are diagnosed with the condition, while only around 7 percent of women have it. The highest risk age group for women appears to be between 40 and 60.

It is not uncommon for young adults and athletes to have slower than normal heart rates. Although this is still considered bradycardia, it is not viewed as a health problem. In others, a more damaging issue concerning the electrical impulses that regulate the speed at which blood is pumped through the heart may cause brady-cardia. High blood pressure, underactive thyroid functions, heart infections, inflammatory diseases (including rheumatoid arthritis), congenital heart defects (heart problems from birth), aging heart tissue, metabolic problems, and electrolyte imbalances are among the possible causes of bradycardia. Additionally, bradycardia can begin with problems in the sinus node, which is considered the heart's natural pacemaker, and it can be caused by obstructive sleep apnea, which is a condition that occurs when the airway becomes blocked or narrowed while a person is asleep.

Some people with bradycardia never experience symptoms or complications; however, when the condition is severe enough, it can mean that the heart does not pump enough oxygenated blood through the body and can lead to a host of health problems. Common symptoms of bradycardia include fatigue, dizziness, chest pains, light-headedness, and shortness of breath. A person with bradycardia may also experience mental confusion or might tire easily while exercising. If the condition is severe and left untreated, it may result in frequent fainting episodes, heart failure, and possibly even sudden cardiac arrest and death.

Bradycardia is diagnosed through a series of tests and exams used to measure the heart rate and determine underlying causes of the issue. An electrocardiogram, or EKG, is typically performed to evaluate the heart rate, and an exercise test may be recommended to determine how the heart rate changes during exertion. Blood tests and other exams may be ordered if there is suspicion of infection or other such factors contributing to the bradycardia. Once a diagnosis is made, treatment for bradycardia varies depending on what is causing the issue and how severe the problem is. For some, an artificial pacemaker to regulate the heart rhythm is recommended. This battery-operated device is implanted below the collarbone and wired into the heart to control the electrical impulses there. For others, treatment consists of changing medications or lowering dosage on medications that may interfere with the heart's operating system. If an underlying condition or ailment like obstructive sleep apnea is the root of the problem, treatment will most likely involve addressing this issue first to see if that corrects the bradycardia.

Bradycardia has been a known issue for many years. Yet, new information about the condition is still being learned. In the 1980s, it was discovered that severe sinus bradycardia has a high mortality rate without the aid of an artificial pacemaker. In 2006, researchers in Italy found a genetic mutation in the sinus node that may be partially responsible for bradycardia; the discovery holds great potential for the possibility of finding improved ways to address the issue in the future.

Tamar Burris

See also: Arrhythmias/Dysrhythmias; Congenital Heart Disease; High Blood Pressure; Inflammation; Rheumatoid Arthritis; Thyroid Disease

Further Reading

Attar, S. (1985). *New Developments in Cardiac Assist Devices.* Westport, CT: Praeger.
Byrne, D. G. (1987). *The Behavioral Management of the Cardiac Patient.* Westport, CT: Praeger.
Johns Hopkins Medicine. (2015). Bradycardia. Retrieved from http://www.hopkinsmedicine .org/healthlibrary/conditions/cardiovascular_diseases/bradycardia_22,Bradycardia/.
Mayo Clinic. (2015). Bradycardia. Retrieved from http://www.mayoclinic.org/diseases -conditions/bradycardia/basics/definition/con-20028373.

BRAIN CANCER

Brain cancer is the abnormal, malignant growth of masses of cells, called tumors, in the brain. Brain cancer tumors can grow and spread rapidly and uncontrollably, frequently leading to death. The cancerous cells cause illness by taking over the space normally occupied by healthy brain cells, robbing the healthy cells of their blood and nutrients. The aggressive, dangerous growth and spread of cancer distinguishes malignant brain tumors from benign, noncancerous brain tumors.

Types

Brain cancer can take various forms. Primary brain cancer originates within the brain when brain cells undergo abnormal transformations. The name given to any particular type of brain tumor is usually based on its site of origin—such as gliomas, meningiomas, pituitary adenomas, and vestibular schwannomas. Cancer originating in the brain can spread to other parts of the body. In contrast to primary brain cancer, metastatic brain cancer originates in other parts of the body and later spreads to the brain through the blood or the lymphatic system. Metastatic brain cancer is more common than primary brain cancer.

Prevalence and Mortality

Brain cancer is one of the less common forms of cancer, though it is also among the more fatal forms. There are approximately 23,000 newly diagnosed cases of brain cancer, with 13,000 deaths, each year in the United States. Worldwide, about 250,000 people are diagnosed with brain cancer each year.

Survival rates for patients with brain cancer depend on various factors, including age, general health, site of the cancer's origin, extent of the cancer's spread, and promptness of treatment. Reported survival rates longer than five years range from less than 10 percent to more than 30 percent for adults. The five-year survival rate for children is about 75 percent.

Risk Factors

Scientists believe that a number of factors play roles in causing brain cancer—though the precise cause in any individual patient is usually unknown. Among the factors that may increase an individual's risk of brain cancer are exposure to certain toxic chemicals, exposure of the head to radiation, cigarette smoking, and infection with HIV.

Toxic chemical exposure is believed to be a factor behind the increased prevalence of brain cancer among individuals in certain professions, such as people who work in the oil and rubber industries, people who handle jet fuel, chemists, and embalmers. Although the prevalence of brain cancer is unusually high in some families, scientists have not found any particular genetic factor linked to the disease.

The artificial sweetener aspartame is sometimes blamed for brain cancer in reports in the popular press. However, based on a review of clinical studies, the U.S. Food and Drug Administration (FDA) does not link aspartame to this disease. Another factor commonly linked to brain cancer is the long-term use of cell phones. Clinical studies disagree regarding the merits of this association, and research into this matter is ongoing.

Symptoms and Diagnosis

People with brain cancer usually experience several troubling symptoms as a result of intracranial pressure and swelling caused by the tumor. Large tumors can cause problems by obstructing the flow of blood and cerebrospinal fluid. Symptoms may include headaches; weakness and sleepiness; vomiting; clumsiness; difficulties in walking and talking; vision and hearing abnormalities; problems in thinking, concentrating, and remembering; and stroke-like seizures.

Although these symptoms and findings of a physical examination may suggest the presence of brain cancer, many of these physical and mental symptoms could also suggest other diseases and conditions. Thus, a diagnosis must be confirmed with certain tests. One of these diagnostic tests is magnetic resonance imaging (MRI), which can reveal the presence of a tumor inside the brain as an area that is colored differently than surrounding tissues. Computed tomography (CT) scans are also used to reveal abnormalities in the brain.

A number of laboratory analytical tests may be used to detect biochemical and metabolic signs of brain cancer. These tests include analyses of white blood cell numbers, electrolyte levels, cerebrospinal fluid characteristics, and liver function.

A biopsy is sometimes performed to confirm the malignant nature of a detected tumor. In a biopsy, a surgeon removes either a portion of the tumor or the entire tumor. To obtain a biopsy sample, the skull may need to be opened in some cases; in other cases, the sample can be collected with a needle inserted through a hole drilled into the skull. Malignant cells can be distinguished from benign cells through a microscopic examination.

Treatment

Treatment for brain cancer is designed to prolong survival and minimize symptoms. Most individuals with brain cancer are treated with some combination of surgery to remove the tumor, radiation therapy to kill the cancer cells, and chemotherapy to interfere with the multiplication and spread of the cancer cells. Because of advanced age or certain health conditions, brain surgery may be considered too risky for some patients. In such cases, treatment will likely be restricted to radiation and drugs.

Surgical removal of the entire tumor may be done at the same time as the biopsy, if possible. If the tumor is benign, removal of the tumor will probably put an end to all of the patient's symptoms. However, if the tumor is malignant, the patient will probably need to undergo radiation and chemotherapy.

Radiation therapy for brain cancer can be done with different techniques. In external radiation, beams of radiation travel through the skin, skull, and healthy tissue to reach the tumor. Several treatments of external radiation are typically necessary. In internal, or implant, radiation, a small radioactive capsule in inserted inside the tumor. The radioactivity of the capsule gradually becomes depleted. In stereotactic radiosurgery, a single large dose of radiation is targeted at the tumor from different angles.

Chemotherapy is typically administered in cycles of treatment interspersed with rest periods, during which the patient's condition is evaluated. Besides anti-cancer drugs, drug therapy for brain cancer may include medications to relieve specific symptoms, such as anticonvulsant drugs to prevent seizures.

As with all forms of cancer, both chemotherapy and radiation therapy for brain cancer involve a number of adverse effects, including nausea, vomiting, and hair loss.

A. J. Smuskiewicz

See also: Cancer; Pituitary Disorders; Vestibular Diseases

Further Reading

American Brain Tumor Association. (2015). Brain tumor information. Retrieved from http://www.abta.org/brain-tumor-information/.

Black, P. (2006). *Living with a Brain Tumor: Dr. Peter Black's Guide to Taking Control of Your Treatment.* New York: Holt Paperbacks.

Johns Hopkins Medicine, Neurology and Neurosurgery. (2015). About brain tumors. Retrieved from http://www.hopkinsmedicine.org/neurology_neurosurgery/centers_clinics/brain_tumor/about-brain-tumors/.

National Cancer Institute. (2015). Brain cancer. Retrieved from http://www.cancer.gov/cancertopics/types/brain.

Start-Vance, V. (2010). *100 Questions & Answers About Brain Tumors.* Burlington, MA: Jones & Bartlett Learning.

Taylor, L. P., Umphrey, A. B. P., & Richard, D. (2012). *Navigating Life with a Brain Tumor.* New York: Oxford University Press.

BRAIN DISEASES

Overview

The brain is the control center of the complex human nervous system, which includes the spinal cord and all the nerves and neurons that control and implement the daily functions: regulating and controlling bodily activities, receiving and interpreting incoming messages, and transmitting information to the muscles and body organs. The most complex organ in the body, the brain is the seat of consciousness, thought, memory, and emotion.

Brain diseases, or the physical and mental conditions that affect the brain, can take many different many different forms, and the causes are as varied as the multitude of the diseases. Many are chronic and incurable conditions with disabling effects that can continue for many years or decades. The effects of the diseases depend on their type and severity, as well the affected area of the brain. Some diseases present painful and serious symptoms, while others develop slowly without obvious symptoms, making them difficult to diagnose and treat.

They can affect anyone at any age, but developmental brain disorders usually appear in early childhood; depression and schizophrenia typically first appear in young adults; and aging increases susceptibility to Alzheimer's disease, Parkinson's disease, and stroke. Surgery, medication, and physical therapy are common treatments that can a disease or improve symptoms and the outcome. But some conditions result in permanent brain damage or death.

Types of Brain Diseases

Because there are so many, brain diseases are grouped in large categories. The category of brain diseases caused by infections includes meningitis, an inflammation of the lining of the brain or spinal cord; encephalitis, inflammation of brain tissue; and brain abscess. The seizure category includes epilepsy, or recurring seizures caused by abnormal, excessive electrical brain activity in the brain. The trauma, or injury, category includes concussion, traumatic brain injury, and hemorrhage, which is bleeding inside the brain.

Brain diseases are also categorized by malignant and benign tumors, masses, and hydrocephalus, which is an abnormal amount of fluid inside the skull, other abnormal pressure inside the brain. The diseases associated with vascular conditions include stroke or any other interruption of blood flow and oxygen to the brain; aneurysm; hematoma, or brain bleeding; and edema, or swelling. Autoimmune brain diseases include vasculitis, or inflammation of the blood vessels in the brain; and multiple sclerosis, in which the body's immune system mistakenly attacks and damages the nerves. Those in the neurodegenerative category include Alzheimer's disease and dementia, Parkinson's disease, Huntington's disease, and amyotrophic lateral sclerosis (ALS). Common chronic psychiatric diseases include anxiety disorders, depression, bipolar disorder, and schizophrenia.

Symptoms

Brain disorders affect the areas of the brain controlling movement, thinking, and behavior. Although each disease has specific symptoms, many are present in one or many. Some common symptoms may include confusion, disorientation, or problems concentrating; stiffness in the neck, limbs, or trunk; fever; headaches, including migraines; seizures or convulsions; memory or cognitive impairment or loss; changes in speech or vision; loss of muscle control, muscle spasm, tremors, numbness, fatigue, or weakness; difficulty swallowing, unstable posture or unsteady walking; dizziness; nausea or vomiting; noticeable changes in personality or behavior, and mental faculty, which may include irritation, mood swings, or depression.

Causes and Risk Factors

The causes of brain disorders vary with the type of disorder, and many are the result of a combination of causes. The most common causes of brain diseases include trauma to the head or brain, which can change the brain's electrical pathways, including how the brain communicates with the rest of the body; stroke; seizures; infections that cause inflammation and swelling; autoimmune disorders; disease and cancer, including tumors and other abnormal growths that prevent proper blood circulation in the brain; inherited genetic conditions; and changes in the brain's electrical pathways. Risk factors include blunt trauma to the head, family history of brain disorders or diseases, viral infections, stroke, tobacco smoking, and any sudden injury or condition that prevents oxygen from reaching the brain.

Diagnosis

A neurologist, or specialist in treating nervous system diseases, may conduct an exam to check vision, hearing, and balance. Common diagnostic tools for brain diseases include a computed tomography (CT) scan, magnetic resonance imaging (MRI), and positron emission tomography (PET). Samples of tissue or fluid from the brain or spinal cord can aid in identifying causes or locations of bleeding in the brain, infections, and other abnormal symptoms.

Treatments

Treatment is based on a specific diagnosis and depends on the severity of symptoms and a person's overall health. Surgery is performed to remove tumors, as well as control or improve the symptoms of epilepsy, head injury, and other diseases. Brain surgery is often performed to repair the effects of trauma, infections and inflammation, bleeding, blood clots, abnormal blood vessels, damage to brain tissues, and pressure following a stroke. Radiation therapy, including radiosurgery, is also used to a kill tumor cells and treat other brain abnormalities due to disease.

Many medications have been developed for brain diseases; they are prescribed to reduce brain swelling and inflammation and the loss of muscle control or degeneration, to prevent seizures, as well as to combat brain tumors and improve vascular conditions and autoimmune disorders that affect the brain. Mental illnesses often require medications to reduce or manage symptoms. Deep brain stimulation is used treat Parkinson's disease and other causes of tremors, and it is under study for epilepsy, depression, and other conditions.

Physical therapy may be prescribed to help regain muscle strength and motor skills, along with speech and occupational therapy.

Prognosis and Outcomes

Most brain diseases require long-term management of symptoms and treatment to prevent future complications. Prognosis depends on the type of disease and severity, as well as overall health, which includes any underlying or co-occurring disorders.

Future

Announced in 2013, the Brain Research through Advancing Innovative Neurotechnologies (BRAIN) Initiative is a broad, collaborative research effort focused on revolutionizing scientific understanding of the human brain. The primary goal of BRAIN is to help researchers uncover the mysteries of brain disorders and discover new ways to treat, cure, and prevent brain disorders.

Ray Marks

See also: Alzheimer's Disease; Anxiety; Bipolar Disorder; Depression; Epilepsy; Huntington's Disease; Mental Disorders; Parkinson's Disease; Schizophrenia; Stroke; Vascular Disorders

Further Reading

BrainFacts.org. (2015). Neurological diseases & disorders A-Z from NINDS. Retrieved from http://www.brainfacts.org/diseases-disorders/diseases-a-to-z-from-ninds/.

Healthline. (2012, July 16). Brain disorders. Retrieved from http://www.healthline.com/health/brain-disorders#Overview1.

National Institute of Health. (2015, September 17). The BRAIN Initiative. Retrieved from http://braininitiative.nih.gov/about.htm.

National Institute of Mental Health. (2015). Brain basics. Retrieved from http://www.nimh.nih.gov/health/educational-resources/brain-basics/brain-basics.shtml.

BREAST CANCER

Breast cancer is a malignant tumor that forms in the cells of the breasts, which may spread (metastasize) into surrounding tissue or to other parts of the body. Each breast is made up of lobules (milk-producing glands), ducts (tiny tubes that carry the milk from the lobules to the nipple), and stroma (fatty and connective tissue). The kind of breast cancer depends on which cells in the breast turn into cancer.

According to the National Cancer Institute (2014), breast cancer is the most common nonskin cancer and the second-leading cause of cancer-related death in women in the United States (lung cancer is the leading cause of cancer death in women). Substantial disparities exist between black and white women in their breast cancer experience. The incidence is highest in white women, but African American women have higher breast cancer mortality rates than women of any other racial or ethnic group in the United States.

Types of Breast Cancer

Most breast cancers are invasive carcinomas, which means they have already grown beyond the layer of cells where it started. The most common type of breast cancer starts with cells in the milk-producing ducts and is called invasive ductal carcinoma (IDC). Breast cancer may also begin in the milk-producing glands, which is known as invasive lobular carcinoma (ILC). Less commonly, breast cancer can begin in the fatty and fibrous connective tissues of the breast.

Symptoms

Early breast cancer usually doesn't cause symptoms. But as the tumor grows, it can change how the breast looks or feels. Different people have different warning signs for breast cancer. Some people do not have any signs or symptoms at all. Possible signs of breast cancer include:

- Painless lump in the breast or armpit
- Thickening or swelling in any part of the breast
- Changes in breast size or shape
- Skin irritation or dimpling
- Breast or nipple pain
- Nipple abnormalities (discharge, erosion, or inversion)
- Scaly, red or swollen skin on the breast or nipple

Risk Factors

Some factors influence risk for breast cancer, which can change over time, due to factors such as aging or lifestyle. They include:

- Early age at first menstrual period (before age 12)
- Late age at menopause (after age 55)
- Never given birth or giving birth for the first time after age 30
- Increasing age
- High breast tissue density
- Personal history of breast cancer or some noncancerous breast diseases
- An above-average exposure to the hormone estrogen
- Family history of breast cancer (mother, sister, daughter)
- Treatment with radiation therapy to the breast/chest
- Being overweight (increases risk for breast cancer after menopause)

- Long-term use of hormone replacement therapy (estrogen and progesterone combined)
- Genetic predisposition (BRCA1 or BRCA2 genes)
- Drinking alcohol (more than one drink a day)
- Not getting regular exercise

Diagnosis

Breast cancer screening involves checking a woman's breasts for cancer before there are signs or symptoms of the disease. Doctors recommend that women have regular mammograms, and in most cases, clinical breast exams to find breast cancer early.

Since 2009, however, there has been controversy about how often and between what ages mammograms should be performed. Before 2009, women over 40 years old were advised to get an annual mammogram. Then, an influential panel called the U.S. Preventive Services Task Force—an independent board of doctors and other experts appointed by the Department of Health and Human Services to evaluate breast cancer screening—recommended that, for women of average risk (without the risk factors listed earlier), screening does not need to be done until the age of 50, and after that, only every other year. The task force also said that after age 74, there was not enough evidence to recommend routine screening. After their first recommendations in 2009, the group continued to make the same recommendations in early 2016 (Grady 2016).

Many doctors, cancer organizations, and women expressed dismay over these recommendations, with the common fear expressed that a malignant tumor might be missed without routine mammograms. The American Cancer Society, which initially was one of the opponents of the U.S. Preventive Services Task Force 2009 guidelines, loosened its recommendations somewhat in 2015, recommending that women of average risk begin with mammograms at age 45 and continue once a year until 54, then every other year for as long as they are healthy and likely to live another 10 years.

Tests and procedures used to diagnose breast cancer include:

Clinical breast examination (CBE). A physical examination of the breasts by a health care provider who uses his or her hands to feel for lumps or other abnormalities.

Mammogram. An x-ray of the breast taken from different angles to look for breast disease in women who appear to have no breast problems. *Diagnostic* mammograms are used for taking more images of any area under concern and are used to diagnose breast disease in women who have breast symptoms (such as a lump or nipple discharge) or other abnormal result on a screening mammogram.

Breast self-examination (BSE). A self-examination of one's own breasts for lumps, changes in size or shape of the breast, or any other changes in the breasts or underarm.

Breast ultrasound. A picture taken of the breast using sound waves to determine whether a breast abnormality is likely to be a fluid-filled cyst or a solid mass, which may be either benign or cancerous. These are particularly helpful for women with dense breast tissue.

Magnetic resonance imaging (MRI). A type of body scan that uses radio waves and strong magnets linked to a computer to create pictures of the interior of the breast. These pictures can show the difference between normal and diseased tissue.

Biopsy. This is a test that removes tissue or fluid from the breast to be looked at under a microscope to determine whether cells are cancerous.

Benefits and Risks of Screening

Every test or procedure carries benefits and risks. As noted in the preceding discussion of the schedule for mammograms, benefits of regular screening include early detection of cancer, better chance of survival, less harmful treatments, more choices for treatment, less time spent recovering, reduction in anxiety of "not knowing," and improved quality of life.

But, there are risks of regular screening, including false positive and false negative results. False positive results: When test results suggest cancer even though cancer is not present. False positives can result in anxiety, stress, and possibly painful and unnecessary tests, such as biopsies, to rule out cancer. False negative results: When cancer is not detected by the test even though it is present. False negative results can cause women or their physicians to ignore other symptoms that suggest the presence of cancer, causing a delay in diagnosis and treatment.

Diagnosis of Breast Cancer

There are many types of breast cancer, but some of them are quite rare. Most breast cancers begin in the cells that line the ducts (ductal cancers). Some begin in the cells that line the lobules (lobular cancers), while a small number start in other tissues. If the cancer cells have not spread, they are called in situ because they are still in one site. When breast cancer spreads out of the duct or lobule, it is called invasive cancer.

In some cases, a single breast tumor can be a combination of types or a mixture of invasive and in situ (noninvasive) cancer.

Ductal carcinoma in situ (DCIS) is the most common type of noninvasive breast cancer, which is confined to the lining of the milk ducts. About one in five new breast cancer cases will be DCIS.

Lobular carcinoma in situ (LCIS) is a kind of breast cancer found only in the lobules of the milk-producing glands of the breast.

Invasive (or infiltrating) ductal carcinoma (IDC) is the most common type of breast cancer that starts in a milk passage (duct) of the breast, breaks through the wall of the duct, and grows into the fatty tissue of the breast. It may be able to spread (metastasize) to other parts of the body through the lymphatic system and bloodstream. About 8 of 10 invasive breast cancers are infiltrating ductal carcinomas.

Invasive (or infiltrating) lobular carcinoma (ILC) starts in the milk-producing lobules and can spread (metastasize) to other parts of the body. About 1 in 10 invasive breast cancers is an ILC.

Staging

Once breast cancer is diagnosed, the cancer will be given a stage and a grade. The stage of a cancer is one of the most important factors in determining prognosis and treatment options. It is based on whether the cancer is invasive or noninvasive, the size of the tumor, how many lymph nodes are involved, and if it has spread to other parts of the body. The stage is usually expressed as a number on a scale of 0 through IV—with stage 0 describing noninvasive cancers and stage IV describing invasive cancers that have spread outside the breast to other parts of the body. Staging may involve blood tests and other tests.

Stage 0 (least advanced stage). Cancer cells are within the lining of a milk duct (DCIS) or lobule (LCIS) and have not invaded into the surrounding fatty breast tissue.

Stage 1, II, and III. The cancer is distinguished by the size of the tumor and whether it has spread to the chest wall or skin or to lymph nodes near the breast.

Stage IV (most advanced stage). The cancer has spread (metastasized) to other organs or to lymph nodes far from the breast.

Tests and procedures used to stage breast cancer may include:

- Blood tests, such as a complete blood count
- Mammogram of the other breast to look for signs of cancer
- Chest x-ray
- Breast MRI
- Bone scan
- Computerized tomography (CT) scan
- Positron emission tomography (PET) scan

Grade

To find out the grade of a tumor, a biopsy sample is examined under a microscope. A grade is given based on how the cancer cells look and behave compared with normal cells. The grade can help predict prognosis. As noted by the American Cancer Society, in general, a lower grade number indicates a slower-growing cancer that is less likely to spread, while a higher number indicates a faster-growing cancer that is more likely to spread. The tumor grade is one factor in deciding if further treatment is needed after surgery. This system of grading is used for invasive cancers but not for in situ cancers.

Grade 1 (well differentiated) cancers have relatively normal-looking cells that do not appear to be growing rapidly and are arranged in small tubules.

Grade 2 (moderately differentiated) cancers have features between grades 1 and 3.

Grade 3 (poorly differentiated) cancers, the highest grade, lack normal features and tend to grow and spread more aggressively (American Cancer Society 2016).

Treatments

Breast cancer treatment options are based on the type of breast cancer, its stage, whether the cancer cells are sensitive to hormones and one's overall health and preferences. Treatments can be classified into local therapy or systemic therapy, based on how they work and when they are used. Local therapy is intended to treat a tumor at the site without affecting the rest of the body. Surgery and radiation therapy are examples of local therapies. Systemic therapy refers to drugs which can be given by mouth or directly into the bloodstream to reach cancer cells anywhere in the body. Chemotherapy, hormone therapy, and targeted therapy are systemic therapies. Most women undergo surgery for breast cancer and also receive additional treatment.

Breast Cancer Surgery

Surgery is the most common treatment for breast cancer and the type of surgery depends on the size of tumor and where it is. Operations used to treat breast cancer include:

Lumpectomy, which is surgical removal of only the breast lump and a surrounding margin of normal tissue.

Partial (or segmental) mastectomy, or surgical removal of more of the breast tissue than a lumpectomy with much of the breast in place.

Mastectomy, which is surgery to remove the entire breast with removal of some of auxiliary (underarm) lymph nodes.

Double (or bilateral) mastectomy is the surgical removal of both breasts.

Therapies

Radiation therapy is treatment using high-powered beams of energy (radiation) to destroy cancer cells. Radiation to the breast is often given after breast-conserving surgery to help lower the chance that the cancer will come back in the breast or nearby lymph nodes. There are two types of radiation therapy.

External beam radiation is the most common type of radiation therapy where radiation is focused from a machine outside the body on the area affected by the cancer. The extent of radiation depends on whether a lumpectomy or mastectomy was done and whether or not lymph nodes are involved.

Internal radiation (also known as brachytherapy) uses radioactive seeds or pellets that are inserted into the breast tissue next to the cancer. It is often used to add extra radiation to the tumor site (and also with external radiation to the whole breast), although it may also be used by itself.

Chemotherapy is treatment with cancer-killing drugs that may be given intravenously (injected into a vein) or taken as a pill. It is given in cycles, with each period of treatment followed by a recovery period.

Hormonal therapy is a treatment that removes hormones from the body or blocks their action and stops cancer cells from growing. Drugs, surgery, or radiation therapy can be used to change hormone levels. Hormone therapy keeps cancer cells from getting or using the natural hormones (estrogen and progesterone) they need to grow.

Biological therapy is a treatment that works with the body's immune system to help it fight cancer or to control side effects from other cancer treatments.

Targeted therapy uses drugs that block the growth of breast cancer cells.

Prevention

Women can help lower their risk of breast cancer in the following ways:

- Being screened for breast cancer regularly. As noted, the American Cancer Society (2015) now recommends yearly mammograms starting at age 45 through 54 and for every two years after that for women, as long as they are in good health. They also state, however, that women of average risk should have the option of yearly mammograms starting at age 40, and after 54 years.
- Having clinical breast examinations and doing breast self-examinations. The American Cancer Society, however, notes that there is not good evidence that these exams are beneficial, although they do stress that women should be familiar with how their breasts look and feel in order to notice if something looks or feels different.
- Controlling weight by making healthy choices and stay active with exercise.
- Knowing family history of breast cancer so preventive steps can be taken for more screening, and possibly genetic testing.
- Finding out the risks and benefits of hormone replacement therapy (HRT) to see if it is right for them.
- Limiting the amount of alcohol to less than one drink a day.

These techniques may help women and their doctors find breast cancer in its earliest and more treatable stages.

Leah Sultan-Khan

See also: Breast Diseases; Cancer; Male Breast Cancer; Physical Activity; Women's Health

Further Reading

American Cancer Society. (2016). Overview: Breast cancer. Retrieved from http://www.cancer .org/cancer/breastcancer/overviewguide/.

American Cancer Society. (2015). American Cancer Society recommendations for early breast cancer detection in women without breast symptoms. Retrieved from http://www .cancer.org/cancer/breastcancer/moreinformation/breastcancerearlydetection/breast -cancer-early-detection-acs-recs.

Breastcancer.org. (2016). Retrieved from http://www.breastcancer.org/.

Canadian Cancer Society. (2016). What is breast cancer? Retrieved from http://www.cancer .ca/en/cancer-information/cancer-type/breast/breast-cancer/?region=on.

Centers for Disease Control and Prevention. (2016). Breast cancer. Retrieved from http:// www.cdc.gov/cancer/breast/.

Grady, D. (2016, January 12). Panel reasserts mammogram advice that triggered breast cancer debate. *New York Times*, p. A15.

Hartmann, L. C., & Loprinzi, C. L., eds. (2012). *The Mayo Clinic Breast Cancer Book.* Intercourse, PA: Good Books.

Mayo Clinic. (2015). Breast cancer. Retrieved from http://www.mayoclinic.org/diseases -conditions/breast-cancer/basics/definition/con-20029275.

National Cancer Institute. (2014). A snapshot of breast cancer. Retrieved from http://www .cancer.gov/research/progress/snapshots/breast.

National Cancer Institute. (2012). What you need to know about breast cancer? Retrieved from http://www.cancer.gov/publications/patient-education/wyntk-breast-cancer.

Smigal, C., Jemal, A., Ward, E., Cokkinides, V., Smith, R., Howe, H. L., & Thun, M. (2006). Trends in breast cancer by race and ethnicity: Update 2006. *A Cancer Journal for Clinicians*, 56(3), 168–183.

Susan G. Komen for the Cure. (2016). Retrieved from http://ww5.komen.org/.

U.S. Department of Health and Human Services. (2009). Breast cancer: A resource guide for minority women. Retrieved from http://minorityhealth.hhs.gov/assets/pdf/checked/bcrg2005.pdf.

BREAST DISEASES
See also Breast Cancer

Overview

The female breast serves as a source of milk for the newborn infant and thus plays an important role in certain life stages. It may undergo many changes during her lifetime, and it is important to recognize any form of abnormality early on.

One of the most common health conditions affecting the breast is the infiltration of breast tissue by tumors that can become cancerous. The male breast and breasts of children can also develop breast related problems, and these can be either benign or noncancerous or malignant or cancerous. These problems all fall under the broad heading of breast diseases.

Types of disorders mentioned in various sources include:

- Atypical hyperplasia—or the development of abnormal cells in the breast duct
- Benign breast masses
- Breast abscesses
- Breast cancer
- Breast cysts
  - Fibrocystic breast condition—associated with lumpiness, thickening and swelling, often associated with a woman's period
  - Cysts—fluid-filled lumps
- Fibroadenoma—solid, round, rubbery lumps that move easily when pushed, occurring most in younger women
- Hyperplasia—an overgrowth of cells in the breast ducts or lobules where milk is produced that may increase the chance of breast cancer later on
- Intraductal papillomas—benign growths similar to warts near the nipple
- Blocked or clogged milk ducts
- Milk production when a woman is not breastfeeding
- Injury
- Mastitis—an infection of breast tissues
- Paget's disease—a type of breast cancer

Types of Symptoms Associated with Breast Diseases

Discharge
Irritation

Lump
Pain
Redness
Swelling
Tenderness

Causes and risk factors for breast diseases include age, exposure to ionizing radiation, hormone changes, and medications. Diagnostic tools include breast biopsy, breast ultrasound, family history, and mammogram.

Treatments may involve medication for pain and surgery. Prevention includes breast self-exams, leading a healthy lifestyle, avoiding tobacco, avoiding too much sun exposure, and eating healthfully and exercising.

Ray Marks

See also: Cancer; Male Breast Cancer; Paget's Disease of the Breast; Physical Activity; Women's Health

Further Reading

American Cancer Society. (2015). Non-cancerous breast conditions. http://www.cancer.org/healthy/findcancerearly/womenshealth/non-cancerousbreastconditions/non-cancerous-breast-conditions-toc.

Cleveland Clinic. (2014, February 27). Understanding benign breast disease. Retrieved from https://my.clevelandclinic.org/health/diseases_conditions/hic_Breast_Cancer_An_Overview/hic_The_Diagnosis_is_Breast_Cancer/hic_Understanding_Benign_Breast_Disease.

Guray, M., & Sahin, A. A. (2006). Benign breast diseases: Classification, diagnosis, and management. *The Oncologist*, 5, 435–449. doi: 10.1634/theoncologist.11-5-435.

Mayo Clinic. (2013, March 8). Fibrocystic breasts. Retrieved from http://www.mayoclinic.org/diseases-conditions/fibrocystic-breasts/basics/definition/con-20034681.

Patient. (2013, July 13). Benign breast disease. Retrieved from http://patient.info/doctor/benign-breast-disease.

Susan G. Komen. (2015, July 3). Benign breast conditions. Retrieved from http://ww5.komen.org/BreastCancer/BenignConditions.html.

BROCHIECTASIS

Brochiectasis is a chronic lung condition that involves destruction and widening of one or more of the large lung airways of one or both lungs or bronchi. These are tubes that transport air in and out of the lungs, and if they are inflamed or infected so that the smooth muscles in their walls are destroyed, the tubes lose their elasticity. This causes them to become abnormally widened, flabby and scarred, easily susceptible to recurrent infections, ulcerated, and collapsible, which can block the clearing of secretions normally made by lung tissue. The condition can be present at birth, and this form is known as *congenital bronchiectasis*, or it can develop later on in life, where it is termed *acquired bronchiectasis*.

The disease mostly affects children, more so boys than girls, but can affect people of all ages.

The disease was first described in 1819, and in the late 1800s was described in more detail by Sir William Osler. In the 1950s, the description was further refined by Reid according to Luce (1994). It is a form of chronic obstructive pulmonary disease (COPD) and one that is relatively uncommon today in the United States.

There are three primary types of bronchiectasis as follows:

1. *Cylindrical bronchiectasis*, which is the mildest form, involves loss of the normal tapering structure of the airways.
2. *Saccular bronchiectasis* is more severe, with greater distortion of the airways.
3. *Cystic bronchiectasis* is the most severe form.

Symptoms

Symptoms may develop gradually over many months or years and may include the following, depending on the type of disease:

- Abnormal chest sounds
- Bluish skin color
- Breath odor
- Chronic or recurrent coughing
- Clubbing of the fingers
- Coughing of blood
- Cough that gets worse when lying on one side
- Decreased ability to effectively expel mucus from the lower airways
- Fatigue
- Impaired clearance of lung or mucus secretions that is often discolored
- Paleness
- Respiratory failure in severe cases
- Shortness of breath that increases with exercise
- Weakness
- Weight loss
- Wheezing

Key Causes and Risk Factors

The main causes of bronchiectasis are thought to be excess alcohol use, drug abuse, a condition called allergic bronchopulmonary aspergillosis, hypersensitivity to an inhaled organism called Aspergillus, and the presence of a bronchial obstruction. Other causes are the presence of congenital anatomic defects, connective tissue disorders, a health condition called cystic fibrosis, exposure to pollutants, and immunodeficiency syndromes. Also categorized as risk factors are inflammatory disorders, lung injuries, pediatric lung infections, lack of appropriate care or access to care, pneumonia, reoccurring inflammations of the airways, smoking, toxic gas, secondhand smoke exposure, and tuberculosis.

Diagnosis

The diagnosis of the condition will be made on the basis of a medical history, a physical examination, blood tests, chest x-rays, chest CT scans, genetic testing, pulmonary function, and sputum culture tests.

Treatments

Treatment is very important and is aimed at controlling infections and bronchial secretions, minimizing obstruction of the airways, and preventing complications through:

Medications to keep airways clear and prevent infection such as antibiotics, expectorants, and steroids
Regular daily draining of the airways using exercises, or a form of postural drainage
Bronchodilators
Chest physical therapy
Nasal sprays
Surgery, as required

Prognosis

Although there is no cure for the condition, if treated appropriately, most people with this condition can lead a fairly normal existence.

Complications include heart problems, respiratory failure, a collapse of the affected lung, recurrent pneumonia or breathing difficulties.

The risk of bronchiectasis can be reduced by treating infections, avoiding upper respiratory infections, smoking, and pollution, as well as by early diagnosis and treatment, and leading a healthy lifestyle.

Seek immediate attention if you have difficulty breathing or if you have this disease and are experiencing severe symptoms.

Ray Marks

See also: Alcoholism; COPD (Chronic Obstructive Pulmonary Disease); Lung Diseases; Pneumonia; Secondhand Smoke

Further Reading

American Lung Association. (2011). Bronchiectasis. Retrieved from http://www.lungusa/lung
    -disease/bronchiectasis/.
Luce, J. M. (1994). Bronchiectasis. In J.F. Murray, and J. A. Nadel. (Eds.). *Textbook of Respiratory Medicine*, 2nd ed. Philadelphia, PA: WB Saunders and Co., 1398–1417.
National Heart Lung and Blood Institute. (2014). What is bronchiectasis? U.S. Department of Health and Human Services. Retrieved from http://www.nhlbi.nih.gov/health/health
    -topics/topics/brn/.
UCSF Medical Center. (2015). Bronchiectasis. Retrieved from http://ucsfhealth.org
    /conditions/bronchiectasis/index.html.

BRONCHITIS

Description

Bronchitis is a condition that is associated with inflammation and irritation of the airways that carry air to the lungs called bronchi and their smaller branches called bronchioles. It results in excess mucus secretions and tissue swelling in these tubes that may narrow or block them. *Chronic bronchitis* is defined as a persistent cough occurring everyday with mucus production, which lasts for at least three months, two years in a row. Once it occurs, it does not go away completely but keeps reoccurring over time, and it is an ongoing serious health condition. It is grouped among lung diseases that are known as chronic obstructive pulmonary disease (COPD). Like other chronic obstructive pulmonary disease conditions, chronic bronchitis can be accompanied by episodes where symptoms get worse very quickly. These episodes are termed *exacerbations* and can vary in degree of severity. They can be triggered by upper- or lower-airway infections, such as colds or flu. Heart problems, as well as infections elsewhere in body, can worsen the symptoms. These flare-up episodes can be serious and often are life-threatening.

Those most affected are likely to be 45 years of age or older, and women are more likely than men to be affected.

Signs and Symptoms

Chest tightness
Coughing
Mucus production that plugs airways and makes breathing difficult
Shortness of breath
Uncomfortable tight feeling in the chest
Wheezing

Causes

The major causes of chronic bronchitis are smoking, secondhand smoke, and air pollution. Other causes are the following

- Bronchial irritants that are commonly inhaled by the affected individual. They include ozone, nitrogen dioxide, sulfur dioxide, hydrogen sulfide, bromine, strong acids, ammonia, some organic solvents, chlorine, coal dust, and grain dust.
- Airborne chemicals, fumes, or dust can produce chronic bronchitis as well.
- Bacteria and viruses can irritate the bronchial tubes, as can allergies and infections.
- Cold weather, dampness, and factors that irritate the lungs can result in chronic bronchitis.
- Recurrent respiratory tract infections during infancy or early childhood can also lead to chronic bronchitis.
- Certain jobs increase the risk of chronic bronchitis, such as manufacturing; coal mining; and jobs involving livestock, grain, textiles, chemical fumes, and gas vapors.

Smoking causes the airways in the lungs to become constricted, or narrowed, and paralyzes the cilia or hair-like cells that line the lung passages, which are designed to remove irritating particles and keep germs and irritants out of the lungs. Smoke in the lungs also causes the lung surfactant, which is the fluid that lings the lung passages and help keep them expanded, to become inactive, and the more one smokes, the more damage is done to the cilia.

When the cilia do not function adequately, mucus stays trapped in the lungs, causing the walls of the bronchial tubes to become irritated, swell, and narrow. The bronchial tubes are less able to expand when the body needs more oxygen. Mucus that remains stuck in the smaller passages can then cause stale air to be trapped in the lungs instead of exhaled. This causes increasing breathing difficulties over time and damage to the air sacs walls in the lungs as the problems progress. If air sacs or alveoli are destroyed, the lungs have greater difficulty in transporting oxygen to the blood stream.

Diagnosis

Diagnosis is done by a physical exam and clinical history, as well as a family history, history of environmental and occupational exposures, and smoking history.

Other tests include x-rays, pulmonary function tests, CT scanning, arterial blood gases, and complete blood counts.

Treatment

Treatment may include exercise, physical therapy, postural drainage, pulmonary rehabilitation, and/or respiratory therapy. Treatment especially involves trying to help the affected person quit smoking or reduce his or her exposure to irritants—for example, by wearing a mask over the nose and mouth or leaving the workplace for another job. Medical treatments include antibiotics, bronchodilators, steroids, medicine called theophylline, and oxygen therapy.

Healthy lifestyle practices—including handwashing; drinking plenty of fluids, especially water; following a well-balanced diet; getting plenty of rest; and not smoking—can reduce the risk of chronic bronchitis and improve symptoms in those affected.

Prognosis

If the disease is diagnosed early, the individual may have better health outcomes than those diagnosed later on in the process. A flu shot every year is recommended for people who have chronic bronchitis. Some people develop bronchitis that only lasts for a short period of time, but if this occurs more often, they may develop a chronic irreversible problem. A person who develops chronic bronchitis in conjunction with another type of illness, such as emphysema, is said to have chronic obstructive pulmonary disease.

If chronic bronchitis is not dealt with in a timely way, a patient may have to undergo surgery to remove part of the damaged lung or undergo a lung transplant.

Ray Marks

See also: COPD (Chronic Obstructive Pulmonary Disorder); Lung Diseases; Pollution; Secondhand Smoke

Further Reading

FamilyDoctor.Org. (2014, February). Chronic bronchitis. Retrieved from http://familydoctor.org/familydoctor/en/diseases-conditions/chronic-bronchitis.printerview.all.html.

Mayo Clinic. (2014, April 1). Bronchitis. Retrieved from http://www.mayoclinic.org/diseases-conditions/bronchitis/basics/definition/con-20014956.

National Heart Lung and Blood Institute. (2011, August 4). What is bronchitis? Retrieved from http://www.nhlbi.nih.gov/health/health-topics/topics/brnchi/.

BRUXISM

Bruxism (tooth grinding) is a condition in which a person grinds or clenches his or her teeth excessively. Statistics show that somewhere between 5 and 20 percent of people in the United States have bruxism, though up to 80 percent of them may be unaware of the problem. This is because the habit is not done consciously and also because many people grind or clench their teeth at night while they are asleep.

There is no agreed-upon cause of bruxism, but there are several factors that may lead to the condition. Prolonged anxiety, stress, tension, or other emotions are among these possible factors. The problem can also manifest as a complication of disease such as Parkinson's disease. If the condition occurs at night (called sleep bruxism), it may be a symptom of other sleep ailments. Bruxism can also be a response to pain from an ear infection or other issue, and in rare cases, it is a side effect of certain medications.

Ingesting stimulating substances, including caffeinated beverages or illicit drugs like methamphetamine, can increase the risk of bruxism. In some cases, people may never realize they have bruxism and the condition does not bother them. In other situations, the condition may cause pain and other problems. Such factors as the amount of stress a person is under, diet, alignment of the teeth, and how long or tightly he or she clenches or grinds the teeth all play a role in whether a case of bruxism is mild or severe.

Although a person is often unaware of grinding or clenching the teeth, symptoms of bruxism can include flattened, chipped, or loose teeth, as well as worn tooth enamel. Seeing indentations in the tongue or experiencing dull headaches that originate in the temple area may also indicate bruxism, as can soreness in the jaw or face or tired and aching jaw muscles. If the problem is severe and is left untreated, it can lead to extensive damage to the teeth or jaw or ongoing tension-type headaches. It can also create disorders in the temporomandibular joints—the joints directly in front of the ears—and may create regular clicking sounds or problems in which the jaw gets temporarily "locked" in place in an open or closed position.

Dental professionals often check for signs of bruxism during routine dental exams. If the condition is suspected, further x-rays may be conducted to determine the extent of the damage. In most cases, little to no medical intervention is required. Some people with bruxism are asked to wear mouth guards to protect the teeth from further damage, particularly at night, while others may be prescribed muscle relaxants to relieve sleep stress. In more severe instances, oral surgery may be recommended to correct damage from bruxism, and if a psychological component or sleep-related disorder is thought to be part of the problem, a patient may also be referred to a sleep specialist or psychologist for further evaluation.

Although the first discovery of bruxism is unknown, reported cases of the ailment date as far back as the 17th century and the term *bruxism* was coined in the early 1900s. Much research has since been conducted on the condition, with many scientists focusing on the psychological components of the problem and experimenting with behavioral adjustments to correct it.

Tamar Burris

See also: Diet and Nutrition; Sleep Disturbances and Sleep Disorders; Stress

Further Reading

Attanasio, R., & Bailey, D. R. (2009). *Dental Management of Sleep Disorders*. Boston, MA: Wiley-Blackwell.

Finestone, H. M. (2009). *The Pain Detective, Every Ache Tells a Story: Understanding How Stress and Emotional Hurt Become Chronic Physical Pain*. Westport, CT: Praeger.

Foldvary-Schaefer, N. (2009). *The Cleveland Clinic Guide to Sleep Disorders*. New York: Kaplan Publishing.

Huynh, N., Manzini, C., Rompré, P. H., & Lavigne, G. J. (2007, October). Weighing the potential effectiveness of various treatments for sleep bruxism. *Journal of the Canadian Dental Association, 73*(8), 727–730.

Mayo Clinic. (2015). Bruxism. Retrieved from http://www.mayoclinic.org/diseases-conditions /bruxism/resources/con-20029395.

Sexton-Radek, K., & Graci, G. (2008). *Combatting Sleep Disorders*. Westport, CT: Praeger, 2008.

BUERGER'S DISEASE

Overview and Facts

Buerger's disease is a rare disease involving narrowing or blockage of the small and medium-sized blood vessels of the hands and feet and commonly affecting two or more limbs. If severe, the reoccurring swelling or inflammation of the arteries and veins of the arms and legs can produce damage of the skin tissues, infection, blood clots that block the blood vessels, and gangrene or tissue death if the blood to the skin cannot supply it with nutrients and oxygen. The problem, which starts in the hands and feet, can spread to the arms and legs.

It is uncommon to find Buerger's disease in the United States but more common to find this in the Middle East and Far East, especially among smokers. Commonly, the legs are more affected than the arms. It is also known as thromboangiitis obliterans (TAO), inflammatory occlusive vascular disease, and occlusive peripheral vascular disease.

History

The first case of thromboangiitis oblierans was published in 1879 in Germany by von Winiwarter. Later, Leo Buerger in New York published a detailed description of the disease, which he depicted as presenile spontaneous gangrene.

Causes

The disease is caused by recurrent inflammation of the blood vessels of the hands and feet, which can tighten and become completely blocked by the development of blood clots. This disease affects adults 35 years and older and is more common among men.

Smoking or chewing tobacco is an important risk factor for this condition, although there may also be a genetic basis for this condition.

Symptoms

Hands or feet may feel cold
Hands or feet may look blue, red, black, or pale
Inflammation of a vein below the skin's surface
Leg burning
Leg numbness
Leg tingling
Pulse may be weak or absent
Hands or feet may be very painful, either at rest or when walking (known as claudication)
Limping because of pain
Skin ulcers may not heal well or changes in the skin of the hands or feet may be present

Complications

Blocked leg arteries
Finger ulcers
Leg blood clots
Toe ulcers
Toe gangrene

Diagnostic Tests

Allen's test to check blood flow to hands
Angiography or arteriography of the limbs to examine condition of arteries

Blood tests
Doppler ultrasound of the limbs

Treatment

The treatment goal is to control symptoms and may include medications, intermittent compression of the arms and legs to increase extremity blood flow, spinal cord stimulation, or sympathectomy or cutting of nerves to promote blood flow and control pain.

Patient should stop any tobacco usage and avoid cold and secondhand smoke.
Exercises and application of warmth to affected areas may help.
Medications may help as indicated.
Amputation may be indicated in severe cases.

Summary

Buerger's disease is an inflammatory condition of the small and medium-sized arteries of the hands and feet. It can produce tingling, numbness, pain, skin ulcers; if severe, it can produce gangrene.

Ray Marks

See also: Inflammation; Vascular Disorders

Further Reading

Arkkila, P. E. T. (2006). Thromboangiitis obliterans (Buerger's disease). *Orphanet Journal of Rare Diseases, 1,* 14. doi:10.1186/1750-1172-1-14.
Healthline. (2012, July 25). Buerger's disease. Retrieved from http://www.healthline.com /health/thromboangiitis-obliterans#Overview1.
Mayo Clinic. (2013, February 1). Buerger's disease. Retrieved from http://www.mayoclinic .org/diseases-conditions/buergers-disease/basics/definition/con-20029501.
National Heart Lung and Blood Institute. (2014, September 23). Types of vasculitis. Retrieved from http://www.nhlbi.nih.gov/health/health-topics/topics/vas/types/.

BURSITIS

Bursitis is a term used to describe either an acute or a chronic, recurrent, longstanding inflammation of the bursa or fluid-filled sac that lies between the tendon of the joint and the skin or between a tendon and a bone in order to assist smooth friction free movement of a joint.

The most common sites are the shoulder, elbow, and hip.

Other joints that can be affected are the knee, heel, and base of the big toe areas.

Inflammation, which is a process involving swelling, and pain in the inflamed area can make it difficult for the person to sit or lie down comfortable or place pressure on the affected area and can disrupt sleep and activities of daily living.

Causes

Bursitis can be caused by an injury or impact to a localized area of the body, by chronic or repetitive overuse of a joint, by gout, by infections, or as a result of inflammatory joint diseases such as rheumatoid arthritis.

If an acute bout of bursitis does not resolve, or if there is repetitive strain applied to the affected bursa, the inflammation can become chronic or long-standing.

Chronic bursitis is more common with aging, certain occupations or hobbies, medical conditions such as diabetes, and thyroid disorders.

Symptoms

The most common problem associated with bursitis is pain and tenderness around the affected joint area. Especially in long-standing cases, the joint may feel stiff and sore to move, and there may be swelling, redness, or warmth or tenderness over the affected joint areas.

The symptoms may be localized to the affected area but can also radiate from the affected area to cause pain in adjacent areas of the body.

Pain and stiffness may be worse at night and in the early morning.

Diagnostic Tests

Tests include a medical history, x-rays to rule out other causes or identify calcifications in the bursae, ultrasound or magnetic resonance imaging, and laboratory tests.

Treatments

Treatments depend on whether the problem is caused by infection or some other cause.

For causes other than infection, treatments may involve rest, gentle exercise, and medications to reduce inflammation and pain.

Physical therapy may be employed to treat chronic as well as acute bursitis to ensure the joint does not lose its range of motion or its muscle strength.

Cortisone injections into the joint or affected bursa or splints may help to reduce the pain and inflammation.

If there is excess fluid in the joint, this may be removed by a process called joint aspiration, and if infected, the bursa may have to be drained surgically.

Surgical removal of the bursa may be indicated in severe cases.

Avoiding activities that place stress on the joint and protecting joint from trauma or infection is advocated as well.

Infectious bursitis requires aggressive medical treatment, and on occasion, septic bursitis requires intravenous antibiotic treatment.

Repeated removal of joint fluid or surgical drainage and removal of the bursa sac may be necessary in severe cases.

Summary

If there are symptoms of pain in a joint or joint swelling or redness for more than two weeks, especially when using the joint, or after treating the joint for inflammation or injury with over-the-counter drugs and ice, a doctor should be consulted.

Ray Marks

See also: Arthritis; Bone Diseases; Inflammation; Joint Disorders

Further Reading

American College of Rheumatology. (2015, May). Tendinitis (bursitis). Retrieved from http://www.rheumatology.org/I-Am-A/Patient-Caregiver/Diseases-Conditions/Tendinitis-Bursitis.

Arthritis Foundation. (2015). Bursitis. Retrieved from http://www.arthritis.org/about-arthritis/types/bursitis/.

Mayo Clinic. (2011). Bursitis. Retrieved from http://mayoclinic.com/health/bursitis/DS00032.

National Institute of Arthritis and Musculoskeletal and Skin Diseases. (2013, June). Questions and answers about bursitis and tendinitis. Retrieved from http://www.niams.nih.gov/Health_Info/Bursitis/default.asp.

C

CANCER

Cancer is any of about 100 diseases characterized by the uncontrolled multiplication of abnormal cells, which destroy healthy tissues in the body and put the individual's life in danger. All parts of the body can be affected by cancer, either as a site in which the disease originates (the primary site) or as a site to which the cancer spreads. Cancer spreads—or metastasizes—the most when it circulates through the blood or lymph systems. Oncologists are doctors who specialize in cancer treatment.

Types

The most common primary sites of cancer development include the skin (melanoma); the breasts (mainly in women), digestive organs (such as the esophagus, stomach, liver, pancreas, colon, and rectum), respiratory organs (the larynx and lungs), reproductive and urinary organs (such as the bladder, kidneys, prostate, testes, ovaries, cervix, and uterus), blood tissues (leukemia), and lymph tissues (lymphoma). Among the many other parts of the body that could become affected by cancer are the brain, the head and neck, and the thyroid gland.

Cancer can strike people of any age. However, children and adults tend to get different types of cancer. Among the cancers that are most common in children are certain kinds that strike nervous tissues, bones, the eyes, and the kidneys.

Causes and Characteristics

Different cancers are caused by different factors, including carcinogens (cancer-causing substances) in the environment, in tobacco products, or in certain foods. Some cancers are caused by excessive exposure to radiation, such as x-rays or ultraviolet (UV) radiation. Other cancers are associated with certain viral infections. Some cancers are linked to inherited genetic factors that raise an individual's risk for the cancer. The causes of many cancers are unknown or little understood.

Cancer begins to grow and spread when the carcinogen or other cause leads to mutations in certain genes (unless the mutations are inherited from parents). Mutations can affect cells in any of several ways. The cells may divide abnormally, they may cease to function, they may die, or they may invade healthy tissues. When a type of gene called a *proto-oncogene* is transformed into an overactive form called an *oncogene*, the cell is directed to multiply excessively. When a gene called a *suppressor gene* becomes mutated, the "stop signal" that directs a cell to stop multiplying no longer functions.

Diagnosis

The earlier cancer is diagnosed, the more likely treatment will be successful. However, many types of cancer do not have noticeable symptoms until later in the disease process, after they have metastasized into less treatable conditions. Thus, people should visit physicians for regular (at least once every three years) cancer-related checkups—especially people who are at risk for certain kinds of cancer. Such routine checkups typically include a thorough physical examination, a blood test (which can reveal early biochemical signs of cancer), and other types of screening tests for specific cancers.

After a preliminary diagnosis indicates that an abnormal tissue growth might be cancer, a conclusive diagnosis must be made to determine whether the growth is malignant (cancerous) or benign (noncancerous). This conclusive diagnosis usually involves a biopsy, in which a tissue sample is examined under a microscope to look for cancerous cells. After a malignancy is discovered, the stage of cancer development is determined with additional tests. Physicians decide on the best treatment approach based on the diagnosed stage.

Treatment

Treatments can be tailored to best match the individual patient and his or her cancer type. For many cases, comprehensive, multifaceted therapy is used, incorporating various forms of physical therapy combined with psychological therapy. Physical treatments involve chemotherapy, radiation therapy, and/or surgery.

In chemotherapy, medications are used to kill malignant cells or slow their spread. Different drugs are available for different cancers. Physicians typically tailor a special combination of drugs for each patient. Most kinds of chemotherapy kill some healthy cells, resulting in severe side effects, such as hair loss and fatigue.

In radiation therapy, or radiotherapy, high-energy x-rays or other forms of radioactive rays are focused on the malignant tissue to kill the cancer cells. One common variety of radiotherapy is external beam radiotherapy, in which the radiation is sent into the body from a machine outside the body. This traditional type of radiotherapy inadvertently destroys some healthy tissue along with the malignant tissue, leading to side effects similar to those resulting from chemotherapy. More advanced form of radiotherapy—such as three-dimensional conformal radiation (radiation shaped like the tumor), stereotactic radiosurgery (targeted gamma rays), and brachytherapy (radioactive implants)—are now available to minimize the damage to healthy tissue.

Surgery entails removal of the known cancerous tissue, as well as any other tissue that the surgeon suspects might be affected.

Some patients seek alternative forms of treatment for their cancer. These treatments include such approaches as acupuncture, herbal therapy, homeopathy, and vitamin and dietary supplements.

Prognosis

Many kinds of cancer are fatal unless they are diagnosed and treated early in the disease process—before they spread beyond the primary site. Certain cancers, such as lung and liver cancers, are seldom successfully treated, resulting in very high mortality rates. Lung cancer kills more people than any other cancer. For such advanced, aggressive cancers, all that physicians may be able to offer to the patient is palliative care, to minimize pain and prolong life as long as possible. However, other cancers, such as breast and prostate cancers, can frequently be cured when diagnosed early.

On average, approximately half of all cancer patients survive five or more years with treatment. In some patients, cancer eventually recurs after apparently disappearing or going into remission. Additional treatment is necessary in such cases.

Research

Despite much progress in treating various kinds of cancer, about 8 million people around the globe continue to die every year from cancer. Researchers are always working to develop more successful treatments, and public health officials are seeking ways to make such treatments more widely available. Ongoing research focuses on a wide range of approaches, including the development of new drugs, genetic factors and molecular mechanisms behind cancer, and strategies to prevent cancer. On January 12, 2016, in his State of the Union address, President Barack Obama announced a major initiative, headed by Vice President Joe Biden, to cure cancer, comparing it to a "moonshot," when the U.S. government put significant resources and research into getting a human being on the moon.

A. J. Smuskiewicz

See also: Blood Cancers; Bone Cancer; Brain Cancer; Breast Cancer; Childhood Cancer; Colon Cancer; Kidney Cancer; Leukemia; Liver Cancer; Lung Cancer; Neoplasms; Non-Hodgkin Lymphoma; Pancreatic Cancer; Skin Cancer

Further Reading

DeVita, V. T., Jr., & DeVita-Raeburn, E. (2015). *The Death of Cancer: After 50 Years on the Front Lines of Medicine, a Pioneering Oncologist Reveals Why the War on Cancer Is Winnable & How We Can Get There.* New York: Sarah Crichton Books/Farrar Straus and Giroux.

Mukherjee, S. (2010). *The Emperor of All Maladies: A Biography of Cancer.* New York: Scribner.

National Cancer Institute. (2016). Retrieved from http://www.cancer.gov.

National Cancer Institute. (2016). Cancer stat fact sheets. Surveillance, Epidemiology, and End Results Program. Retrieved from http://seer.cancer.gov/statfacts/.

Srivastava, R. (2015). *A Cancer Companion: An Oncologist's Advice on Diagnosis, Treatment, and Recovery.* Chicago, IL: The University of Chicago Press.

World Health Organization. (2015). Media centre: cancer. http://www.who.int/mediacentre/factsheets/fs297/en/.

CANCER SURVIVORSHIP

Cancer survivors are individuals who have been diagnosed with cancer, from the time of their diagnosis throughout their life. The impact of cancer on family members, friends, and caregivers of survivors is also a component of survivorship. Prior to the establishment of the National Coalition for Cancer Survivorship (NCCS) in 1985, the medical community commonly restricted use of the term *survivor* to individuals with cancer who remained disease free for a minimum of five years.

Cancer Survivorship at a Glance. The majority of cancer survivors in the United States are women over the age of 65; however, many children, young adult, and adults are cancer survivors. Of the nearly 12 million cancer survivors in 2007, 7 million were 65 years or older, 6.3 million were women, and 4.7 were diagnosed 10 years earlier or more. Additionally, the three largest groups of cancer survivors include breast (22 percent), prostate (19 percent), and colorectal cancer (10 percent).

Cancer Survivors and Age. Because cancer risk increases with age, a larger portion of cancer survivors are 65 years of age or older.

More Women Survivors. In general, women survive cancer longer than men. This is due to the fact that cancers among women, such as breast and cervical cancer, are often diagnosed at a younger age, tumors can be found early, and treatment is often successful. On the other hand, prostate cancer, a common contributor of male cancer survivors, is more commonly diagnosed in older men who have a shorter expected lifespan when diagnosed.

Disparities. Disparities in health care affect cancer survival rates. Low-income men and women who have no health care or insufficient coverage are more likely to be diagnosed with cancer at later stages, when fewer treatment options are available and survival rates are not as optimistic.

Cancer Survivorship on the Rise. People who are diagnosed with cancer live for many years after diagnosis because of significant advances in the medical arena—such as better detection methods, more accurate diagnosis, and more effective treatments—coupled with better clinical follow-up care after treatment, fewer deaths from other causes, and an aging population. In fact, cancer survivorship is on the rise, with an estimated 66 percent of people diagnosed with cancer expected to live at least five years after diagnosis. According to the National Cancer Institute's (NCI) Surveillance, Epidemiology and End Results Program, which reports the number of new cases and follow-up data, and the U.S. Census data from 2006 and 2007, in 2007 there were 11.7 million cancer survivors living in the United States. That is a significant increase compared to the 9.8 million survivors in 2001 and the 3 million in 1971. Additionally, in 2007 more than 1 million people were alive after being diagnosed with cancer at least 25 years earlier.

Lifestyle after Cancer. Even though a particular cancer is treated and cured, cancer survivors can experience a recurrence of cancer. This is when the cancer returns in the spot where it was originally detected. Also, because of treatment effects, unhealthy lifestyle behaviors, genetics, or other risk factors, cancer survivors are at an increased risk of developing a second cancer. Because of this, it is critical that cancer survivors pay close attention to their health and practice healthy lifestyle behaviors. Cancer survivors may find themselves motivated to make significant changes to their lifestyle in hopes of improving and preserving their health and quality of life. Because of this natural heightened sense of health awareness, medical professionals should take advantage of this "teachable moment" to talk with their patients about important health behavior changes that may help prevent subsequent disease. Health care providers can highlight the benefits of positive behavior changes and discourage the continuation of unhealthy behaviors because such unhealthy behaviors may increase cancer risk and recurrence. Additionally, which may not be as clear a connection as with cancer survivors, an experience with cancer may provide an opportunity to promote the health of one or more family members of survivors. Because many of these family members may be at an increased risk for cancer because of shared cancer-causing genes, a similar lifestyle, and/or common toxic exposures, recognizing and addressing the health needs of these secondary survivors may give way to improving the well-being of an extended group of people, thus potentially reducing the overall cancer burden.

Risks, Issues, and Concerns of Cancer Survivors. Although many individuals are cured of cancer and are considered "cancer free," this does not mean that survivors are free of the effects of their illness. Some side effects are short-lived, including hair loss and nausea; some may persist for weeks or months, including fatigue and memory loss; others may become permanent, including lymphedema and infertility; and some may appear months or years after treatment and can be life-threatening, including recurrence and osteoporosis. Some of these concerns are insignificant and disappear with time. However, some can have potentially devastating effects on patient's physical health, cognitive, and emotional well-being, as well as their social adaption and economic status. Because of this, it is critical that the unique needs of cancer survivors are met in a timely manner, before more significant, irreversible effects occur.

Reoccurrence. Worrying about a cancer reoccurrence is likely the most common and lasting fear among cancer survivors and often occurs for years after treatment, if not for the survivor's entire lifetime. This phenomenon is so common that it is referred to as the Damocles syndrome, after the Greek mythology figure. Cancer survivors are often interested in knowing what they can do to reduce their risk of having a cancer reoccurrence and to improve their overall health and well-being. This gives them a sense of control over their future health, and often, they have less fear of cancer recurrence compared to those who make no behavior modifications.

Organization Hard at Work to Promote Life Beyond Cancer. A variety of organizations work tirelessly researching the common issues, both physical and psychological, surrounding cancer survivorship to enhance the quality of life and minimize adverse effects from a cancer diagnosis for survivors, their family, friends, and caregivers. The following organizations are just a few that have strived to recognize and address the unique and important needs of cancer survivors:

- 1988: Natalie Davis Spingarn, a cancer survivor, created the "The Cancer Survivor's Bill of Right's," which was formally recognized by the American Cancer Society in 1988.
- 1996: The Office of Cancer Survivorship (OCS), a branch of the National Cancer Institute (NCI), was established and charged with scientifically evaluating the unique and poorly understood needs of the rapidly increasing number of Americans who were surviving cancer.
- 1997: LIVESTRONG (formerly the Lance Armstrong Foundation) was established with the mission of improving the quality of life among cancer survivors by promoting their physical, psychological, and social recovery and that of their loved ones.
- 2004: The Centers for Disease Control and Prevention (CDC) Division of Cancer Prevention and Control (DCPC), in collaboration with LIVESTRONG and nearly 100 experts in cancer survivorship and public health, released "A National Action Plan for Cancer Survivorship: Advancing Public Health Strategies." This action plan established goals, activities, and priorities to address the issues facing the growing number of cancer survivors in the United States. The CDC has also partnered with national organizations to address several of the cancer survivorship priority needs cited in the action plan. Their goal is to improve care and quality of life for cancer patients, their family, friends, and caregivers, as well as participate in initiatives to increase survivorship of underserved populations.
- 2004: The President's Cancer Panel (PCP), an advocacy group established by Congress to report on the progress and struggles in the nation's effort to reduce the cancer burden, released a report entitled "Living Beyond Cancer: Finding a New Balance." The recommendations put forth in this report were aimed at individuals and groups who have an impact on the quality of life of cancer survivors and their loved ones, including policymakers, scientific and medical communities, employers, insurers, and advocates of cancer survivors.

Cancer, which was once considered a death sentence, has become a controllable and treatable disease in many circumstances. Individuals with cancer are living longer because of better screening tests and improved care. The number of cancer survivors will likely increase with the development of more sophisticated screening tools and more effective surgery and treatment procedures. Because cancer survivors are becoming a larger proportion of the U.S. population, addressing the needs of this population is a necessity in order to improve their quality of life and that of their loved ones and caregivers. It is understood that significantly more research is needed in the area of cancer survivorship in order to effectively address the special needs of this unique population.

Cathy Hogstrom Stiller

See also: Cancer; Diet and Nutrition; Social Health; Spirituality; Wellness

Further Reading

American Cancer Society. (2016). Survivorship: During and after treatment. http://www .cancer.org/treatment/survivorshipduringandaftertreatment/

Centers for Disease Control and Prevention (CDC). (2011). Cancer survivors—United States, 2007. *MMWR*, *60*(9), 269–272. Retrieved from http://www.cdc.gov/cancer/survivorship /what_cdc_is_doing/research/survivors_article.htm.

Feuerstein, M., & Findley, P. (2006). *The Cancer Survivor's Guide: The Essential Handbook to Life after Cancer*. New York: Marlowe & Co.

Hawkins, A., Smith, T., Zhao, L., Rodriquez, J., Berkowtiz, Z., & Stein, K. (2010). Health-related behavior change after cancer: Results of the American Cancer Society's studies of cancer survivors (SCS). *Journal of Cancer Survivorship*, *4*, 20–32.

The National Action Plan for Cancer Survivorship: Advancing Public Health Strategies. (2004). Retrieved from http://www.cdc.gov/cancer/survivorship/what_cdc_is_doing /action_plan.htm.

National Cancer Institute. (2011). US cancer survivors grows to nearly 12 million. Retrieved from http://www.cancer.gov/newscenter/pressreleases/2011/survivorshipMMWR2011.

Pollack, L., Greer, G., Rowland, J., Miller, A., Doneski, D., Coughlin, S. S., & Ulman, D. (2005). Cancer survivorship: A new challenge in comprehensive cancer control. *Cancer Causes and Control*, *16*(Suppl), 51–59.

CANCERS, CHILDHOOD

Cancer develops when the cells in the body begin growing abnormally. Cancer can affect anyone often without warning. Childhood cancer is rare; nevertheless, it exits. The National Cancer Institute (NCI 2014) reported that over the past several decades, the rate of cancer among children has risen slightly. *Healthy People 2020* established an overall objective to reduce cancer mortality by 10 percent in the United States. Three common types of childhood cancer are addressed here: leukemia, brain cancer, and lymphoma.

Background

Leukemia was first diagnosed in 1845. The word *leukemia* comes from the Greek words "leukos" and "heima" meaning "white blood" (McGlauflin et al. 2005). The function of the white blood cell is to protect the body against diseases and infections. When cancer cells are present, white blood cells become overwhelmed, no longer able to perform their primary function.

In 1913, leukemia was classified into four types: chronic lymphocytic leukemia, chronic myelogenous leukemia, acute lymphocytic leukemia, and acute myelogenous leukemia. Childhood cancers are reported as being rare due to increase in survival rates and significant advances in treatment and long term-remission (NCI 2014). McGlauflin and colleagues suggest the increase of cancer in the 20th century is because people who would have died from infectious diseases are now living longer and, further, that "cancer" may not have been diagnosed.

Though lymphoma was not the first cancer to be identified, it is the first in which treatment was successful. In 1894, Fawlor's solution was identified as the first chemotherapeutic agent for treatment of lymphoma. Less than a quarter of a century later, physicians discovered that soldiers who were exposed to mustard gas poisoning experienced dissolution of lymphoid tissue, thus furthering the use and development of chemotherapy as treatment.

Facts and Figures

About 15,780 children are diagnosed with cancer each year in the United States (NCI 2014), or less than 1 percent of all cases of cancer diagnosed. According to the National Cancer Institute (2014) and the American Cancer Society (ACS 2016), there are 12 major types of childhood cancer. Leukemia accounts for 30 percent of childhood cancers. The highest pediatric leukemia incidence rate is among children aged 1–4. The two most common types of leukemia are acute lymphocytic leukemia (ALL) and acute myelogenous leukemia (AML). About 98 percent of leukemia is diagnosed as acute. Approximately 60 percent of children with leukemia have type ALL and 38 percent have type AML (ACS 2015).

Brain Cancer

Brain cancer, usually occurring as a tumor, is a mass cause by abnormal or uncontrolled growth of cells. Tumors are categorized by several factors, including location, cell involvement, and reproduction rate. The American Cancer Society (2016) reports that brain and central nervous system tumors account for 26 percent of childhood cancers.

There are two primary brain tumors categories: *benign* (noncancerous) and *malignant* (cancerous). Typically, benign tumors do not spread to other parts of the body and rarely reoccur after removal. In other parts of the body, the benign tumor is "almost never life-threatening." The process of cancer cells traveling from one part of the body to another is called *metastasis*. Malignant tumors are serious and often life-threatening.

Lymphoma

Lymphoma typically begins in the lymph nodes, tonsils, and thymus. It can also spread to the bone marrow and other organs. *KidsHealth* (2016) reported that about 1,700 kids, younger than age 20, are diagnosed with lymphoma annually, either as Hodgkin lymphoma and non-Hodgkin lymphoma. In Hodgkin lymphoma, there is the presence of malignant cells, called Reed-Sternberg cells. Non-Hodgkin lymphoma also begins in the cells of the immune system. While considered rare before the age of three, some 500 new cases in the United States are reported each year (*KidsHealth* 2016).

Symptoms, Treatment, and Outcomes

All cancers have one thing in common: the replication of abnormal cells. Despite this similarity, cancers differ in symptoms, treatment and outcomes.

One of the many symptoms associated with leukemia is anemia. Leukemia affects bone marrow and impairs its ability to produce the oxygen-carrying red blood cells. Children suffering with leukemia develop hemorrhaging, high fevers, and bruising and excessive bleeding. Other symptoms include dizziness, pain in the joints, swollen lymph nodes in the neck area or groin, and poor appetite. Left untreated, these symptoms can cause death.

Brain tumors that press directly on the surrounding brain cause varied symptoms. The type and severity of the symptoms vary with the age of the child, the type of mass and its location. The more common brain tumors in children begin in the lower part of the brain causing headaches; vomiting; seizures; weakness in the face, etc. In Hodgkin lymphoma, symptoms are similar to leukemia and include, swollen lymph nodes (neck or groin), abdominal pain, itching and hives, poor appetite, weakness, and fatigue (American Childhood Cancer Organization [ACCO] 2016; *KidsHealth* 2016). Symptoms of non-Hodgkin lymphoma mirror other immune-suppressed illnesses (e.g., HIV/AIDS).

Treatment

According to McGlauflin et al. (2005), Thomas Fowler created Fowler's solution, "A combination of arsenic trioxide and potassium bicarbonate which became the remedy for treatment of anemia, Hodgkin's disease and leukemia." The use of arsenic fell out favors when radiation therapy was discovered. Both chemotherapy and radiation remain the primary forms of treatment of childhood leukemia. Because the goal of treatment is remission, chemotherapy is recommended for a period of two to three years.

Children diagnosed with ALL receive chemotherapy drugs in differing combinations. Children's bodies respond to chemotherapy allowing treatments at higher dosages than adults. Sometimes a bone marrow transplant may be necessary, either in addition to or instead of chemotherapy. Extensive treatment provides doctor with a better chance of treating effectively (ACS 2015).

Brain Cancer

Because the brain is responsible for all functions and senses, treatments for brain tumor are more complicated than the rest of the childhood cancers (*KidsHealth* 2016; ACCO 2016). Most patients require a combination of treatments such as surgery, radiation, and chemotherapy. Over the years, advancement in all treatments has resulted in better outcomes (Bracken 2010). Surgery is frequently the recommended treatment for brain tumors; pediatric neurosurgeons have greater success curing children with brain tumors because of advance diagnostic technologies. Instead of trying to take a whole tumor out, doctors will take out a partial of the tumor and use radiation or chemotherapy to help shrink the remaining part; some patients have a second surgery to remove the shrunken tumor.

Lymphoma

Treatment for lymphoma is based on the staging, which determines how extensive the cancer is. The primary treatment for lymphoma is chemotherapy and, in some cases, radiation. In severe cases, where there is a likelihood the cancer will reoccur, physicians use bone marrow and stem cell transplant therapies. When healthy bone marrow/stem cells are introduced in the body, the white blood cells are supported in their primary function: to protect the body against diseases and infections.

New forms of treatment are being developed to treat childhood lymphoma; these therapies incorporate immune therapies.

Outcomes

The survival rate for leukemia, lymphoma, and brain cancers has improved significantly. According to American Cancer Society (2016), the overall survival rate for children with all types of cancers improved from 58 percent in 1977 to 80 percent in 2004. Taken individually, the ACS (2015), Centers for Disease Control and Prevention (CDC 2009), and NCI (2014), report survival rates of nearly 90 percent for acute lymphoblastic leukemia (compared with only 10 percent survival for the same disease in the 1960s), 71 percent for brain and other nervous system tumors, 95 percent for Hodgkin lymphomas, and 85 percent for non-Hodgkin lymphoma.

As important as the improved survival rates is the reduction in the associated death rates. According to the CDC, from 1990 to 2004, childhood leukemia death rates fell by 3 percent each year. Brain tumors and other nervous system tumors went down by 1 percent per year; all other childhood cancer went down by 1.3 percent (2009).

Linda R. Barley

See also: Brain Cancer; Cancer Survivorship; Hodgkin Disease; Leukemia; Lymphoma; Non-Hodgkin Lymphoma

Further Reading

American Cancer Society. (2015). Brain and spinal cord tumors in children. Retrieved from http://www.cancer.org/acs/groups/cid/documents/webcontent/003089-pdf.pdf.

American Cancer Society. (2015). Childhood leukemia. Retrieved from http://www.cancer.org/acs/groups/cid/documents/webcontent/003095-pdf.pdf.

American Cancer Society. (2016). Cancer in children. Retrieved from http://www.cancer.org/cancer/cancerinchildren/.

American Childhood Cancer Organization (ACCO). (2016). Get the facts about childhood cancer. Retrieved from http://www.acco.org/about-childhood-cancer/.

Bracken, J. M. (2010). *Children with Cancer: A Reference Guide for Parents,* revised and updated edition. New York: Oxford University Press.

Centers for Disease Control and Prevention (CDC). (2009). Cancer in children. Retrieved from http://www.cdc.gov/Features/dsCancerInChildren.

KidsHealth. (2016). Cancer Basics (for parents). Retrieved from http://kidshealth.org/en/parents/center/cancer-center.html?ref=search.

McGlauflin, S., Munger, J., & Nelson, R. (2005). History of leukemia. Retrieved from http://rebeccanelson.com/leukemia/history.html.

National Cancer Institute. (2014). Factsheet: Childhood cancers. Retrieved from http://www.cancer.gov/types/childhood-cancers/child-adolescent-cancers-fact-sheet.

United States SEER Program, 1975–1995. Cancer incidence and survival among children and adolescents. Retrieved from http://seer.cancer.gov/publications/childhood.

CANCERS, OCCUPATIONAL

Occupational cancers refer to a collection of different diseases that are influenced by exposures to harmful substances in the workplace. Millions of workers in the United States and elsewhere may develop cancer-related illnesses as a result of factors that put them at risk in the workplace environment. These cancer-causing agents can be chemicals, such as benzene and diesel fumes; minerals, such as asbestos; wood dust; secondhand smoke; viruses; and ultraviolet radiation. Different forms of cancer that can be attributed in part or as a whole to workplace carcinogens are lung cancer, bladder cancer, leukemia, laryngeal cancer, skin cancer, kidney cancer, and liver cancer. Occupational cancers are the leading cause of death in the workplace.

Influencing Factors

Factors influencing the development of occupational cancers include the job type, age, ethnicity, gender, and general health status. As for other forms of cancer, people may be at higher risk for occupational cancers due to their lifestyles and behaviors, their family history, their health status, and the type of chemical(s) they are exposed to. Occupations that may put workers at risk include bartenders, painters, miners, truck drivers, welders, and masonry workers.

Symptoms and Tests

Symptoms may include fever, weight loss, general weakness, appetite loss, fatigue, abnormal swallowing, abnormal bleeding, shortness of breath, and lumps in parts of the body. There are methods for protecting workers from exposure to harmful carcinogens, and reducing exposure is very important. Unfortunately, some companies do not always take proper precautions, and it may be only after employees develop occupational cancers that companies implement changes, often as a result of bad publicity and lawsuits.

Regulation

In the United States, the Department of Labor's Office of Safety and Health Administration (OSHA), regulates substances and conditions that can cause cancer and other harm. On its website, companies and workers can find much information, including lists of substances and the limits to which workers should be exposed, as well as complaint forms and anti-whistleblower information (https://www.osha .gov/index.html). In Canada, the Occupational Cancer Research Centre and Canadian Centre for Occupational Health and Safety regulates and researches occupational cancers.

Ray Marks

See also: Bladder Cancer; Cancer; Kidney Cancer; Laryngeal Cancer; Leukemia; Liver Cancer; Lung Cancer; Skin Cancer

Further Reading

Canadian Centre for Occupational Health and Safety. (2015). Occupation cancer: OSH answers. Retrieved from http://www.ccohs.ca/oshanswers/diseases/occupational_cancer.html.

Centers for Disease Control and Prevention, National Institute for Occupational Safety and Health (NIOSH). (2016). Occupational cancer. Retrieved from http://www.cdc.gov/niosh/topics/cancer/.

Occupational Cancer Research Centre. (2015). Retrieved from http://occupationalcancer/ca.

Occupational Safety & Health Administration (OSHA). Department of Labor. (2016). Retrieved from https://www.osha.gov/index.html.

Robinson, C. F., Sullivan, P. A., Li, J., & Walker, J. T. (2011). Occupational lung cancer in US women, 1984–1998. *American Journal of Industrial Medicine, 54*(2), 102–117. doi: 10.1002/ajim.20905.

World Health Organization (WHO). (2011). Environmental and occupational cancers. http://www.who.int/mediacentre/factsheets/fs350/en/.

CARDIOMYOPATHY

Cardiomyopathy is a term used to describe a group of diseases that affect the heart, in particular, the heart muscle. Often progressive, the damage caused by this disease can result in the damaged heart being less efficient at pumping blood and maintaining a normal electrical rhythm, and it is usually due to enlargement of the heart muscle or thickening or rigidity of the heart muscle. If this progresses to a point where the blood flow to the body is severely affected, the disease may become life-threatening because the body cannot receive adequate amounts of oxygen or nutrients. It has also been found that people with this condition may also experience heart failure, irregular heartbeats, known as arrhythmias, and fluid can build up in the lungs, ankles, feet, legs, or abdomen as a result of heart failure. The heart lining can also become inflamed, leading to a condition called endocarditis. In rare cases, the heart muscle may be replaced with scar tissue. Cardiomyopathy is also termed dilated cardiomyopathy, hypertrophic cardiomyopathy, and restrictive cardiomyopathy.

There are two major types of cardiomyopathy, and these can be acquired or inherited. These are classified as *ischemic* and *nonischemic* types.

The *ischemic* type represents those forms of cardiomyopathy that result from decreased blood to the heart muscle as a result of coronary artery disease and its affect on the arteries supplying the heart with blood, which become narrower.

The *nonischemic* type refers to all those forms of cardiomyopathy that are not caused by coronary artery disease. This type of problem is less common that the ischemic type and there are three main types that can occur as follows:

1. Dilated type
2. Hypertrophic type
3. Restrictive type

In the dilated type, the damage of the heart muscle leads to an enlarged floppy heart, and the heart cannot pump blood adequately. This is the most common type. As more blood stays in the heart after each heartbeat, the heart muscle keeps on stretching and gets even weaker. This type is most common in middle-aged people, especially men.

In the hypertrophic type, the heart muscle fibers enlarge abnormally, and the heart wall thickens. This makes it harder for blood to leave the heart. This type can develop at any age but is more severe if it starts in childhood.

In the restrictive type, portions of the wall of the heart become stiff and lose their flexibility, and cannot fill adequately with blood. This type can occur at any age, but tends to affect older people.

Complications of cardiomyopathy include:

Heart failure
Blood clots
Heart murmurs
Cardiac arrest and sudden death
Stroke

Common Risk Factors for Cardiomyopathy

The factors that can increase the chances of developing cardiomyopathy may include:

Abuse of cocaine or antidepressant medications
Alcoholism
Certain drugs such as chemotherapy drugs used to treat cancer
Chronic rapid heart rate
Coronary artery disease
Diabetes
End-stage kidney disease
Genetic factors/defects/abnormalities
Heart attacks
High blood pressure
Heart valve disease or problems
Heart tissue damage from a previous heart attack
Hypertension
Infections
Inflammation of the heart muscle
Nutritional deficiencies such as vitamin B1, selenium, magnesium, calcium
Obesity
Pregnancy, or in the first five months afterward, where it is termed peripartum
    cardiomyopathy
Systemic lupus erythematosus

Possible Causes of Nonischemic Cardiomyopathy

Dilated Type

- Chronic exposure to toxins, including alcohol and some chemotherapy drugs
- Illnesses such as rheumatoid arthritis, diabetes, or thyroid disease
- Ischemic heart disease with decreased blood flow to the heart

- On occasion, pregnancy or childbirth
- Viral infections

Hypertrophic Type

- Aging
- Genetics or family history

Restrictive Type

Illnesses such as:

- Amyloidosis—resulting in the depositing of fibers that collect in the heart muscle
- Hemochromatosis—a condition where there is too much iron in the body
- Sarcoidosis—or small inflammatory granules or masses that can collect in the heart and other organs

Symptoms

The symptoms of cardiomyopathy vary and depend on its type and severity. While some people have no symptoms and need no treatment, cardiomyopathy can lead, in the long run, to heart failure and can develop quickly.
Symptoms include:

Abnormal heart sounds and heart murmurs
Bloating of the abdomen due to fluid buildup
Blood clots
Breathlessness with exertion
Coughing
Chest pain
Dizziness, light-headedness, fainting
Fatigue
Irregular heart beat
Palpitations
Shortness of breath
Swelling of the feet or legs
Weakness
Weight gain

On occasion, a person may have no symptoms but may experience sudden cardiac death if he or she has hypertrophic cardiomyopathy.

In dilated cardiomyopathy, blood clots may form, and if they are deposited to other parts of the body such as the brain, this may be the first sign the person has a heart condition.

Diagnostic Tests

The diagnostic process may include a medical examination where the doctor can listen to the heart with a stethoscope.

Other methods that may be applied include:

Blood tests
Cardiac catheterization—insertion of a tube into a blood vessel to help identify problems with the heart
Chest x-rays
Electrocardiograms—record the heart's electrical activity
Echocardiograms—use high-frequency sound waves to describe the heart structure
Heart biopsy
Stress tests

Treatments

For heart muscle failure due to coronary artery disease, treatments may include angioplasty surgery, stent placement, or coronary artery bypass surgery to improve the heart function and decrease the symptoms of the condition.

For most patients, treatment is aimed at relieving symptoms and preventing further damage, and the condition will get worse than necessary without treatment.

The main treatment approaches are:

Lifestyle Modification, Medications, and Surgery

Avoid alcohol
Lose weight if this is indicated
Eat a low-fat diet
Limit salt intake
Following a moderate approved exercise regimen

Medications
These may include

ACE inhibitors to relax blood vessels, lower blood pressure, and decrease load on heart
Anti-arrhythmia agents to prevent irregular heart rhythms
Beta blockers to slow the heart and limit disease progression
Calcium channel blockers to lower blood pressure and relax the heart
Diuretics to eliminate excess fluid

Surgery
The types of surgery that may be indicated include

- Implantation of a pacemaker or defibrillator to improve the heart beat
- Surgery to reduce the thickening of the heart muscle wall
- Replacement of a heart valve
- Heart transplants

Prevention

Treating blood pressure and trying to reduce the risk of coronary heart disease through diet and lifestyle may help to prevent cardiomyopathy. People with a family history of heart problems should be screened and started on an appropriate exercise and diet program as early as possible.

If you have any of the signs or symptoms listed or chest pain that lasts longer than two minutes, contact your physician or call 911.

Summary

Cardiomyopathy is a health condition that affects the heart muscle, and this often affects blood flow as a result. The outlook is determined by the type of condition, the cause of the condition, and severity of the condition, as well as the ability of the individual to respond to treatment.

Ray Marks

See also: Arrhythmias/Dysrhythmias; Coronary Artery Disease; Heart Diseases; Heart Murmur; High Blood Pressure; Stroke

Further Reading

American College of Cardiology. (2012). CardioSmart. Retrieved from http://www.cardiosmart.org/HeartDisease/CTT.aspx?id=204.

Cardiomyopathy Association website. Retrieved from http://www.cardiomyopathy.org/.

Lifescript, Healthy Living for Women. (2011). Cardiomyopathy. Retrieved from http://www.lifescript.com/health/a-z/conditions_a-z/conditions/c/cardiomyopathy.aspx?p=1.

Mathews, R. J. (2012). Cardiomyopathy. Retrieved from http://www.rjmatthewsmd.com/Definitions/cardiomyopathy.htm.

Mayo Clinic. (2011). Cardiomyopathy. Retrieved from http://www.mayoclinic.com/health/cardiomyopathy/DS00519.

National Heart, Lung, and Blood Institute. (2011). What is cardiomyopathy? Retrieved from http://ww.nhlbi.nih.gov/health/health-topics/topics/cm.

YouTube. (2011). Cardiomyopathy. Retrieved from http://www.youtube.com/watch?v=rXyVzOmyWfo.

CARDIOVASCULAR DISEASE

Cardiovascular disease, also known as heart disease, refers to a wide range of diseases that affect the heart. These diseases include coronary heart disease, cerebrovascular disease, congenital heart defects, and heart arrhythmias. While all of these diseases differ, they generally involve the blockage or narrowing of blood vessels that supply blood to the heart, brain, or extremities. If the narrowing or blockage of blood vessels is not reversed, it can potentially cause a heart attack or stroke. Cardiovascular disease is the number-one cause of death in the United States, with an estimated 600,000 deaths from the disease every year.

The most common cardiovascular disease is *coronary heart disease*, a condition that involves the buildup of a substance called plaque within the coronary arteries, which deliver blood and oxygen to the heart. This buildup of plaque, known as atherosclerosis, can take many years and may eventually harden, which narrows the coronary arteries. This narrowing reduces the amount of blood and oxygen the heart receives and increases the risk that the plaque will rupture. If the plaque ruptures and a blood clot forms that blocks the flow of blood to the heart, that portion of the heart begins to die due to a lack of blood and oxygen, triggering a heart attack.

Another common cardiovascular disease is cerebrovascular disease, which encompasses a group of medical conditions that involve the supply of blood to the brain being restricted, known as *ischemia*. This restriction takes place when plaque builds up in the carotid and vertebral arteries, which supply blood to the brain. If the plaque buildup becomes severe enough that it blocks the flow of blood to the brain, it can cause an ischemic stroke. The buildup of plaque in the carotid and vertebral arteries can also cause them to rupture, which causes bleeding and can lead to a hemorrhagic stroke.

Congenial heart defects, another type of cardiovascular disease, are a group of medical conditions that involve structural problems with the heart that are present at birth. These defects can include the arteries, veins, the valves of the heart, or the walls of the heart. Congenial heart defects generally disrupt the flow of blood through the heart, although the severity of the disruption depends on the specific defect.

Heart arrhythmias are another type of cardiovascular disease that causes the electrical impulses that regulate heartbeat to not work properly. If the electrical impulses are not working correctly, it can cause the heart to beat too slow or too fast. While heart arrhythmias are usually harmless, they can cause irritating symptoms and become potentially life-threatening.

The cause of most types of cardiovascular disease is *atherosclerosis*, which involves the buildup of plaque in the arteries. The buildup of plaque increases the pressure on the arteries and, over time, can cause them to thicken and become stiff. Atherosclerosis is commonly caused by a lack of exercise, an unhealthy diet, or smoking. Heart arrhythmias have several causes, including heart defects, high blood pressure, diabetes, coronary heart disease, and smoking. Heart defects usually occur while the baby is still developing in the womb and can be caused by genes, medications, and some medical conditions. Several factors can increase an individual's risk of developing cardiovascular disease including age, family history, stress, high blood pressure, and high blood cholesterol levels.

The symptoms and effects of cardiovascular disease vary, depending on the type of cardiovascular condition an individual has. Coronary heart disease can cause chest pain, shortness of breath, and pain or numbness in the extremities. More severe effects include heart attack, stroke, heart failure, and potentially death if the artery blockage is not reversed. Cerebrovascular disease can cause numbness to the face or extremities, difficulty speaking, difficulty seeing, severe headaches, and fainting. More severe effects include stroke, which can cause neurological damage or death. Heart arrhythmias can cause a quick or slow heartbeat, a fluttering sensation in the chest, shortness of breath, and chest pain. Symptoms of congenital heart defects can range from easily tiring and shortness of breath to more serious symptoms such as swelling in the legs or around the eyes and gray- or blue-colored skin due to a lack of oxygen saturation.

In order to diagnose cardiovascular disease, a health care professional will begin by performing a standard physical exam and asking the patient about his or her personal and family medical history. Further testing will depend on the specific type of cardiovascular disease the medical professional believes the patient has. Blood tests can be used to determine if the patient has substances in the blood that indicate heart disease, such as cholesterol and triglyceride levels. An electrocardiogram (ECG) is a test where probes are placed on the chest to record the electrical impulses that cause the heart to beat, which can detect if the heart has an irregular rhythm. An echocardiogram is a noninvasive test where an ultrasound is taken of the chest using sound waves that are transmitted through the heart by a transducer. The echoes of the sound waves produce moving pictures of the heart that provide a more detailed picture than an x-ray. Doctors may also use a cardiac catheterization, in which dye is inserted into an artery through a tube and viewed on an x-ray to check if blood is flowing through the heart normally. X-rays, CT scans, and MRIs can also be taken of the heart to check for irregularities.

There are several treatments available for individuals with cardiovascular disease, most of which focus on opening up arteries that have been narrowed or blocked by plaque. Lifestyle changes such as increased exercise, a diet low in sodium and fat, and quitting smoking can help to reverse artery blockage. Medications are also available to lower blood pressure and cholesterol levels, as well as help thin the blood. If medications are unsuccessful, doctors may recommend surgery to clear blockages in the arteries. The most common procedure is a coronary angioplasty, during which a catheter is placed in the artery and a small balloon is threaded through and inflated to remove the blockage. Individuals with heart arrhythmias may have pacemakers or implantable cardioverter defibrillators (ICDs) inserted to regulate heartbeat.

Symptoms of cardiovascular disease have been traced back as far as ancient Egypt. In the 18th century, German physician Friedrich Hoffman became one of the first doctors to discover the link between blockages in the coronary arteries and cardiovascular disease. During the late 18th century, cardiologist William Osler discovered that angina, the chest tightening associated with cardiovascular disease, was a symptom of the disease and not a unique medical condition. In 1912, American cardiologist James B. Herrick discovered that angina was caused by the narrowing of the coronary arteries and invented the term "heart attack." The Association for the Prevention and Relief of Heart Disease was founded in 1915 by a group of doctors to study the disease and would go on to become the American Heart Association in 1924. By 1948, the National Heart Institute had launched the Framingham Heart Study, which was the first major study into the causes and treatment of cardiovascular disease. In 1950, researcher John Gofman identified low-density lipoprotein (LDL) and high-density lipoprotein (HDL), as well as the importance of maintaining the levels of these types of cholesterol through diet.

Heart disease remains the number-one cause of death in the United States, with coronary heart disease being the most common type, killing around 380,000 people each year. Men are generally at a greater risk for developing cardiovascular disease than women, and the disease is the leading cause of death for African Americans, whites, and Latinos. Due to the prevalence of cardiovascular disease in the United States, 720,000 Americans suffer from a heart attack each year.

Renee Dubie

See also: Arrhythmias/Dysrhythmias; Atherosclerosis; Cerebral Vascular Disease; Congenital Heart Disease; Coronary Artery Disease; Heart Diseases; Stroke

Further Reading

American Heart Association. (2015). Heart conditions. Retrieved from http://www.heart.org /HEARTORG/Conditions/Conditions_UCM_001087_SubHomePage.jsp.

American Heart Association. (2015). What is cardiovascular disease? Retrieved from http:// www.heart.org/HEARTORG/Caregiver/Resources/WhatisCardiovascularDisease/What -is-Cardiovascular-Disease_UCM_301852_Article.jsp#.Vri8YlJGNro.

Centers for Disease Control and Prevention. (2015). About heart disease. Retrieved from http://www.cdc.gov/heartdisease/about.htm.

DeSilva, R. A. (2013). *Heart Disease*. Santa Barbara, CA: Greenwood.

Esselstyn Jr., C. B. (2007). *Prevent and Reverse Heart Disease: The Revolutionary, Scientifically Proven, Nutrition-Based Cure*. New York: Avery-Penguin.

Gillinov, M., & Nissen, S. (2012). *Heart 411: The Only Guide to Heart Health You'll Ever Need*. New York: Three Rivers Press.

Granato, J. E., MD. (2008). *Living with Coronary Heart Disease: A Guide for Patients and Families (A Johns Hopkins Press Health Book)*. Baltimore, MD: Johns Hopkins University Press.

Mayo Clinic. (2012). *Healthy Heart for Life!* New York: Time Home Entertainment.

Mayo Clinic. (2015). Heart disease. Retrieved from http://www.mayoclinic.org/diseases -conditions/heart-disease/basics/definition/con-20034056.

Pampel, F. C., & Pauley, S. (2013). *Progress Against Heart Disease*. Santa Barbara, CA: Praeger.

World Heart Federation. (2015). Heart disease. Retrieved from http://www.world-heart -federation.org/cardiovascular-health/heart-disease/.

CAREGIVING AND CAREGIVERS

Overview

A caregiver is anyone who provides help to another person in need, usually involved in assisting those who are disabled or limited in one or more aspects of their daily lives. Nearly half of all adults in the United States suffer from one or more chronic diseases, so as this population ages, they will require help from professional and lay caregivers, who will assist them in managing their daily activities and help prevent their illnesses from becoming worse.

Some of the chronic diseases that require intensive caregiving include Alzheimer's disease and other types of dementia, stroke, HIV/AIDS, terminal cancers, Parkinson's disease, and many other conditions.

The Caregivers

Key professional caregivers are nurses, nurse practitioners, social workers, and physical and occupational therapists. Other caregivers commonly include parents, spouses, children, nonfamily members, nursing and home health care aides, and human services personnel. Some are paid (professionals); some are not (family members).

Caregivers take care of adults and children. Women are most likely to be caregivers, but many may have long-term health care needs of their own.

Caregiving Services

Caregivers perform many tasks, among them are cooking and feeding; bathing, dressing, and toileting; grocery and other shopping; house cleaning; making appointments; assisting with medication; screening for alcohol misuse and depression; social and emotional support; and transportation. Caregivers may also be called on to handle legal and financial matters, paying bills, and related issues.

Companies set up for caregiving services offer transportation, meal delivery, nursing care at home, housekeeping and other home care, and home modifications, which enable people to perform daily tasks otherwise impossible.

Symptoms of Caregiver Stress

Although caregiving can be rewarding, the responsibilities, challenges, and demands on time faced by caregivers, especially those who are family members, can lead to stress. In turn, stress can increase the risk of poor health for the caregiver, or it can cause caregiver burnout.

Caregiver stress, or the physical and emotional strain of caregiving, can take many forms, including alcohol or drug abuse, anger, anxiety or depression, denial, dissatisfaction, exhaustion, headaches, irritability, loneliness, and feeling sad, frustrated, or guilty. Although most caregivers may be in good health, it is not uncommon for them to develop heart disease, cancer, diabetes, arthritis, and other serious health problems.

Prevention

To prevent stress, it can be helpful to take regular breaks throughout the day; eat healthful meals; exercise regularly; stay active socially; join a caregiver support group; and get professional help from a doctor, counselor, psychologist, or other mental health provider.

Respite services that provide a temporary substitute for caregivers can help reduce stress. Examples include in-home services, adult day care, short-term nursing homes or rehabilitation facilities, and daytime hospital stays.

Assistance from caregivers and caregiving services are available. Elder care specialists are experts in aging-related issues; they can assess the needs of an older adult and make recommendations for meeting those needs. Doctors, nurses, nurse practitioners, social workers, and other professionals can also provide help.

Ray Marks

See also: AIDS; Alzheimer's Disease; Cancer; Parkinson's Disease; Stroke

Further Reading

Administration for Community Living. (2014, June 6). Caregivers. Retrieved from http://www.acl.gov/Get_Help/Help_Caregivers/Index.aspx.
Family Caregiver Alliance. (2015). Women and caregiving: Facts and figures. Retrieved from http:// https://caregiver.org/women-and-caregiving-facts-and-figures.
KidsHealth. (2015). Taking care of you: Support for caregivers. Retrieved from http://kidshealth.org/parent/system/ill/caregivers.html.
Womenshealth.gov. (2012, July 16). Caregiver stress fact sheet. Retrieved from http://www.womenshealth.gov/publications/our-publications/fact-sheet/caregiver-stress.cfm.

CARPAL TUNNEL SYNDROME

Carpal tunnel syndrome (CTS) is a health condition occurring in one to three of every 1,000 adults in the population per year in the United States and worldwide and is associated with characteristic symptoms and signs that result from abnormal compression or excess pressure on the median nerve of the hand within the carpal tunnel at the wrist. According to a report in *The Rheumatologist*, approximately 10 million Americans suffer from this syndrome, which is also called median nerve entrapment.

The median nerve and several tendons supplying the hand run down the forearm to the hand through a small passageway in the wrist known as the carpal tunnel. This nerve helps to controls movement and feeling in the thumb and the first three fingers, and pressure in the tightly spaced carpal tunnel from swelling of the nerve or tendons or narrowing of the carpal tunnel can cause problems of sensation and pain that can affect the ability of the hand to function normally.

Carpal tunnel syndrome is not fatal, but it can lead progressively to complete, irreversible damage of the median nerve and result in a severe loss of hand function, if it is not treated.

It occurs more readily in females than males, ages 30 to 60 years, and more readily in Caucasians than African Americans.

Causes

Although the cause may not be known, excessive repetitive movements or trauma may be involved.

Jobs related to carpal tunnel syndrome include sewing, driving, assembly line work, hairdressing, data entry or repetitive keyboard use, cleaning, manufacturing, and fish or meat packing jobs.

Risk Factors

Although no definite cause for carpal tunnel syndrome exists, several risk factors— including genetic, medical, social, work, sports-related, and demographic factors— have been identified.

The shape of the wrist and wrist bone structures, which can be inherited or altered by injury; underlying health problems, such as diabetes and alcoholism; inflammatory conditions such as rheumatoid arthritis, bone spurs, and kidney failure; workplace factors; and pattern of hand usage are among the most common risk factors.

Other health conditions associated with carpal tunnel syndrome are:

- Obesity
- Pregnancy due to fluid retention
- Hypothyroidism
- Infections
- Tenosynovitis of inflammation of the flexor tendons of the wrist joint
- Trauma, including joint dislocations, wrist fractures
- Amyloidosis
- Sarcoidosis
- Multiple myeloma

Symptoms

The usual symptoms of carpal tunnel syndrome include numbness, tingling, or pins and needles in the fingers or hand, plus weakness, and vague or burning pain of the affected hand. These symptoms may or may not be accompanied by changes in sensation and hand strength, as well as loss of function of the hand and wrist.

The symptoms occur most often in the thumb, index finger, middle finger, and half of the ring finger, and in some cases there may be pain in the arm between the hand and the elbow and a tendency to drop objects or difficulty feeling or handling small objects.

The symptoms may occur at night at first, may be worse at night, and may be relieved by shaking the hand(s).

Diagnostic Tests and Investigative Approaches

If a person is complaining of the symptoms of carpal tunnel syndrome, first, the physician may examine the person's overall medical history, as well as any history of trauma, or history related to the person's work and sporting activities. The physician may also conduct certain tests and ask about the presence of specific health problems associated with carpal tunnel syndrome. During the exam, the physician may check the person's wrist sensation, wrist and hand strength, and range of motion and may visually or manually inspect overall upper limb function.

Further tests may include:

Phalen's test for carpal tunnel syndrome, examining Tinel's sign, or:
- Blood tests to see if any health problems might be causing your symptoms
- Nerve conduction tests to find out if the median nerve is working as it should
- X-rays (which may be helpful)
- Electromyogram or electrodiagnostic tests to measure the muscle function at the wrist

Treatments

Mild symptoms usually can often be treated at home. The sooner treatment is started, the better the chances of stopping symptoms and preventing long-term nerve damage.

There are two types of treatment approaches. These include nonsurgical and surgical approaches.

Nonsurgical procedures may include wrist splinting and the use of steroids in the form of local injections or oral steroids as a secondary option.

Nonsteroidal anti-inflammatory medications may also be used in conjunction with the preceding options, as may the use of therapeutic ultrasound or infrared treatments using infrared therapy gloves directed at the inflamed area, along with certain therapeutic exercises.

Other interventions include acupuncture, use of diuretics, pyridoxine, massage therapy, ice, yoga, and nerve and tendon gliding exercises, as well as changing the way the hand is used, ergonomically changing how the hand is used, or changing the need to perform repetitive movements may be helpful.

The underlying health conditions should be rigorously treated at the outset.

Surgical procedures may include an open carpal tunnel release using a relatively large longitudinal incision, endoscopic carpal tunnel release surgery using an endoscope or arthroscopic device, a full-open endoscopic carpal tunnel release, or a mini-open carpal tunnel release using a short-incision procedure.

Prevention

A healthy lifestyle, maintaining a healthy weight, and regular exercising may be beneficial as a whole.

Modifications of the worksite or workstation, avoiding repetitive movements, and taking breaks periodically may be helpful as well.

Keep hands warm, use correct postures, wear fingerless gloves, and avoid placing the body or hands in stressful positions or excessive vibration of the hands.

Ray Marks

See also: Alcoholism; Diabetes, Type 1; Hypothyroidism; Kidney Failure; Multiple Myeloma; Rheumatoid Arthritis

Further Reading

American College of Rheumatology. (2013, September). Carpal tunnel syndrome. Retrieved from http://www.rheumatology.org/I-Am-A/Patient-Caregiver/Diseases-Conditions/Carpal-Tunnel-Syndrome.

American Society of Hand Surgery. (2015). Carpal tunnel syndrome. Retrieved from http://www.assh.org/handcare/hand-arm-conditions/carpal-tunnel/.

Mayo Clinic. (2014, April 2). Retrieved from http://www.mayoclinic.org/diseases-conditions/carpal-tunnel-syndrome/basics/definition/con-20030332.

National Institute of Neurological Disorders and Stroke (2015, April 17). Carpal tunnel syndrome fact sheet. Retrieved from http://www.ninds.nih.gov/disorders/carpal_tunnel/detail_carpal_tunnel.htm.

The Rheumatologist. (2012). Patient fact sheet: Carpal tunnel syndrome. Retrieved from http://www.the-rheumatologist.org/article/patient-fact-sheet-carpal-tunnel-syndrome/.

CELIAC DISEASE

Description

Celiac disease is a chronic immune disease affecting the digestive system and one in which the affected individual cannot eat gluten-based products because they damage the small intestine and make it difficult for the small intestine to absorb nutrients and minerals properly. Gluten is a protein found in wheat, rye, and barley, and possibly in oats; it may also be used in products such as vitamin and nutrient supplements, lip balms, and some medicines.

The disease can occur at any point in time in the person's life and affects as many as 2 million Americans, including children as well as adults, men and women. Yet, 97 percent of cases with celiac disease may go undiagnosed.

The disease is caused by an immune reaction to foods or substances containing gluten.

It is also termed celiac sprue and gluten intolerance.

Signs and Symptoms

There may be no symptoms to tell if an individual has a problem, and if there are symptoms of celiac disease, this may vary. Common symptoms include:

- Abdominal bloating and pain
- Arthritis
- Bone or joint pain
- Bone loss or osteoporosis
- Canker sores in the mouth
- Chronic diarrhea
- Constipation
- Depression or anxiety
- Extreme tiredness
- Gas
- Infertility or recurrent miscarriage
- Itchy skin rash with blisters
- Mood changes
- Seizures

- Slowed growth
- Stomach pain
- Tingling numbness in hands and feet
- Unexplained iron deficiency anemia
- Vomiting
- Weight loss

Children who have celiac disease may commonly be very irritable because they cannot absorb the nutrients needed to allow them to thrive. They may show delayed growth, short stature, delayed puberty, and dental enamel defects of the permanent teeth.

Causes

The disease is commonly hereditary.

The disease may be influenced by length of time person was breast fed, age when the person started to eat gluten-based foods, amount of gluten in the foods, age, and degree of damage to the small intestine.

Other health conditions associated with celiac disease include:

Addison's disease
Autoimmune thyroid disease
Autoimmune liver disease
Rheumatoid arthritis
Sjögren's syndrome
Type I diabetes

Diagnosis

Blood tests or intestinal and skin biopsies may be used to establish if a person has celiac disease.

Treatment

The only treatment for celiac disease is a gluten-free diet. As noted by the Celiac Disease Foundation (2016), the foods that cause problems are grains with gluten, including wheat, rye, and barley. But the following are safe: rice, cassava, corn (maize), soy, potato, tapioca, beans, sorghum, quinoa, millet, buckwheat groats (also known as kasha), arrowroot, amaranth, teff, flax, chia, yucca, gluten-free oats, and nut flours. But, whole foods from other food groups are safe: dairy and eggs, meats and fish, and fruits and vegetables are good, unless any of these foods is processed with a gluten substance.

Prognosis or Outcome

Celiac disease can be very serious if it causes long-lasting digestive problems and keeps your body from getting all the nutrition it needs. Over time, celiac disease can cause anemia, infertility, weak and brittle bones, an itchy skin rash, and other health problems. If left untreated, complications that can arise include malnutrition, loss of calcium and bone density, lactose intolerance, cancer, or neurological complications.

A dietician can help with the choice of foods and how to manage the disease.

Ray Marks

See also: Addison's Disease; Autoimmune Disease; Dermatitis; Diabetes, Type 1; Rheumatoid Arthritis; Sjögren's Syndrome

Further Reading

Academy of Nutrition and Dietetics. (2015). Celiac disease. Retrieved from http://www .cureceliacdisease.org/.

Celiac Disease Foundation. (2016). Celiac disease. Retrieved from https://celiac.org/celiac -disease/.

Green, P. H. R., & Jones, R. (2010). *Celiac Disease: A Hidden Epidemic,* revised and updated edition. New York, NY: William Morrow.

Mayo Clinic. (2013, May 22). Celiac disease. Retrieved from http://www.mayoclinic.org /diseases-conditions/celiac-disease/basics/definition/con-20030410.

National Institute of Diabetes and Digestive and Kidney Diseases. (2015, June 25). Celiac disease. Retrieved from http://www.niddk.nih.gov/health-information/health-topics /digestive-diseases/celiac-disease/Pages/facts.aspx.

Thompson, T. (2006). *Celiac Disease Nutrition Guide*, 2nd ed. Chicago: American Dietetic Association.

University of Chicago Celiac Disease Center. (2015). Patients and caregivers guide to celiac disease. Retrieved from http://www.cureceliacdisease.org/living-with-celiac/guide.

CELLULITIS

Background

Cellulitis is a common, noncontagious skin condition that arises as a result of bacterial infection that can spread rapidly and affect the soft tissues underneath the skin.

The skin sites most often affected are those in the lower legs, but the condition can occur anywhere on the body, including the face.

The condition may simply be localized to the skin surface, but cellulitis can also affect tissues under the skin and can spread to the lymph nodes and blood stream. On occasion, small red spots may appear on top of the affected skin area, and less commonly, there may be small blisters that form that can burst.

Recurrent episodes of cellulitis often occur with fungal infections and may result in damage to the lymphatic drainage system, and such episodes can cause long-standing swelling of the affected part of the body.

If this form of infection is not treated, this may pose a threat to the individual in regard to his or her health. And if cellulitis on the face is not treated, it can spread to the brain and cause a dangerous infection called meningitis. Cellulitis can also cause other problems, such as blood clots in the legs known as thrombophlebitis.

Symptoms and Signs

A person with cellulitis will usually have one or more areas of the skin that are red or inflamed and feel hot and tender, and the skin may look swollen.

Other symptoms may include:

Drainage or leakage of yellow clear fluid or pus from the skin
Large blisters
Skin tenderness
Tender or swollen lymph nodes near the affected area
Tight and glossy stretched appearance of the skin
Pain
Fever
Chills or shaking
Fatigue
General ill feeling
Muscle aches and pains
Sweating
Hair loss at site of infection
Joint stiffness caused by tissue swelling over joint
Nausea and vomiting

Key Causes

Cellulitis commonly occurs when bacteria enter the skin through a crack or skin lesion. This can occur as a result of a wound, ulcer, abrasion, athlete's foot or dermatitis, skin lesions such as chickenpox, severe acne, or skin disruptions or infections following surgery, as well as following insect or spider bites.

People who handle fish, meat, poultry, or soil without gloves may be susceptible. People who are morbidly obese can develop cellulites in the abdominal skin region.

Risk factors include:

- Animal bites
- Chronic swelling of the arms or legs known as lymphedema
- Circulatory problems that result in inadequate blood flow to the limbs and poor venous or lymphatic drainage
- Cracks in the skin
- Foreign objects in the skin
- Having a weakened immune system
- Having certain skin conditions such as eczema, psoriasis
- Injected illegal drugs under the skin
- infection of the bone under the skin
- Intravenous drug use
- Known injuries to the skin

- Medical problems such as diabetes
- Liver diseases such as chronic hepatitis or cirrhosis
- Use of corticosteroid medications or medications that suppress the immune system

Diagnostic Procedures

Health care providers can conduct a physical examination of the skin and related lymph nodes. They may run tests to examine blood for infections, by using a blood culture. They may also order a complete blood count or a culture of any fluid or material inside the affected area.

Treatments

Analgesics
Antibiotics
Elevating the infected area higher than the heart to reduce swelling
Hospitalization with antibiotics delivered intravenously if the individual is very ill, has an immune deficiency, or has an infection around the eyes
Rest
Surgery on occasion

Prevention

If you have a skin wound, this should be kept clean by washing the area gently with soap and water each day.

Antibiotic creams or ointments can be applied to the skin surface for protection, covered with a bandage, and changed every day until a scab forms. People with diabetes and those with circulation problems should try to prevent skin wounds and treat any abrasions or cuts as soon as possible.

Prognosis

The outlook for cellulitis depends on the cause, but antibiotics are normally successful in clearing up the condition in a short space of time. Longer treatments may be needed if the person has a chronic disease or a deficient immune system. Complications that may occur are blood infections, bone infections, heart inflammation, lymph vessel inflammation, meningitis, shock, and tissue death or gangrene.

Ray Marks

See also: Eczema; Meningitis; Obesity, Morbid; Psoriasis; Skin Conditions; Thrombophlebitis

Further Reading
Mayo Clinic. (2015, February 11). Cellulitis. Retrieved from http://www.mayoclinic.org /diseases-conditions/cellulitis/basics/definition/con-20023471.

MedlinePlus. (2015, May 10). Cellulitis. Retrieved from https://www.nlm.nih.gov/medline plus/cellulitis.html.

National Institute of Allergy and Infectious Diseases. (2013, November 8). Cellulitis and erysipelas. Retrieved from http://www.niaid.nih.gov/topics/cellulitiserysipelas/Pages /default.aspx.

CENTERS FOR DISEASE CONTROL AND PREVENTION (CDC)

The Centers for Disease Control and Prevention (CDC) is an agency of the U.S. federal government based in Atlanta, Georgia, focused on health promotion, prevention, and emergency preparedness activities. As the primary public health agency within the United States responsible for protecting the nation's health, the CDC works on prevention and control initiatives in several key areas, including infectious and chronic disease, occupational safety, environmental health, injuries, and disabilities. The CDC is responsible for working collaboratively with state and local health departments to manage health data and to investigate epidemics and disease outbreaks. CDC is also responsible for conducting research to prevent health problems and for developing health policies to protect the public from health risks. CDC celebrated its 65th anniversary in 2011.

CDC is the primary agency of the U.S. federal government responsible for implementing *Healthy People,* the national set of science-based health goals and objectives. CDC has been a key agency in implementing some of the most notable public health advancements in the past 100 years, including the control and eradication of several infectious diseases, the recognition of tobacco smoking as a health hazard, the monitoring of the HIV epidemic in the United States and abroad, and the response to potential acts of bioterrorism, such as the 2001 anthrax attack in the United States.

Founder Dr. Joseph W. Mountin first opened CDC on July 1, 1946, as the Communicable Disease Center, where its early efforts were directed toward malaria control. Three years later when the United States was declared free of malaria, CDC redirected its efforts toward disease surveillance, focusing first on polio. During the 1950s, CDC began working on the prevention of other infectious diseases, including rabies and influenza, and due largely in part to the Korean War, began work to prepare the United States against manmade epidemics and biological warfare. This work led to the creation of the Epidemiology Intelligence Service (EIS), a program of CDC still in existence today that is responsible for working domestically and internationally.

In 1960, CDC assumed responsibility of the Tuberculosis Program from the U.S. Public Health Service. Throughout this decade, CDC was involved in a number of significant public health achievements, including playing a key role in the eradication of smallpox, the expansion of the National Surveillance Program to include several new infectious diseases, the initiation of a national measles eradication campaign, and the investigation of what was later identified as Legionnaires' disease. To protect scientists while working with infectious and potentially lethal pathogens, CDC built its first "biocontaminant lab" in 1969.

As the scope of CDC's work continued to expand beyond that of infectious disease, in 1970 the Communicable Disease Center was renamed the Center for Disease Control (and in 1981, Center became Centers). In the following years, CDC further extended its reach globally by assisting Sierra Leone battle an outbreak of the lethal viral disease Lassa fever and investigating two outbreaks of hemorrhagic fever in Zaire and Sudan, later identified to be caused by the Ebola virus. However, during the 2014 cases of Americans who returned to the United States having contracted the Ebola virus, the CDC received criticism for not being ready to fight the disease and, in particular, for not ensuring that American hospitals were ready to handle Ebola. They then instituted new guidelines.

While CDC remained focused on infectious disease monitoring and prevention (particularly in relation to the emerging HIV virus), the 1980s was a period of considerable growth for CDC, specifically in the areas of chronic disease and injury prevention. In recognition of the considerable impact of child abuse, homicide, and suicide, in 1983 CDC established its Violence Epidemiology Branch. Three years later, CDC assumed responsibility for the Office on Smoking and Health and in 1988, the National Center for Chronic Disease Prevention and Health Promotion was established. In 1992, CDC became known as the Centers for Disease Control and Prevention; however, the well-known, three-letter acronym CDC was retained.

CDC continues to conduct public health investigations and research studies that have national and global reach, mostly notably through initiatives aimed at preventing international disease transmission. Since 1990, CDC has continued work in virtually all areas of disease prevention and health promotion. CDC investigates outbreaks of new and reemerging diseases. CDC investigated a new infectious illness in southwestern United States in 1993 (later identified as Hantavirus), and in 2003, CDC provided guidance for the emerging Sudden Acute Respiratory Syndrome (SARS) epidemic in Asia. More recently, CDC detected and investigated multistate outbreaks of food borne illness, and in 2009, CDC demonstrated its singular ability to assist with emerging infectious agents when it identified the novel H1N1 influenza virus.

CDC is a leader in the improvement of maternal and child health outcomes, including the recommendation to offer HIV testing to all pregnant women and the monitoring of the significant decline in U.S. children born with HIV infection. In order to better understand the burdens associated with pregnancy, birth, and motherhood, CDC established the program Safe Motherhood under the Children's Health Act of 2000.

In addition to implementation disease prevention programs, CDC collaborates with state health departments and other key agencies to provide a comprehensive disease and bioterrorism monitoring system. CDC maintains national health statistics and publishes the *Morbidity and Mortality Weekly Report* (MMWR), which contains data on notifiable diseases reported by state and territorial health departments, surveillance data on chronic and infectious diseases, and short reports on topics of interest to readers.

CDC's National Center for Chronic Disease Prevention and Health Promotion (NCCDPHP) develops strategic prevention initiatives that support a vision of "all people living healthy lives free from the devastation of chronic diseases." Major program areas include arthritis, diabetes, healthy aging, heart disease and stroke, and tobacco, among others. Through its programmatic efforts, NCCD-PHP also directly addresses four modifiable behavioral risk factors identified as common causes of chronic disease, including lack of physical activity, poor nutrition, excessive consumption of alcohol, and tobacco use. CDC targets chronic disease prevention through the lifespan, with programs such as *Healthy Youth*, *Healthy Communities*, and *Healthy Aging*. CDC publishes the weekly online peer-reviewed journal *Preventing Chronic Disease: Public Health Research, Practice and Policy*.

As one of the major operating units of the U.S. Department of Health and Human Services, CDC employs more than 15,000 employees in locations spanning more than 50 countries worldwide. CDC is organized under a number of offices, centers, and institutes, including the Office of the Director, the National Institute for Occupational Safety and Health, and the Center for Global Health. Specific CDC programs are organized under several coordinating offices: the Office for State, Tribal, Local and Territorial Support; the Office of Public Health Preparedness and Response; the Office of Surveillance, Epidemiology, and Laboratory Services; the Office of Noncommunicable Diseases, Injury and Environmental Health; and the Office of Infectious Disease. While each individual unit implements programs and responses within its area of expertise, the organizational structure provides significant opportunity for intra-organizational support and resource sharing.

Today, CDC's goal—"to protect the health of all people"—is reinforced through its commitment to the following five strategic focus areas: (1) increasing support to local and state health departments, (2) improving global health, (3) decreasing leading causes of death, (4) strengthening surveillance and epidemiology, and (5) reforming health policies.

William D. Kernan

See also: Public Health; World Health Organization

Further Reading

Centers for Disease Control and Prevention. 1600 Clifton Rd, Atlanta, GA 30333, (800) 232–4636, www.cdc.gov.

Centers for Disease Control and Prevention. (2016, February 25). About CDC 24-7: CDC fact sheet. Retrieved from http://www.cdc.gov/about/facts/cdcfastfacts/.

Centers for Disease Control and Prevention. (2015, June 30). About the Center. Retrieved from http://www.cdc.gov/chronicdisease/about/.

Centers for Disease Control and Prevention. (2015, July 22). Our history, our story. Retrieved from http://www.cdc.gov/about/history/ourstory.htm.

Reagan, P. A., & Brookins-Fisher, J. (2002). *Community Health in the 21st Century*. San Francisco, CA: Benjamin Cummings.

Riegelman, R. (2010). *Public Health 101: Healthy People, Healthy Populations*. Sudbury, MA: Jones & Bartlett Learning.

CEREBROVASCULAR DISEASE

Cerebrovascular disease refers to any of several disorders of the blood vessels that supply the brain—the carotid arteries (in the front of the neck) and the vertebral arteries (on the sides of the spinal column). These disorders are caused primarily by atherosclerosis, in which cholesterol plaque builds up along the artery walls, damaging the lining of the blood vessels, narrowing and stiffening the vessels (known as stenosis), and making the vessels susceptible to fluctuations in blood pressure.

Cerebrovascular disease is most common among elderly individuals and among people with Type 2 diabetes, ischemic heart disease, obesity, a history of smoking, and the use of hormone replacement therapy. More than 130,000 deaths related to cerebrovascular disease occur every year in the United States. The vast majority of those deaths are among people aged 65 and older. Cerebrovascular disease is more prevalent among men than women. Genetic factors play a role in determining one's risk of cerebrovascular disease, with blacks generally being at a greater risk than whites.

The main manifestation of cerebrovascular disease is stroke, a major cause of serious long-term disability and the third leading cause of death in the United States. More than 6 million American adults—almost 3 percent of the adult population—have had a stroke. Every year, about 800,000 Americans have a stroke.

Most strokes occur when blood flow to the brain is substantially reduced or stopped, a condition known as ischemia. This blood blockage could be caused by a thrombus (blood clot) or an embolus (a piece of blood clot, fatty plaque, tumor, air, or other substance that travels through a blood vessel until it stops when reaching a narrow point). Certain drugs and medical conditions increase the risk of thrombus and embolus. Different parts of the brain can be affected, depending on the areas deprived of blood.

Some strokes occur as a result of intracranial hemorrhage, when a sudden spike in blood pressure—perhaps because of emotional excitement, hypertension, or a drug reaction—causes blood vessels in or around the brain to rupture. This bleeding is usually life-threatening. Other types of cerebrovascular disease involve aneurysms, which are weak, bulging areas in the arteries leading to the brain. These areas can eventually burst, causing bleeding and hemorrhagic stroke.

Thrombosis strokes make up approximately 40 percent of all cerebrovascular diseases, embolisms make up about 30 percent of cerebrovascular diseases, and hemorrhages make up about 20 percent of cerebrovascular diseases.

Diagnosis and Treatment

Unfortunately, cerebrovascular disease often goes undiagnosed until a patient has a stroke or other major cerebrovascular event. A physician identifies cerebrovascular problems and diagnoses cerebrovascular disease partly with a physical examination, including using a stethoscope to listen for sounds of abnormal blood flow, known as bruit. The examination may also involve checks for neurological, muscular, and sensory deficiencies, such as changes in vision, eye movements, and reflexes.

Imaging technologies are also important in diagnosis. One such diagnostic imaging technique is angiography, in which a catheter is guided into the arteries of the neck. A contrast dye is injected into the arteries through the catheter. X-rays of the procedure reveal abnormalities in the arteries. Ultrasonography focuses high-frequency sound waves on blood vessels to examine them for sign of abnormalities. Computed tomography scans are used to help diagnose hemorrhagic strokes. Magnetic resonance imaging can reveal signs of previous TIAs.

Patients who have been diagnosed as having cerebrovascular disease can be given blood platelet inhibitors—such as aspirin, clopidogrel, dipyridamole, sulfinpyrazone, or ticlopidine—to reduce their risk for a first stroke or a recurrence of stroke. Approximately 25 percent of patients who recover from a first stroke will have another stroke within five years. Individuals who have had ischemic stroke can be given a drug called tissue plasminogen activator within three hours from the onset of symptoms to limit damage.

Surgical procedures may be used in the treatment of some cases of cerebrovascular disease. In carotid endarterectomy, an incision is made into a carotid artery to remove the plaque and improve blood flow. In carotid angioplasty, a balloon-tipped catheter is inserted into the artery. The balloon is then inflated to press the plaque against the artery walls, reopening the vessel. A metal mesh tube, called a stent, may be inserted into the artery to help keep it open.

Treatment for hemorrhagic stroke often includes surgery to relieve intracranial pressure resulting from the bleeding. The defective blood vessel must be sealed off, and blood flow must be redirected to other vessels.

Prevention

Practicing certain simple behaviors can help a person prevent the development of cerebrovascular disease. These behaviors include not smoking; exercising regularly; avoiding obesity; controlling blood pressure; eating a healthy diet; and avoiding anger, stress, and other strong negative emotions.

Less Common Cerebrovascular Conditions

Vascular malformations are abnormal connections between, or malformations of, arteries or veins. Arteriovenous malformations are tangles of abnormally formed arteries or veins, with a high rate for bleeding. In moyamoya disease, the carotid arteries and their branches may become irreversibly blocked. Venous angiomas are benign tumors in veins. A vein of Galen malformation is an abnormal connection between arteries and veins that develops in the brain during embryonic growth.

A. J. Smuskiewicz

See also: Arrhythmias/Dysrhythmias; Arteriovenous Malformations; Atherosclerosis; Cardiovascular Disease; Congenital Heart Disease; Coronary Artery Disease; Heart Diseases; Stroke; Venous Disorders

Further Reading

American Association of Neurological Surgeons. (2005, December). Patient information: Cerebrovascular disease. Retrieved from http://www.aans.org/Patient%20Information /Conditions%20and%20Treatments/Cerebrovascular%20Disease.aspx.

Centers for Disease Control and Prevention. (2015). Cerebrovascular disease or stroke. Retrieved from http://www.cdc.gov/nchs/fastats/stroke.htm#.

Cleveland Clinic. (2015). Cerebrovascular occlusive disease: Overview. Retrieved from https://my.clevelandclinic.org/services/heart/disorders/carotid-artery/cerebrovascular -occlusive-disease.

LifeBridge Health. (2015). Cerebrovascular disease. Retrieved from http://www.lifebridge health.org/Main/CerebrovascularDisease.aspx.

Taylor, J. B. (2008). *My Stroke of Insight: A Brain Scientist's Personal Journey*. New York: Plume-Penguin.

CERVICAL CANCER

Cervical cancer is cancer of the cervix, the lower part of the uterus. This cancer can affect either of the two main types of cells in the cervix—the squamous cells in the exocervix (near the vagina) or the glandular cells in the endocervix (near the main body of the uterus). These two cell types meet in an area called the transformation zone.

Approximately 90 percent of cervical cancers affect squamous cells. Such cancer is known as squamous cell carcinoma, and it usually begins to develop in the transformation zone. Most other types of cervical cancer, known as adenocarcinoma, affect the glandular cells. This cancer usually develops in the mucus-producing cells of the cervix. Some types of cervical cancer affect both squamous and glandular cells.

According to the American Cancer Society (2015), about 12,900 new cases of cervical cancer are diagnosed, and about 4,100 women die from cervical cancer, each year in the United States.

Risk Factors

The risk for cervical cancer increases between the ages of 20 and 50, when most cases are diagnosed. Risk is also related to ethnicity, with Hispanic women at the greatest risk, followed by—in descending order—African Americans, Asians and Pacific Islanders, whites, and Native Americans. Research suggests that some cases are associated with an inherited condition that makes a woman's immune system less able to resist infection with human papilloma virus (HPV). Infection with certain strains of this sexually transmitted disease (STD), which can cause genital warts in both men and women, is the greatest risk factor for cervical cancer. In fact, most researchers believe that HPV infection—especially the strains HPV 16 and 18—is necessary for cervical cancer to develop. Other sexually transmitted infections that raise the risk of cervical cancer are chlamydia and HIV, the virus that causes AIDS.

Certain lifestyle factors are associated with increased risk for cervical cancer, including smoking, a diet low in fruits and vegetables, being overweight, and long-term use of birth control pills. In addition, women are at elevated risk if they have had three or more pregnancies, if they were younger than 17 during their first pregnancy, and if their mothers were given the drug diethylstilbestrol (DES) when they were pregnant. DES was used between 1940 and 1971 to prevent miscarriage.

Symptoms

Cervical cancer usually does not produce noticeable symptoms in its early stages. But after the cancer establishes itself in a relatively large area of the cervix, symptoms commonly develop. These symptoms may include abnormal vaginal bleeding and other unusual vaginal discharges and pain during intercourse. Because identical symptoms could be caused by other conditions, a medical diagnosis is necessary to determine the cause.

Diagnosis

Doctors advise women to get regular Pap tests, or Pap smears, so that cellular changes in cervical tissue can be found and addressed in either pre-cancerous or early cancerous stages. Although not all pre-cancerous conditions develop into cancer, doctors usually recommend treatment at the pre-cancerous stage to minimize the risk. Pap tests can also detect HPV infection.

If a Pap test reveals suspicious results in the form of abnormal cervical cells, additional tests are needed to arrive at a definitive diagnosis. In a colposcopy pelvic examination, the interior of the cervix is inspected with a magnifying instrument called a colposcope, and a small piece of tissue is removed for a biopsy. Biopsies of cervical tissue can reveal clear evidence of squamous cell carcinoma, adenocarcinoma, or other cervical cancer under microscopic examination.

If cancer is confirmed, various imaging tests can be performed to determine the stage of cancer development and, thus, the most appropriate treatment strategy. Such tests could include computed tomography (CT), magnetic resonance imaging (MRI), and positron emission tomography (PET).

Prevention and Treatment

Because HPV infection is the greatest risk for cervical cancer, preventing HPV infection is crucial to preventing cervical cancer. Thus, condoms should be used and other protective measures should be taken regarding sexual intercourse. Vaccinations against HPV are recommended for all children at age 11 or 12, before they are exposed to the virus. If not vaccinated at that age, females can be vaccinated through age 26 and males through age 21.

Treatment for cervical cancer is most successful when begun in its early stages. As previously indicated, the early stages of this cancer can be detected by getting regular Pap tests. The use of the Pap test as a screening tool is credited with reducing the death rate from cervical cancer by more than 50 percent from 1985 to 2015.

Cervical cancer development is classified into nine stages, with five-year survival rates for these stages ranging from 93 percent to 15 percent.

Once cancer is diagnosed and its stage of development is determined, a treatment strategy can be initiated. The four main treatment options are surgery, radiation therapy, chemotherapy, and targeted therapy. Some combination of these therapies is usually used.

Many kinds of surgical procedures are available. These procedures range from destruction of abnormal tissue with a focused laser beam to removal of the uterus and adjoining tissues in a radical hysterectomy. In advanced cases, in which the cancer has spread widely, even more radical surgery—involving removal of the vagina, bladder, rectum, and part of the colon—may be necessary.

Radiation therapy might be administered in the form of external beams or as an internal radiation source placed near the cancerous tissue. Medications commonly used in general cervical cancer treatment include cisplatin, carboplatin, and paclitaxel. In targeted therapy, medications are selected for their effectiveness in targeting specific biological changes that occur in cervical cancer. For example, drugs known as angiogenesis inhibitors block the development of new blood vessels that cancer tumors need to grow.

A. J. Smuskiewicz

See also: HPV (Human Papillomavirus); Sexually Transmitted Diseases; Squamous Cell Carcinoma; Women's Health

Further Reading

American Cancer Society. (2015). Cervical cancer. Retrieved from http://www.cancer.org/cancer/cervicalcancer/.

Centers for Disease Control and Prevention (CDC). (2015, October 28). Cervical cancer. Retrieved from http://www.cdc.gov/cancer/cervical/.

Mayo Clinic. (2015, January 31). Cervical cancer. Retrieved from http://www.mayoclinic.org/diseases-conditions/cervical-cancer/basics/definition/con-20030522.

McCormick, C. C., & Giuntoli II, R. L. (2010). *Johns Hopkins Patients' Guide to Cervical Cancer.* Burlington, MA: Jones & Bartlett Learning.

National Cancer Institute. (2015). Cervical cancer—for patients. Retrieved from http://www.cancer.gov/types/cervical.

WomensHealth.gov. (2014, April 21). Cervical cancer. Retrieved from http://www.womenshealth.gov/publications/our-publications/fact-sheet/cervical-cancer.html.

CHARCOT-MARIE-TOOTH DISEASE

Charcot-Marie-Tooth (CMT) disease is a term that represents a group of hereditary disorders that affect nerves of the arms and legs. The condition is associated with muscle weakness, decreased muscle mass, and often decreased sensation, and it is the most common inherited neurologic disorder. It is also known as hereditary motor and sensory neuropathy, hereditary peroneal nerve dysfunction, progressive neuropathic (peroneal) muscular atrophy, and neuropathy-peroneal (hereditary).

The different types of CMT are the following:

CMT type 1 is due to abnormalities in the protective sheath of the nerve cell.
CMT type 2 is due to abnormalities in the nerve fiber.
CMT type 3 abnormality is related to severe problems with the nerve sheath that is present in infancy and causes very severe muscle wasting, weakness, and problems with sensation.
CMT 4 includes several different types of nerve associated muscle and sensory problems.
CMT X caused by mutations in the X chromosome.
There are approximately 125,000 cases of CMT in the United States.

History

In 1886, the French Professor Jean Martin Charcot and his student Pierre Marie published the first description of a condition called peroneal muscular atrophy, where they observed a form of muscle weakness and wasting that began in the legs.

In 1886, Professor Howard Henry Tooth, who was at Cambridge, described the condition called peroneal muscular atrophy in his dissertation.

In 1968, the disease was divided into two types, based on differences in pathology and physiology; since then Charcot-Marie-Tooth disease has been further divided based on its genetic causes.

Symptoms and Signs

The symptoms of CMT can appear in mid-childhood, early adulthood, or adolescence, but it can also occur later in life. The symptoms vary widely, even among the same family members, and generally worsen over time.

The symptoms may first begin in the feet and legs and may eventually affect the hands, arms, and thighs. There may be no pain involved initially, although later pain can range from mild to severe.

Often, foot deformities develop and muscle weakness can make it difficult to balance when walking.

Key symptoms and features of the disease include:

Aching or burning sensations in the feet and lower legs
Awkward walking pattern because of a higher than normal stepping pattern
Claw-like hand[s]
Curled toes
Decreased leg and foot sensation
Decreased running ability
Decreased sensitivity to touch, heat, and cold
Dropped foot or problem lifting the ankle upward or holding it up
Fatigue with activities that require strength and mobility
Foot deformities
Frequent tripping or falling
Gradual hearing loss, deafness, or loss of vision in rare cases

Hand and arm weakness
High foot arches
Loss of muscle mass in the feet and legs
Numbness of the legs and feet
Pain
Poor handwriting
Respiratory weakness in rare cases
Slapping gait or walking pattern
Weakness of the feet, legs, or hips

Key Causes and Risk Factors

The key cause of Charcot-Marie-Tooth disease is genetic due to mutations in genes that control the structure and function of the nerves to the lower and upper limbs.

The nerve damage that results produces weaker impulses to the muscles of the limbs, and at the same time, the brain may not receive pain messages from the limbs as a result.

A person who has a family member with this disease is at greater risk for the condition.

Other related causes include neuropathies, such as diabetes.

Diagnostic Procedures

A physical exam, nerve conduction studies, electromyography to test the function of the muscles, muscle and nerve biopsies, and genetic testing are examples of the diagnostic procedures used to detect CMT.

Treatments

Medications for pain if necessary might be recommended, along with physical therapy, occupational therapy, orthopedic devices such as braces or orthopedic shoes, or surgery.

Exercises—especially stretching exercises, exercises to build aerobic endurance, and strength, balance, and mobility exercises—might be helpful.

Assistive devices, such as walker or cane, and good lighting to void stumbling and falling are also indicated for the person unsteady on his or her feet because falls can lead to serious injury.

Foot care is also important to prevent complications and can include daily foot inspections to prevent ulcers, wounds, and infections and careful cutting of the nails.

Wearing the right footwear and keeping the feet moisturized and pliable helps to reduce pain and discomfort from the condition.

Prognosis

The outlook for the disease depends on its severity, and appropriate treatments can help the affected person to manage the disease.

Although the disease may not affect life expectancy, there may be progressive muscle weakness and difficulty walking, with injuries to the body because of lack of adequate sensation.

Research may help to prevent the condition or to better treat this condition and may involve gene therapy or the use of hormones that promote nerve growth and possibly prevent nerve degeneration in the future.

Ray Marks

See also: Diabetes, Type 1; Neurological Diseases; Neuromuscular Disorders; Physical Therapy

Further Reading

Charcot-Marie-Tooth Association. (2015). What is CMT? Retrieved from http://www.cmtausa.org/understanding-cmt/what-is-cmt/.
Genetics Home Reference. (2015, October 26). What is Charcot-Marie-Tooth disease? Retrieved from http://ghr.nlm.nih.gov/condition/charcot-marie-tooth-disease.
Mayo Clinic. (2013, February 14). Charcot-Marie-Tooth disease. Retrieved from http://www.mayoclinic.org/diseases-conditions/charcot-marie-tooth-disease/basics/definition/con-20029920.
National Institute of Neurological Disorders and Stroke. (2015, July 17). Charcot-Marie-Tooth disease fact sheet. Retrieved from http://www.ninds.nih.gov/disorders/charcot_marie_tooth/detail_charcot_marie_tooth.htm.

CHOLESTEROL

Overview

Found in every cell in the body, cholesterol is a waxy substance produced mainly in the liver; it also comes from eating dairy products, eggs, and meat. The body produces the cholesterol it needs to produce vitamin D and some hormones and to insulate nerve fibers and maintain healthy cells. But too much cholesterol can cause heart disease, heart attack, atherosclerosis, and stroke, and too little may suggest an underlying chronic disorder.

Cholesterol travels through the blood by attaching to lipoproteins—a type of a protein. Low-density lipoproteins (LDL), often called bad cholesterol, can clog arteries and increase the risk of heart disease. High-density lipoproteins (HDL) are called good cholesterol because they help the body clear arteries, which reduces the risk of heart disease. Triglycerides are another type of fat circulating through the body attached to lipoproteins. Stored in the fat cells, they convert calories to energy, but excess calories can lead to high triglycerides, or hypertriglyceridemia, a condition also associated with a greater risk of heart disease.

Age and sex (men 45 years and older, women 55 years and older), being overweight or obese, eating a high-fat diet, family history, inactivity, smoking (which can reduce HDL cholesterol), diabetes and other diseases, and some medications are known to cause or contribute to potentially harmful high cholesterol levels.

Types of Cholesterol Disorders

Dyslipidemia refers to disorders that have lipid, or fat, levels in the blood that are too high or too low. The most common types of dyslipidemia are high levels of LDL cholesterol, low levels of HDL cholesterol, and high levels of triglycerides. The most prevalent common is hyperlipidemia (also called hyperlipoproteinemia because the fat is attached to proteins in the blood and high blood cholesterol), which is an excess of cholesterol and triglycerides. Increasing the risk for many health problems, hyperlipidemia can be further categorized into two disorders: hypercholesterolemia, or high level of cholesterol, and hypertriglyceridemia, a high level of triglycerides.

Much less common is the disorder hypolipidemia, otherwise known as low blood cholesterol, which occurs when the blood has an unusually low level of fat. This condition may indicate an underlying illness such as an overactive thyroid, anemia, cancer, liver disease, chronic infection, malnutrition, and digestion disorders. It may also be the result of rare genetic disorders, which affect growth, eye development, intellectual ability, and digestion.

Nearly 74 million adults in the United States have high LDL cholesterol, and almost 31 million adults have a high total cholesterol level that puts their risk for heart disease at about twice that as people with normal levels. Changes in eating and activity habits can often reduce cholesterol levels, and medications may be prescribed when these measures prove inadequate. Treatment for low cholesterol focuses on the underlying cause.

Symptoms

Regardless of the type of high cholesterol, people usually have no symptoms. Occasionally, deposits of cholesterol form underneath the skin in those with very high levels of cholesterol or who have familial combined hyperlipidemia, a genetic disorder that increases blood fats; when they appear, symptoms may include chest pain, cramping in the calf muscles, sores that do not heal on the toes, and sudden muscle or balance problems similar to a stroke. People who have a high level of triglycerides may experience lesions on their skin, or with extremely high levels, develop inflammation of the pancreas. Low blood cholesterol usually does not show any symptoms, most often resulting from another disorder or illness.

Causes and Risk Factors

Causes of the types of high cholesterol are genetic, as well as age and sex. As both men and women age, LDL cholesterol levels tend to rise; women younger than 55 usually have levels lower than men, but after age 55, their levels often become rise. Other factors that contribute to an increase risk in high cholesterol are eating foods high in saturated and trans fats, being overweight, a large waist circumference, a lack of regular exercise, smoking, and drinking excess alcohol. Diabetes, high-blood pressure, hypothyroidism, Cushing's syndrome, and kidney failure may also increase risk, as well as taking birth control pills, beta-blockers, estrogen, corticosteroids, and some diuretic medications. Low cholesterol can be caused by thyroid and liver diseases, anemia, malnutrition or the inability to absorb food, and rare genetic abnormalities or disorders.

Diagnosis

Medical history, physical examination, and blood tests taken after fasting for 9 to 12 hours can diagnose cholesterol disorders, including the levels of LDL cholesterol, HDL cholesterol, and triglycerides. Blood cholesterol tests indicate the amount of fat in the blood. A total cholesterol level test measures both LDL and HDL levels in milligrams per deciliter (mg/dL); normal target levels are LDL 70 to 130 mg/dL (lower is better), HDL more than 50 mg/dL (higher is better), total cholesterol less than 200 mg/dL (lower is better), and triglycerides 10 to 150 mg/dL (lower is better).

Treatments

Even lacking outward symptoms, high cholesterol does not go away on its own, and it requires action to avoid narrowing and clogging of the arteries, which can lead to heart attacks, chest pain, poor circulation, and stroke, all of which can be life-threatening. After ruling out underlying illnesses or causes, treatment for high cholesterol includes changes in diet, weight reduction, and additional exercise. If necessary, according to individual risk, medications may be prescribed, although they help manage rather than cure high blood cholesterol. The most commonly prescribed drugs are statins; others include selective cholesterol absorption inhibitors, resins, fibrates, and niacin. Low blood cholesterol treatment depends on the underlying cause.

Prevention

Healthful lifestyle habits that can prevent most types of high cholesterol include eating a diet with many vegetables, fruits, and fiber-rich whole grains that is also low in salt and saturated and trans fats; regular exercise; maintaining a healthy weight; not smoking, reducing alcohol; getting adequate sleep; and preventing and treating medical conditions that may contribute to developing high cholesterol. Prevention of abnormally low blood cholesterol depends on its underlying condition.

Prognosis and Outcomes

If untreated, high cholesterol levels can lead to hardening of the arteries, which over time can cause heart disease, stroke, and other diseases. Lifestyle habits, preventive measures, and medications can manage high cholesterol not caused by genetic inheritance, which may be more difficult to control.

Ray Marks

See also: Atherosclerosis; Cardiovascular Disease; Diabetes, Type 2; Diet and Nutrition; Food Guides from the USDA; Heart Diseases; Obesity; Prediabetes; Stroke

Further Reading

American Heart Association. (2015). Confused about cholesterol? Retrieved from http://www.heart.org/HEARTORG/Conditions/Cholesterol/Cholesterol_UCM_001089_Sub HomePage.jsp.

Centers for Disease Control and Prevention. (2015, March 16). Cholesterol. Retrieved from http://www.cdc.gov/cholesterol/index.htm.

Hormone Health Network. (2013, April). Dyslipidemia. Retrieved from http://www.hormone.org/diseases-and-conditions/heart-health-and-metabolism/dyslipidemia.

Mayo Clinic. (2016). High cholesterol. Retrieved from http://www.mayoclinic.org/diseases-conditions/high-blood-cholesterol/home/ovc-20181871.

National Institutes of Health. (2012). High blood cholesterol: What you need to know. Retrieved from http://www.nhlbi.nih.gov/health/public/heart/chol/wyntk.htm.

CHRONIC DISEASE MANAGEMENT

Background

A chronic disease is a medical problem that lasts for a long time, possibly a lifetime. Because people with chronic disease do not get better in the same way as people who have an acute condition that goes away in a reasonable space of time, chronic diseases are very hard to deal with. These diseases require not only that you visit medical providers regularly, but that the affected person be vigilant to avoid situations that can worsen the condition. This is very hard physically, as well as emotionally and socially, especially for young people, and lowers quality of life, in general, because most of these diseases cause pain, fatigue, depression, and disability, and there are periods when these symptoms flare up more than usual and often require multiple hospitalizations if severe.

Indeed, disability and poor quality of life attributable to chronic diseases such as arthritis, diabetes, and heart disease constitute challenging public health problems for American society, as well as most modern societies across the globe. In the absence of any effective cure for these conditions, and others such as cancer, the secondary prevention of complications and improving quality of life and functional capacity through better disease self-management becomes critical and is high among the key objectives of medical practitioners. The organizing focus of such disease self-management should be on improving coping, communication, and control by enhancing self-efficacy for managing one's illness, avoiding complications, and prolonging one's life by making better lifestyle choices.

Management

Among chronic diseases and conditions that require continuous management are

Alzheimer's disease and other dementias
Arthritis
Asthma

Cancer
Chronic obstructive pulmonary disease
Diabetes
Heart disease (or cardiovascular disease)
Osteoporosis

Interventions

The chronic care model (CCM) is a framework to improve care for chronic conditions at both the individual and population level. It encourages more productive interactions between patients and health care providers and stresses the importance of all essential elements of a health care system, including delivery of information and resources that encourage high-quality chronic care, self-management support, and self-management that integrates the skills and choices of patients with the services and support they receive from family, friends, worksites, and organizations and that takes culture, as well as the physical and policy environments of neighborhoods, communities, health care systems, and governments, into account.

To assist with the aforementioned self-management processes that most adults with one or more chronic diseases need to adopt, the Stanford University School of Medicine Chronic Disease Management Program has developed a 2.5-hour workshop, conducted once a week for six weeks in community settings. People with varying chronic diseases can attend together. The workshops are led by two trained facilitators, both of whom are chronic disease suffers.

Topics include but are not limited to:

- Strategies for dealing with frustration, fatigue, pain, and isolation
- Appropriate exercise for maintaining muscle strength and endurance, as well as joint range of motion and flexibility
- Appropriate use of medications
- Approaches for effectively communicating with providers and caregivers, as well as families and friends
- Nutrition and chronic disease management
- Strategies of how to understand whether new treatments are appropriate for the individual

Each participant receives a copy of the book *Living a Healthy Life with Chronic Conditions*, 3rd edition, by Lorig et al. (2006) and an audio relaxation tape, *Time for Healing*, by Catherine Regan.

However, it is especially important to ensure that the poor and disadvantaged in society are exposed to such programs in order to prevent premature death and unnecessary disability. Thus, programs such as that mentioned earlier, plus opportunities for improving one's diet, more physical activity, and tobacco cessation and receiving equitable and good quality health care need to be available to all, even those in the poorest settings. Of the 35 million people who died from chronic disease in 2005, half were under 70 years of age, and 80 percent of these deaths occurred in low and middle income countries (World Health Organization 2015).

In addition, if you are healthy, but your friend or family member has a chronic disease, you should try to understand the challenges he or she faces and be supportive. In particular, many people with chronic disease look healthy, and this makes their struggle especially frustrating.

If you are a chronic disease sufferer and need assistance to manage your health condition more optimally, it is important to request this and discuss this with your medical provider. You may also need to modify your living arrangements, use assistive devices, and work with your employer to maximize your ability to have a high life quality.

Your provider may encourage you to undertake a self-management program aimed at structural behavior change to help you sustain the benefits of the medical and surgical treatments you may be receiving. The best programs should include techniques aimed at behavioral change, be tailored individually, take the patient's perspective into account, and may vary with the course of the patient's disease and comorbidities. These should be preceded by appropriate assessments often by more than one health professional and may involve assessment of the home and family situation.

Other approaches include psychosocial interventions, such as cognitive behavioral therapy, patient education, physical therapy, occupational therapy, respiratory therapy, nursing, electronic prompts, podiatry, and nutrition counseling.

Ray Marks

See also: Depression; Diet and Nutrition; Mental Disorders; Occupational Health; Physical Therapy; Rehabilitation

Further Reading
Baumann, L. C., & Dang, T. T. (2012). Helping patients with chronic conditions overcome barriers to self-care. *Nurse Practitioner, 37*, 32–38.
Centers for Disease Control and Prevention. (2015, August 26). Chronic disease overview. Retrieved from http://www.cdc.gov/chronicdisease/overview/index.htm.
Lorig, K., Holman, H., Sobel, D., & Laurent, D. (2006). *Living a Healthy Life with Chronic Conditions,* 3rd ed. Boulder, CO: Bull Publishing Company.
Marks, R., Allegrante, J. P., & Lorig, K. (2005). A review and synthesis of research evidence for self-efficacy-enhancing interventions for reducing chronic disability: Implications for health education practice (part I). *Health Promotion and Practice, 6*(1), 37–43.
New York City Department of Health. (2015, May). Chronic diseases and conditions. Retrieved from http://www.health.ny.gov/diseases/chronic/.
Palo Alto Medical Foundation. (2013, October). Health problems & chronic diseases. Retrieved from http://www.pamf.org/teen/health/diseases/.
Regan, C., Time for Healing CD: Relaxation for the Mind and Body, 1st ed. Boulder, CO: Bull Publishing Company.
Stanford Medicine. (2015). Chronic disease self-management program. Retrieved from http://patienteducation.stanford.edu/programs/cdsmp.html.
World Health Organization. (2015). Chronic diseases and health promotion. Retrieved from http://www.who.int/chp/en/.

CHRONIC FATIGUE SYNDROME

Background

Chronic fatigue syndrome (CFS) is a complex and debilitating health problem associated with extreme fatigue that is not relieved by resting or sleeping. The fatigue may also be worsened by physical and/or mental fatigue and is generally not explained by any other medical condition. It can be so severe that the person with this condition must remain in bed and may become extremely disabled or challenged with regard to his or her ability to carry out normal activities of daily living. Currently, a name change from CFS to ME/CFS—myalgic encephalopathy/chronic fatigue syndrome—is being proposed because of the belief that the syndrome known as CFS is often associated with misunderstandings or is trivialized by practitioners as well as affected individuals. ME/CFS affects more than a million U.S. citizens. This may be an underestimate because it is difficult to diagnose, and not all people with this condition may seek help. CFS is also known as chronic fatigue and immune system dysfunction, myalgic encephalopathy, or myalgic encephalomyelitis.

Symptoms

The symptoms of CFS are said to have a distinct onset and can affect several body systems and exist in differing intensities. To meet diagnostic criteria for CFS, the individual must have unexplained persistent fatigue for six months or longer and at least four of these signs and symptoms:

    Enlarged neck or armpit lymph nodes
    Extreme exhaustion lasting more than 24 hours after either physical or mental exercise
    Headache that is not like a normal headache in terms of pattern or severity
    Impaired concentration
    Impaired memory
    Muscle aches and pain
    Pain that moves from one joint to the other without any accompanying swelling or redness
    Unrefreshing sleep

Other symptoms may include:

    Confusion
    Fatigue or continued tiredness
    Forgetfulness
    Inability to fall asleep or insomnia
    Irritability
    Mild fever
    Reduced ability to function physically
    Sore throat
    Sudden severe fatigue, especially following a flu-like illness
    Weakness

Other related symptoms can include:

Dry eyes and mouth
Impaired circulation in the hands and feet
Intolerance to alcohol
Irritable bowel syndrome
Painful menstrual periods in women
Visual disturbances

Key Causes and Risk Factors

The cause of CFS is not known, but several theories to explain this syndrome exist. Alone or in combination, these include infectious agents such as the herpes or Epstein-Barr viruses; immune system hyperactivity problems; food allergies and/or metal allergies; abnormal hormone levels and production; having a hereditary predisposition to CFS, especially related to genes involved in the sympathetic nervous system and the hypothalamus-adrenal gland axis that controls the responses of the body to injuries and stresses; and psychological stress-related theories.

As well, experts suspect a syndrome called central sensitization, or hypersensitivity to sensations and pain stimuli, may possibly be to blame, in part, for CFS.

Evidence for the presence of a chronically active immune system as a cause of CFS includes:

- The presence of high levels of pro-inflammatory cellular messengers in the immune system called cytokines
- Decreased functioning of natural killer cells
- Evidence of antibodies in the blood stream or tissues known to be involved in attacking ones own tissues
- Reduced numbers of white blood cells that specifically counter infectious agents

Risk Factors

Age, especially those in the age range 30 to 50 years of age
Brain abnormalities
Environmental factors
Genetic factors
Gender—women are diagnosed more often with CFS than men
Lifestyle—being overweight and inactive may predispose to CFS
Previous illnesses
Stress

Diagnosis

There is no single test that is diagnostic of CFS. Many tests may be performed to rule out any specific underlying health problem.

Symptoms: There must be a proven absence of other causes of chronic fatigue.

Procedures to rule out other conditions can include investigations directed toward examining the presence of a sleep disorder; immune disorders; muscle or nerve diseases; endocrine diseases; medical problems such as anemia, diabetes, underactive thyroid gland, or tumors; and mental and emotional health problems or psychiatric conditions such as depression, anxiety, bipolar disorder, or schizophrenia.

Treatment

Treatment is generally aimed at relieving symptoms and, depending on the severity of the syndrome, may include:

Acupuncture
Biofeedback
Breathing exercises
Combination of gentle exercise and psychological counseling
Controlled or supervised exercising
Dietary changes
Emotional support and counseling for the affected individual and their families/
    friends
Hypnosis
Lifestyle and home remedies including stress reduction, improved sleep habits, pacing
    of activities
Massage

Medications may include:

Anti-anxiety drugs
Antibiotics to activate the immune system
Antidepressants
Antihistamines or allergy medications
Antidepressants, which can relieve depression and at low doses can improve sleep and
    reduce pain
Antivirals such as Ampligen, which may improve the body's use of oxygen
D-ribose, which may improve cellular function, energy, sleep, mental clarity, and pain
Nonsteroidal anti-inflammatory drugs such as Advil
Psychostimulants such as Ritalin to help memory and concentration
Sleeping pills or avoiding caffeine may improve sleep quality and duration
Meditation
Physical therapy
Stress management programs
Therapeutic support groups, which have other people with CFS as members
Yoga or tai-chi

Prognosis

While some people recover in six months to a year, there is no cure for some with CFS, and for those individuals, possible complications may include depression, social isolation, lifestyle restrictions, medication side effects, and increased work absences; therefore, early diagnosis and intervention is strongly indicated.

More research to establish the causes of ME/CFS and the efficacy of different intervention modes are strongly indicated.

Prevention of Flare-Ups

People with CFS may try to avoid doing too much on days they do not feel well or energetic. They may want to balance their activities to include adequate rest and activity periods. They may want to break down chores into small manageable steps. Relaxation techniques that are useful for relieving stress and chronic pain may also be helpful.

Ray Marks

See also: Environment; Genetics and Genomics; Physical Activity

Further Reading

Centers for Disease Control and Prevention. (2015, April 7). Chronic fatigue syndrome (CFS). Retrieved from http://www.cdc.gov/cfs/index.html.

Mayo Clinic. (2014, July 1). Chronic fatigue syndrome. Retrieved from http://www.mayoclinic.org/diseases-conditions/chronic-fatigue-syndrome/basics/definition/con-20022009.

Office on Women's Health. (2014, September 4). Chronic fatigue syndrome. Retrieved from http://womenshealth.gov/publications/our-publications/fact-sheet/chronic-fatigue-syndrome.html.

Solve ME/CFS Initiative. (2015). What is ME/CFS? Retrieved from http://solvecfs.org/.

University of Maryland Medical Center. (2015). Chronic fatigue syndrome—causes. Retrieved from http://umm.edu/health/medical/reports/articles/chronic-fatigue-syndrome.

CIRCULATION DISORDERS

Description

The circulatory system comprises the heart and blood vessels, including arteries, veins, and capillaries. This network carries oxygen and nutrients to all cells of the body with each heartbeat and removes wastes and carbon dioxide. Problems in the circulatory system affect more than 64 million Americans, including teens, and often involve narrowing of the arteries due to plaque buildup or associated risk factors for atherosclerosis such as smoking. These disorders include heart disorders, blood disorders, and blood vessel disorders, and any or all of these can reduce the nutrients and oxygen conveyed to the cells and can allow waste products that cause illness to accumulate in the body. These disorders are also termed vascular disorders.

Common circulatory disorders include angina, arrhythmia, atherosclerosis, cardiomyopathy, hypertension or high blood pressure, coronary artery diseases, peripheral vascular disease. Because the essential requirements of the body will remain unmet if the circulation is less than optimal, several physical and psychological problems can arise.

Common Signs and Symptoms

- Abnormal pulse
- Abnormal blood pressure
- Chest pain
- Claudication or leg pain or cramping after activity
- Coldness of the hands or feet
- Confusion or loss of memory
- Difficulty breathing or shortness of breath
- Dizziness
- Fainting
- Fatigue or lack of energy
- Frequent headaches
- Hair loss because nutrients may not be reaching hair follicles, which then weaken
- Impotence if circulation is severely compromised
- Increased risk of infections due to dysfunction of the immune system
- Lack of stamina in daily life
- Leg cramps after walking or workouts
- Numbness or tingling in the legs, hands, feet, or toes
- Pain, often located in the legs
- Skin color changes, wherein the skin may turn yellowish, blue (cyanosed) or pale
- Skin dryness
- Slow healing of infections, wounds
- Swelling, often in the arms or legs, or around the affected blood vessels
- Weakness

Other problems can include blood clots and pulmonary embolism, a life-threatening condition caused by blockage of an artery in the lung due to a blood clot.

Circulation symptoms can also occur in the head, arms, kidneys, stomach, and other organs.

An interruption of the blood flow to the brain can cause a stroke, while impaired blood flow to the heart may cause a heart attack.

Key Causes and Risk Factors

There are many causes of circulatory disorders, including:

Aging because blood circulation becomes poorer as one ages.

Congenital heart defects or inherited circulatory diseases are risk factors as well.

Having a family history of a vascular or heart disease is a common risk factor, as is pregnancy, excessive sitting, standing, illness, or injury.

Acquired circulatory problems can occur as a result of unhealthy lifestyles, especially smoking, alcoholism, and drug abuse.

Physical inactivity or insufficient exercise, poor eating habits, and certain medical problems also cause circulation problems.

Medical conditions that affect poor blood circulation are diabetes, thyroid disease, high blood pressure, obesity, anemia, and pneumonia and can result in circulatory problems.

Other common conditions causing circulatory problems are aneurysms or localized weaknesses of vessel walls; vascular malformations or abnormal connections between veins and arteries; and Raynaud's disease, where arteries of the fingers go into spasm and deprive the fingers of blood supply.

Occupational exposure such as excessive vibration, or cold, and trauma can cause a circulatory disorder.

Diagnosis

Today, there are home medical diagnostic tests that may be relevant to circulatory disease. These approaches that can also be performed by a physician include:

- Angiogram tests
- Blood pressure tests
- Heart function tests
- Heart electrocardiogram tests

Treatment

Lifestyle changes such as giving up smoking and limiting fats, cholesterol, refined sugars, and salt intake may be helpful as may supervised exercise and losing weight.

Medications such as anti-inflammatory drugs and clot dissolvers as well as those that help in controlling blood pressure or blood glucose, or both, may be helpful.

Surgery may also be useful as indicated.

Prognosis or Outcome

The outlook for a circulatory disorder depends on the cause and duration of the problem, as well as age.

Living a healthy lifestyle of moderation is likely to result in a favorable outcome, if regular medical visits are undertaken and recommendations are followed.

Prevention strategies against circulation disorders are similar to treatment strategies and include having routine check-ups, not smoking or quitting smoking, having a healthy diet, exercising regularly and avoiding excessive stress.

Ray Marks

See also: Angina; Arrhythmias/Dysrhythmias; Atherosclerosis; Cardiomyopathy; Coronary Artery Disease; Heart Diseases; Hypertension; Vascular Disorders

Further Reading

American Heart Association. (2014, September 15). About peripheral artery disease (PAD). Retrieved from http://www.heart.org/HEARTORG/Conditions/More/PeripheralArteryDisease/About-Peripheral-Artery-Disease-PAD_UCM_301301_Article.jsp.

Johns Hopkins Medicine. (2015). Vascular conditions and diseases. Retrieved from http://www.hopkinsmedicine.org/healthlibrary/conditions/adult/cardiovascular_diseases/vascular_conditions_and_diseases_85,p08260/.

National Heart Lung and Blood Institute. (2015). Heart and vascular diseases. Retrieved from http://www.nhlbi.nih.gov/health/resources/heart.

Texas Heart Institute. (2015, August.) Peripheral vascular disease. Retrieved from http://www.texasheart.org/HIC/Topics/Cond/pvd.cfm.

Vascular Cures. (2014). What is vascular disease? Retrieved from http://www.vascularcures.org/about-vascular-disease.

COLON CANCER

Also called colorectal cancer or rectal cancer, colon cancer refers to the presence of cancer in either the colon or rectum, and these two conditions are often discussed together given their common features. The colon and rectum are important components of the digestive system and are involved in storage and expulsion of waste matter from foods.

In the majority of cases, cancer in either of these areas develops slowly, and most start out in the form of abnormal tissue growths that starts in the lining of these structures; these growths are called polyps.

Polyps can be readily detected if present and can either be cancerous or noncancerous (or benign) and can be surgically removed. A type of polyp that can become cancerous is known as an adenoma. These constitute the majority of cancers that form in the colon or rectum. Other types of tumors that can cause colon cancer occur more rarely and include sarcomas, lymphomas, melanomas, and carcinoid tumors.

According to the National Cancer Institute in the United States, the number of new cases and deaths in the United States attributable to colon or rectal cancer is currently 103,120 for colon cancer and 40,290 for new rectal cancer cases. The combined numbers of deaths are 51,690, and colorectal cancer remains the fourth most common cause of cancer-related deaths in the United States. From 2004 to 2008, the median age at diagnosis was 70, and for death from either colon or rectal cancer it was 75 years of age. Blacks were the most commonly affected group, and males generally had higher death rates from these conditions than females.

The five stages of colon cancer are as follows:

Stage 0—very early cancer localized to the innermost layer of the intestine
Stage I—the cancer is located in the inner layers of the colon
Stage II—the cancer has spread to the colon muscle wall
Stage III—cancer has spread to the lymph nodes
Stage IV—cancer has spread to distant sites such as other organs

Symptoms

Symptoms may not be present, but if they occur, they may include:

- Blood in the stool
- Change in bowel habits
- Change in character of stool
- Fatigue
- General stomach discomfort, cramps, or bloating
- Rectal pain
- Small-caliber narrow stools or ribbon-like stools
- Tenderness in the lower abdomen
- Unexplained nausea or vomiting
- Weakness
- Weight loss for no known reason

Key Risk Factors

Key risk factors include the following:

Being African American
Being older than 60 years of age
Diabetes
Diet high in fat or processed and red meats
Excess alcohol usage
Family history of colon cancer and polyps
Genetic syndromes such as familial adenomatous polyposis
Obesity
Personal history of breast, uterine, or ovarian cancer
Personal history of colorectal cancer or polyps
Radiation therapy for cancer
Smoking
Ulcerative colitis or Crohn's disease

Diagnosis

Diagnostic approaches and tools include abdominal exploration, barium enema lower gastrointestinal series investigations, blood tests to detect tumor markers, colonoscopy, complete blood count, digital rectal exam, fecal occult blood tests, fecal immunochemical tests, genetic testing, liver function tests, sigmoidoscopy, or virtual colonoscopy.

Treatment

There are several treatment options for colorectal cancers, including chemotherapy, drug therapy, immunotherapy, radiation therapy, surgery and ileostomy, colostomy, ileoanal reservoir, ostomy and continent ileostomy procedures, and/or vaccine therapy. Treatments can include a combination of one or more of these strategies.

Prognosis

If detected early, the outcome for colorectal cancer is quite positive. Recovery from colon cancer will depend on the extent of the disease before surgery and other treatments that are implemented. The outcome is best for tumors located solely in the inner layers of the colon and worse if the cancer has spread to other organs.

Prevention

Screening that includes imaging technologies, biopsy procedures, and tests for tumors using tumor markers are recommended for those aged 50 and above, until age 75, as well as earlier for high-risk groups. In addition to changing diet and lifestyle to include low-fat, high-fiber diets, drinking alcohol in moderation, exercising, and quitting smoking, colonoscopy screening to find polyps before they become cancerous reduces the risk of premature death.

Seeking medical care if you experience any of the symptoms listed herein and following up visits as recommended by the medical team or doctor is also important.

Ray Marks

See also: Breast Cancer; Cancer; Crohn's Disease; Diabetes, Type 1; Lymphoma; Melanoma; Ovarian Cancer; Ulcerative Colitis; Uterine Cancer

Further Reading

American Cancer Society. (2016). Colon/rectum cancer. Retrieved from http://www.cancer.org/cancer/colonandrectumcancer/.

Jorgenson, C. M., Gelb, B. S., Merritt, T. L., & Seeff, L. S. (2001). CDC's Screen for Life: A national colorectal cancer action campaign. *Journal of Women's Health and Gender-Based Medicine*, *10*(5), 417–422.

Mayo Clinic. (2012). Colon cancer. Retrieved from http://www.mayoclinic.com/health/colon-cancer/DS00035.

National Cancer Institute. (2014). Colorectal cancer screening: Basic fact sheet. Retrieved from http://www.cancer.gov/types/colorectal/screening-fact-sheet.

National Digestive Diseases Information Clearing House. (2012). Colonoscopy. Retrieved from http://digestive.niddk.nih.gov/ddiseases/pubs/colonoscopy/.

PubMed Health. (2012). Colon cancer. A.D.A.M. Medical Encyclopedia. Retrieved from http://www.ncbi.nlm.nih.gov/pubmedhealth/PMH0001308/.

COLOR BLINDNESS

Color blindness is a disorder that is identified by the reduced ability to see certain colors normally. The most common type of color blindness is the inability to distinguish between red and green. Less common is the inability to distinguish between blue and yellow, which affects about 5 percent of those with color blindness. A person who has difficulty seeing blue-yellow colors typically has trouble differentiating between red and green as well. Achromatopsia is the truest form of color blindness; a person with this rare disorder cannot distinguish colors at all. Instead, those who suffer from achromatopsia will picture everything in shades of gray. About 1 in 10 men suffer from some form of color blindness, while only around 1 in 200 women are color blind.

In a normally functioning eye, special photoreceptive nerve cells called cones are used to sense color. These cones contain pigments, which are a natural, light-sensitive substance that allow the eye to detect different colors. If one or more pigments are missing, a person will have some level of color blindness. The most common cause of color blindness is a genetic mutation. Inherited color blindness typically affects both eyes, and the severity of the condition does not change over the course of a lifetime. Such conditions as diabetes, multiple sclerosis, and Parkinson's disease can also cause color blindness. When disease is the cause, color blindness may affect one eye more severely than the other, and there is possibility for improvement when the underlying problem is successfully treated (if treatment is possible). Color blindness may also be a side effect of certain medications used to treat heart conditions and other ailments, and it can also occur as an effect of the aging process. Another possible cause of color blindness is long-term exposure to certain chemicals, including carbon disulfide, a flammable liquid used as a solvent in industrial processes.

Sometimes, parents notice signs of color blindness when a young child is first learning to distinguish colors. Others with more mild forms of color blindness remain unaware that they have a problem until later in life. For example, statistics show that some 40 percent of people with mild color blindness do not discover their condition until after completing high school. The symptoms of color blindness may vary depending on the level of severity. Signs of the condition include having difficulty interpreting color in a normal fashion, having trouble detecting shades of a certain color, or the inability to distinguish between particular colors. In extremely severe cases, a reduced ability to fully see color may be accompanied with jerky, side-to-side movements of the eye.

The inability to distinguish specific colors can affect a person's ability to work in certain fields, including fashion design and interior decorating. People with color blindness may also not be able to work as electricians because they need to be able to see color accurately when dealing with color-coded wires. Additionally, color blindness can affect normal, daily activities such as driving or getting dressed. Color blindness can be detected during an eye exam. While there is no known cure for the condition, it can sometimes be alleviated with special contact lenses or eyewear with colored filters.

The first known scientist to conduct a comprehensive study of color blindness was John Dalton. A late-18th-century British chemist and physicist, Dalton was interested in color blindness because it was a condition that both he and his brother suffered from. Although his theory that the problem lay in a discoloration of the liquid in the eyeball was disproved after his death, his research was so broadly recognized that inherited color blindness came to commonly be referred to as Daltonism within the scientific community. With their theories on color perception, 19th-century European researchers Thomas Young and Hermann von Helmholtz established the basic understanding of how color is interpreted through the eye.

Their Young-Helmholtz theory laid the groundwork for the modern understanding of color blindness. While inherited color blindness is still recognized as a lifelong condition with no cure, scientists are continuing to study gene replacement techniques that may one day be able to restore full color vision to those afflicted by the condition.

Tamar Burris

See also: Eye Diseases; Hyperopia; Myopia

Further Reading

Adams, N. (2014). *Healthy Vision: Prevent and Reverse Eye Disease through Better Nutrition.* Guilford, CT: Lyons Press.

American Academy of Opthalmology. (2013). What is color blindness? Retrieved from http://www.aao.org/eye-health/tips-prevention/what-is-color-blindness.

American Optometric Association. (2015). Color vision deficiency. Retrieved from http://www.aoa.org/patients-and-public/eye-and-vision-problems/glossary-of-eye-and-vision-conditions/color-deficiency?sso=y.

Kitchen, C. K. *Fact and Fiction of Healthy Vision: Eye Care for Adults and Children.* Westport, CT: Praeger, 2007.

Mayo Clinic. (2015). Poor color vision. Retrieved from http://www.mayoclinic.org/diseases-conditions/poor-color-vision/basics/definition/con-20022091.

COMPLEX REGIONAL PAIN SYNDROME

Complex regional pain syndrome (CRPS) is a rare chronic disorder characterized by intense pain in the arms, hands, legs, or feet. Formerly known as reflex sympathetic dystrophy syndrome, it occurs when the nervous system becomes overactive and sends constant pain signals to the brain that result in intense burning or aching pain; swelling; and changes in skin color, temperature, and moisture.

The cause is unknown, but it is usually associated with injury to a nerve or tissue and following surgery or immobilization. Anyone can develop the condition, but it is more common in women, and most people affected are between 25 and 55 years old. Although considered a rare disorder, as many as 200,000 people experience it in the United States in any given year. The earlier the diagnosis is made, the more likely treatment can prevent CRPS from worsening. It has no cure, but medications, other therapies, and surgery can improve symptoms that may lead to remission.

Symptoms

Continuous pain that remains intense is the main symptom of CRPS—specifically, the sensation of burning pain and skin sensitivity to the touch, as well as changes to the skin in temperature (warmer or cooler than elsewhere in the body), color (may by blotchy purple or red), and texture (shiny or sweaty). Additional symptoms include abnormal hair or nail growth patterns, swollen and stiff joints, weakness, and diminished range of motion in the affected area. Pain from the initial injury may spread to other parts of the body and worsen with emotional stress.

Key Causes and Risk Factors

Although the precise cause is unknown, the disorder occurs when the nervous system and the immune system malfunction as they respond to tissue damage from trauma. The nerves misfire, sending constant pain signals to the brain. Risk factors include having had surgery or experienced physical trauma, including cuts, lacerations, fractures, or burns; immobilization of limbs following a stroke or heart attack; and diabetes or hyperthyroidism.

Diagnosis

No one test can confirm CRPS, and a diagnosis is made based on symptoms. In addition to a complete medical history and physical examination, diagnostic tests may include x-rays, MRI, and bone scans, as well as thermography, which measures skin temperature and blood flow, and other nervous system tests that look for disturbances in the sympathetic nervous system.

Treatment

Early diagnosis can lead to the most effective treatment, which improves the possibility of recovery. Treatment is individualized and may require a combination of options. Research and clinical practice provide new information about methods, but the goal of all treatments is relieving pain and restoring function to affected limbs. Depending on the symptoms and their duration, treatments include medications such as topical analgesics, antidepressants, corticosteroids, and opioids; physical and occupational therapy; nerve blocks; spinal cord stimulation; and intrathecal drug pumps that deliver opioids or local anesthetics through the spinal cord; surgery may be needed if a nerve has been compressed.

Prognosis

Because no drug or combination of drugs has produced consistent long-term improvement of symptoms, some people with CRPS will have continual pain and disabilities even with treatment. The prognosis for those with CRPS varies, so others may experience remission. People with chronic symptoms may benefit from psychotherapy because the condition can lead to depression, anxiety, or post-traumatic stress disorder.

Ray Marks

See also: Anxiety Disorders; Depression; Diabetes, Type 1; Heart Diseases; Hyperthyroidism; PTSD (Post-traumatic Stress Disorder)

Further Reading

American Society for Surgery of the Hand (ASSH). (2012). Complex regional pain syndrome (CRPS). Retrieved from http://www.assh.org/handcare/hand-arm-conditions/Complex -Regional-Pain-Syndrome-CRPS.

Mayo Clinic. (2014, April 12). Complex regional pain syndrome. Retrieved from http://www .mayoclinic.org/diseases-conditions/complex-regional-pain-syndrome/basics/definition /con-20022844.

National Institute of Neurological Disorders and Stroke. (2015, September 4). NINDS com- plex regional pain syndrome information page. Retrieved from http://www.ninds.nih .gov/disorders/reflex_sympathetic_dystrophy/reflex_sympathetic_dystrophy.htm.

RSDSA. (2015). Telltale signs and symptoms of CRPS/RSD. Retrieved from http://rsds.org /telltale-signs-and-symptoms-of-crpsrsd/.

CONGENITAL HEART DISEASE

Congenital heart defects are structural abnormalities of the heart that are present at birth. These issues rank as the most common type of birth defect in the world, affecting some 8 out of every 1,000 newborns. In the United States alone, around 35,000 children are born with a congenital heart defect each year.

There are many types of congenital heart defects. These abnormalities can range from problems with the interior walls of the heart to defects within the heart valves or even structural issues in the veins or arteries. Some congenital heart defects are simple and have little to no symptoms, while others are more complex and require advanced surgical procedures in order to be fixed or a lifetime of specialized medi- cal treatment. Common congenital heart defects include aortic valve stenosis, an abnormality in which a heart valve does not open and close properly so that blood may be either leaked from or trapped in the heart; coarctation of the aorta, which is a narrowing of the major artery (aorta) that transports blood to the body; ven- tricular septal defect, an abnormal hole in the wall between two chambers of the heart; and tetralogy of Fallot, which is a complex defect involving four separate problems (a hole in the wall between the lower heart chambers, a blockage between the heart and lungs, a misplaced aorta that lies directly over the hole in the lower chambers, and an overly developed muscle surrounding the lower right heart cham- ber). The causes of congenital heart defects are not fully understood. Some defects are inherited through genes from one or both parents, while others are associated with such separate genetic disorders as Down syndrome. Smoking while pregnant can also contribute to the development of certain congenital heart defects, includ- ing septal problems.

Although many congenital heart defects do not have signs or symptoms, more severe problems will most likely be accompanied with rapid breathing or short- ness of breath, extreme fatigue, poor circulation, and a bluish tinge to the finger- nails, lips, and skin. A heart murmur, which is an unusual or uneven heartbeat, can also be another potential sign of a congenital heart defect; however, murmurs do not necessarily mean there is a defect. It is common that congenital heart de- fects are diagnosed in infancy or even while a fetus is in utero, but because some defects have few to no signs, they may not be diagnosed until a child is older. A physical exam, chest x-rays, and blood tests are all tools used to help pinpoint a defect. Other diagnostic exams include an electrocardiography exam, which is a test used to record the heart's electrical activity; an echocardiogram, which utilizes sound waves via ultrasound to create an image of the heart in motion; and cardiac catheterization, which involves inserting a thin, flexible tube into a vein and then threading it through the heart and then injecting it with special dye to measure the pressure and oxygen levels inside the chambers and blood vessels to see the blood flow through the heart. If a defect is suspected in a fetus, a fetal echocardiography exam can be performed to help a doctor evaluate the problem as well as potential solutions before a baby is born.

The treatment for congenital heart defects depends on the type of defect that has occurred, as well as the severity of the defect and other medical factors, including the age and general health of the person with the defect. Certain defects (including pulmonary artery stenosis, in which a heart valve does not open fully) can be fixed with a catheter procedure. Much like in a cardiac catheterization exam, a thin, flexible tube is threaded through a vein or artery until it reaches the problem area. Then, balloons or other devices are used to fix the issue. Open-heart surgery may be required to fix issues like holes in the heart chambers or to repair complex defects. And, in cases when the defect is too severe and complicated for repair, a heart transplant may be recommended. Such procedures are not without their risks and complications. A person with a congenital heart defect that needs repair is at higher risk of infective endocarditis, which is a life-threatening infection of the inner tissues of the heart. Many people born with congenital heart defects require close medical monitoring throughout their lives to ensure they maintain heart health, even if the defect is repaired at a very young age.

Tamar Burris

See also: Arrhythmias/Dysrhythmias; Atherosclerosis; Cardiovascular Disease; Cerebral Vascular Disease; Coronary Artery Disease; Heart Diseases; Stroke

Further Reading

American Heart Association. (2015). Common types of heart defects. Retrieved from http://www.heart.org/HEARTORG/Conditions/CongenitalHeartDefects/AboutCongenita HeartDefects/Common-Types-of-Heart-Defects_UCM_307017_Article.jsp#.Vrjs81 JGNro.

Centers for Disease Control and Prevention. (2015). Congenital heart defects. Retrieved from http://www.cdc.gov/ncbddd/heartdefects/index.html.

Cleveland Clinic Children's. (2015). Pediatric and congenital heart conditions. Retrieved from https://my.clevelandclinic.org/childrens-hospital/health-info/diseases-conditions /hic-pediatric-congenital-heart-defects.

DeSilva, R. A. (2013). *Heart Disease*. Westport, CT: Greenwood.

Everett, A. D. & Lim, D. S. (2011). *Illustrated Field Guide to Congenital Heart Disease and Repair*. Charlottesville, VA: Scientific Software Solutions.

CONGESTIVE HEART FAILURE

Congestive heart failure, also called congestive cardiac failure, or heart failure, refers to the inability of the heart to function as a pump and supply enough blood and oxygen to the body and its organs. It is a serious condition in which the blood flow is commonly inefficient, and this often causes congestion in the liver, abdomen, lower extremities, and lungs. The condition usually proceeds progressively, and the heart does not necessarily stop beating until it is severely damaged. Four out of five people over age 65 with this condition will survive longer than one year.

For a child to grow and develop, the heart needs to maintain its normal pumping functions in order to provide optimal blood flow throughout the body. However, sometimes the heart of a child may not function normally. Several factors can produce congestive heart failure in either infancy or childhood. These include heart valve obstruction or insufficiency; mechanical obstruction of the heart; internal stresses on the walls of the lower heart chambers or ventricles; high blood in the lungs or general circulation system; inflammation of the heart muscle or oxygen lack; and, finally, certain metabolic disturbances, such as hyperthyroidism or hypothyroidism.

Heart failure can affect the left side or right side of the heart, or both sides, but it typically begins on the left.

Left-sided heart failure causes shortness of breath during either exertion or at rest, or both, fatigue, dizziness, and confusion; while right-sided failure causes swelling of the abdomen, legs, and feet due to fluid accumulation under the skin, enlarged liver, or jaundice.

The term *systolic heart failure* refers to the inability of the left ventricle or heart chamber to contract adequately. *Diastolic heart failure* refers to the inability of the left ventricle of heart chamber to relax or fill completely.

Complications of heart failure include:

Death
Heart valve dysfunction
Heart attack and stroke
Kidney damage
Liver damage

Causes of Chronic and Acute Heart Failure

Congestive heart failure often occurs after other conditions have damaged or weakened the heart.

These conditions include high blood pressure and coronary artery disease.

Other risk factors include the presence of faulty heart valves and diseases or infections that cause damage to the heart muscle such as weakness or stiffening, heart defects, and abnormalities in the heartbeat.

Other diseases associated with heart failure include diabetes, kidney conditions, HIV/AIDS, and alcoholism.

Illnesses associated with heart failure are pneumonia, anemia, or hyperthyroidism, which place extra strains on a heart that is already failing.

Additional risk factors include exposure to chemotherapy drugs, obesity, and chain smoking.

One or more of these conditions or risk factors can exist without a person knowing this, and having more than one risk factor increases the risk.

Acute heart failure can occur due to severe infections, allergic reactions, blood clots in the lungs, and use of certain medications.

Symptoms

Cardiac failure can occur over a prolonged period of time, but it can also start suddenly.

Typical symptoms of chronic heart failure include:

Breathlessness on exertion
Coughing
Difficulty concentrating
Fatigue
Feeling faint
Irregular pulse
Lack of appetite
Nausea
Need to urinate at night
Persistent coughing or wheezing
Rapid or irregular heart beat
Sudden weight gain
Swelling of the abdomen
Swelling of the legs, ankles, and feet
Waking from sleep after a few hours due to breathlessness
Weakness
Weight gain

In acute heart failure, symptoms may be similar to those presenting in people with long-standing heart problems, but they may be more severe and may worsen suddenly.

There may also be a sudden fluid buildup, sudden shortness of breath, and chest pain.

The heart may beat rapidly or irregularly.

Diagnostic Tests

Heart failure is often not diagnosed because no clearly stated definition of this condition exists.

The diagnosis of heart failure can be aided by a medical examination plus:

Blood tests
Cardiac computerized tomography
Chest x-rays
Coronary catheterization or angiogram

Electrocardiograms
Echocardiograms
Magnetic resonance imaging
Stress tests

The results of one or more of these tests can be classified in terms of one of two scales.

a. The *New York Heart Association Scale,* which has four components: Class I heart failure is the mildest form, and Class IV is the most severe.
b. The *American College of Cardiology Scale,* which includes a category for people at risk for developing heart disease and ranges from A to D. Stage A refers to a person who has several risk factors for heart failure, while Stage D refers to a person with end-stage heart failure.

Treatment plans are then constructed on the basis of the category of heart disease that exists.

Treatments

Treatments depend on the cause and may include:
One or more medications may to help reduce the severity of the problem, increase survival rates, and reduce complications.
Heart transplantation, coronary bypass surgery, or support with an artificial heart device, as well as supplemental oxygen usage and hospice care, may be indicated.
In addition, lifestyle changes that involve exercising, reducing salt in the diet, lowering cholesterol, managing stress, treating depression, limiting alcohol intake, and losing weight can be helpful.

Summary

Congestive heart failure is a condition that results in the failure of the heart to pump an adequate amount of blood to the body. Chronic congestive heart failure cannot be reversed and is often fatal. Therefore, people who experience unusual symptoms of chest pain, shortness of breath, weakness, or swelling of the legs or abdomen should visit their physician or an emergency room as soon as possible.

Prevention

Lifestyle changes and elimination or reduction of risk factors may reduce the chances of heart failure. Once diagnosed, working with the doctor and other professionals to develop a treatment plan will be helpful. Those diagnosed with heart failure should have follow-up appointments every three to six months to check the function of the heart.

Ray Marks

See also: Coronary Artery Disease; Environment; Heart Disease; Heart Valve Disorders; Liver Diseases

Further Reading

American Heart Association. (2012). Heart failure in children and adolescents. Retrieved from http://www.heart.org/HEARTORG/Conditions/Heart.

Centers for Disease Control and Prevention. (2011). Heart failure death rates among adults aged 65 years and older, by state, 2006. Heart failure fact sheet. Retrieved from http://www.cdc.gov/dhdsp/data_statistics/fact-sheets/fs_heart_failure.htm.

Heart Failure Society of America. (2012). Retrieved from http://www.hfsa.org.

Kasper, E. K., & Knudson, M. (2010). *Living Well with Heart Failure, the Misnamed, Misunderstood Condition*. Baltimore, MD: Johns Hopkins University Press.

Keith, J. D. (1956). Congestive heart failure. *Pediatrics, 18*(3), 491–500.

Mayo Clinic. (2011). Heart failure. Retrieved from http://mayoclinic.com/health/heart-failure/DS00061.

National Heart, Lung, and Blood Institute. (2012). What is heart failure? Retrieved from http://www.nhlbi.nih.gov/health/health-topics/topics/hf/.

COPD (CHRONIC OBSTRUCTIVE PULMONARY DISEASE)

COPD, which stands for chronic obstructive pulmonary disease, refers to progressive respiratory disorders in which breathing becomes increasingly difficult. The disease is characterized by shortness of breath, chest tightness, wheezing, and coughing up mucus. Advanced cases of COPD often result in an inability to walk and do other routine activities. Most people who have COPD are, or were, heavy smokers. However, other forms of lung irritation, such as exposure to large amounts of chemical fumes and dust, may also contribute to causing the disease.

In people who have COPD, less air flows into and out of the lungs' airways (bronchial tubes and bronchioles) than under normal conditions. The airflow reduction may be caused by reduced elasticity of the airways and air sacs (alveoli) of the lungs, by destruction or inflammation of the walls between air sacs, or by unusually large amounts of mucus in the airways.

Most people who have COPD actually have two individual conditions that are each marked by breathing difficulties. These conditions are emphysema, in which the walls of air sacs break down, and chronic bronchitis, in which the airways become inflamed and filled with mucus.

Millions of people have COPD, which is the third leading cause of death in the United States.

Risk Factors

COPD is most frequently diagnosed in people who are older than age 40. That's because it takes several years for the accumulation of lung irritants—such as tobacco smoke, dust, chemical gases, and air pollution—to reach levels great enough to cause symptoms. Exposure to such airborne substances constitutes the primary risk factor for COPD.

In rare cases, the development of COPD is associated with a genetic condition called alpha-1 antitrypsin deficiency, in which low levels of a particular protein made by the liver places the individual at heightened risk for lung damage from chemical irritants. Such gene-based cases of COPD tend to happen in people younger than 40. In other cases, COPD may develop from a progressively worsening condition of asthma.

Symptoms

Symptoms of COPD typically do not become noticeable until the disease has progressed to a relatively advanced point. When a person has an ongoing cough that produces a lot of mucus, is short of breath after any physical activity, wheezes with each breath, and/or feels an uncomfortable tightness in the chest, he or she should go to a doctor to get checked for COPD. Another sign of COPD is the frequent development of colds and influenza.

If COPD is not promptly addressed with medical care, additional symptoms may develop. These symptoms may include swelling in the legs, ankles, or feet; fatigue in the lower-body muscles; bluish or gray lips or fingernails; mental disorientation; and weight loss. Some of these symptoms are signs that the individual requires emergency medical treatment.

Diagnosis

To confirm that patients with symptoms suggestive of COPD actually have COPD, a number of tests and other medical procedures are required. The first step in diagnosis is to obtain histories of the health backgrounds of the patient and his or her family. To do so, the doctor will usually ask the patient about his or her exposure to tobacco smoke and other lung irritants, as well as whether any family members had COPD. Another important diagnostic step is a physical examination that includes listening to breathing sounds with a stethoscope.

Suspicions of COPD are followed up with tests of lung function, which measure how much air is breathed in and out by the patient and how much oxygen is delivered to the blood. The main lung-function test is spirometry, in which the patient blows into a tube connected to a machine that measures the amount of air breathed out and the rate at which the air is breathed. This test can detect COPD before the patient even notices symptoms.

Additional diagnostic tests may include conventional x-rays of the chest, computed tomography (CT) scans of the chest, and a blood test that measures oxygen levels.

Prevention and Treatment

COPD can best be prevented by avoiding smoking or exposure to other lung irritants. If an individual is a long-term smoker, quitting as soon as possible can still help in reducing risk or disease severity.

There is no cure for COPD. However, various treatments and lifestyle changes can slow the progression of the disease, decrease the risk of complications, and help the individual feel better and remain more active.

Important lifestyle changes are quitting smoking and avoiding other lung irritants (including secondhand smoke), getting proper nutrition, and exercising to strengthen the breathing muscles. Medications that are often effective in treatment are bronchodilators (which relax muscles around the airways) and glucocorticosteroids (which reduce airway inflammation). People with chronic breathing problems can benefit from a comprehensive program of pulmonary rehabilitation—consisting of exercise, nutritional adjustments, and psychological counseling.

Advanced cases of COPD may require the patient to use oxygen therapy, in which oxygen gas from a tank is inhaled through nasal prongs or a mask. The most severe cases may require surgical procedures, ranging from removal of diseased tissues in the lungs to a complete lung transplant.

A. J. Smuskiewicz

See also: Cor Pulmonale; Emphysema; Lung Cancer; Lung Diseases; Pneumonia; Pollution; Secondhand Smoke; Tobacco Addiction

Further Reading

COPD Foundation. (2016). About the COPD Foundation. Retrieved from http://www.copd foundation.org.

Mahler, D. A. (2015). *COPD: Answers to Your Questions*. Minneapolis, MN: Two Harbors Press.

Mayo Clinic. (2015). COPD. Retrieved from http://www.mayoclinic.org/diseases-conditions /copd/basics/definition/con-20032017.

National Heart, Lung, and Blood Institute. (2013). What is COPD? Retrieved from http:// www.nhlbi.nih.gov/health/health-topics/topics/copd.

COR PULMONALE

Overview

The term *cor pulmonale*, also called right-sided heart failure, refers to an alteration in the structure and function of one of the four chambers of the heart, known as the right ventricle. The condition is usually related to a disorder in the breathing or respiratory system due to pulmonary hypertension or high blood pressure in the arteries of the lungs and right ventricle of the heart. The condition develops as a secondary problem in relation to several different forms of disease processes involving both the heart and breathing systems. The condition is usually a slowly developing one with a progressive course, and it can lead to heart failure. It can also occur suddenly, and if it does, this can be very serious and life-threatening.

Symptoms

Symptoms may be present constantly or only intermittently and include shortness of breath during activity, fainting spells, chest pain or discomfort, palpitations, leg and ankle swelling, and coughing or wheezing. Limited exercise tolerance, chest discomfort, and abnormal liver enlargement are other signs.

There may be abnormal heart sounds as well.

Causes and Risk Factors

Any factor causing excess strain on the right ventricle can cause cor pulmonale.

Key causative factors include chronic obstructive pulmonary disease (COPD), chronic bronchitis, and emphysema; blood clots in the lungs or arteries that lead to the lungs; cystic fibrosis; the presence of lung tissue scarring; deformity of the spine that compresses the lungs; mountain sickness; primary pulmonary hypertension; pulmonary vascular disease; neuromuscular diseases such as muscular dystrophy; and sleep apnea or pauses in breathing when a person is trying to sleep. If any of these factors cause the wall of the right ventricle to dilate and bulge, the right ventricle will eventually be unable to function.

Diagnostic Tools

The health care provider may examine the lung and heart and blood pressure systems.

The skin can be checked to see if it is yellow or blue in color.

There may be abdominal swelling, ankle swelling, or swelling of the neck veins that are observable.

Specific lab tests might include blood tests, x-rays, CT scans of the chest, echocardiograms, and, on occasion, lung biopsies, electrocardiographs, lung scans, and heart catheterization tests.

Treatments

The goal of treatment is to control symptoms and typically involves a variety of medications. Blood thinners, oxygen, and surgery in the form of a lung transplant might be needed in severe cases. The cause of the problem should be identified and treated, where possible.

To reduce symptoms, it appears that excessive exercise should be avoided, as should smoking. Traveling to places of high altitude should be avoided.

The outcome depends on how severe the condition is, as well as how adherent the patient is to the recommended regimen. It also depends on the cause of the condition.

Uncontrolled progressive disease may lead to heart failure, severe shortness of breath, severe fluid retention, shock, or death.

Ray Marks

See also: Cystic Fibrosis; Emphysema; Lung Diseases; Neuromuscular Disorders

Further Reading

American Heart Association. (2015, September 30). Types of heart failure. Retrieved from http://www.heart.org/HEARTORG/Conditions/HeartFailure/AboutHeartFailure/Types -of-Heart-Failure_UCM_306323_Article.jsp#.Vjy89GtKjwo.

Mayo Clinic. (2015, August 18). Heart failure causes. Retrieved from http://www.mayoclinic .org/diseases-conditions/heart-failure/basics/causes/con-20029801.

Merck Manual. (2015). Cor pulmonale. Retrieved from http://www.merckmanuals.com /home/SearchResults?query=Cor+Pulmonale&icd9=415.0%3b416.9%3b416.0.

The New York Times. (2008, September 23). Right-sided heart failure. Retrieved from http:// www.nytimes.com/health/guides/disease/right-sided-heart-failure/overview.html.

CREUTZFELDT-JAKOB DISEASE

Creutzfeldt-Jakob, Jakob-Creutzfeldt, Jakob's disease, or subacute spongiform encephalopathy is a very rare degenerative disorder affecting many areas of the brain. It is a human prion disease that causes the sudden onset of symptoms common to other neurological problems or disorders. As the condition progresses, there may be increasing evidence of dementia, and involuntary movements called myoclonus may become apparent. Some may have swallowing difficulties, as well as problems talking, and in the end stages, they may lose all mental and physical capabilities and lapse into a state of unconsciousness or coma.

The disease proceeds rapidly and is normally about four to six months in duration, with 90 percent of cases dying within one year. Most often, it affects older adults who are 60 years or older, but it can affect younger people in its variant form called variant Creutzfeldt-Jakob disease, thought to be related to mad cow disease.

The disease affects one in 1 million people worldwide, and each year, about 200 cases occur in the United States.

Types

The three major types are sporadic, hereditary, and acquired.

History

The disease was diagnosed independently by Hans Gerhard Creutzfeldt and Alfons Maria Jakob in the early 1920s.

Symptoms

The symptoms of the condition may include:

Changes in behavior and personality, agitation, and restlessness
Confusion and problems with memory
Depression
Inability to sleep
Muscle weakness

Loss of muscle mass
Poor coordination
Unusual physical symptoms and writhing movements, especially of the arms and legs
Problems with vision

Causes

Creutzfeldt-Jakob disease and its variants belong to a broad group of diseases termed *transmissible spongiform encephalopathies*. This term is used because the affected brain tissue appears to have spongy holes when seen under a microscope. In most cases, there is no apparent reason for the sudden onset of this condition. Ten percent of cases may be experiencing this condition as a result of hereditary factors. In other cases, infection might be the cause. These infectious organisms may be hard to detect and may have long incubation periods. Another, more accepted, theory is that the disease is caused by a type of protein known as a prion. These may be harmless but may cause disease if they are in an infected form. It is possible that a person can experience a spontaneous change of the prion's normal genetic configuration to become an infectious form. When abnormal prions form clusters or aggregates, it is thought they can produce brain damage and nerve loss. In other cases, it is believed 5 to 10 percent of cases are inherited, and some are caused by contamination after being exposed to infected tissues after medical procedures. Variant Creutzfeldt-Jakob disease is linked to eating beef infected with bovine spongiform encephalopathy.

Diagnosis

There are no definitive tests for the disease. Medical examinations and neurological tests can help rule out other health conditions, however. These include encephalograms or EEGs, computerized tomography or CT scans, as well as magnetic resonance imaging or MRI scans, and brain biopsies. Family history may be helpful in solidifying the diagnosis.

Treatments

There is no effective treatment for Creutzfeldt-Jakob disease. Current treatment is aimed at reducing the symptoms and making the patient as comfortable as possible. Nursing to prevent complications in the later stages of the disease may be needed to prevent bed sores and to deal with loss of bladder control and eating ability.

Prevention

Exposure to infected brain tissue should be avoided.

Prognosis and Outcomes

The prognosis for this condition is poor. Some die within a few weeks, although some may live for several years.

Future

Scientists are studying whether infection is the cause of the condition, as well as what influences prions to become infected. They are also examining how the disorder affects the brain using autopsy material and rat models. It is hoped these studies will help to improve the diagnosis of Creutzfeldt-Jakob disease and help determine what types of treatments might be effective in reducing nerve damage.

Ray Marks

See also: Dementia; Neurological Diseases

Further Resources

Centers for Disease Control and Prevention. (2015, January 13). CJD. (Creutzfeldt-Jakob disease, classic). Retrieved from http://www.cdc.gov/prions/cjd/index.html.

CJD Foundation. (2016). Creutzfeldt-Jakob disease. Retrieved from http://www.cjdfoundation.org/.

National Institutes of Neurological Disorders and Stroke. (2016). Creutzfeldt-Jakob disease fact sheet. Retrieved from http://www.ninds.nih.gov/disorders/cjd/detail_cjd.htm.

Rare Diseases.org. (2012). Creutzfeldt-Jakob disease. Retrieved from http://www.rarediseases.org/rare-disease-information/rare-diseases/byID/33/viewAbstract.

UCSF Medical Center. (2016, November 29). Creutzfeldt-Jakob disease, signs and symptoms. Retrieved from UCSF http://www.ucsfhealth.org/conditions/creutzfeldt-jakob_disease/signs_and_symptoms.html.

World Health Organization. (2012). Variant Creutzfeldt-Jakob disease. Retrieved from http://www.who.int/mediacentre/factsheets/fs180/en/#.

CROHN'S DISEASE

Crohn's disease is a type of inflammatory bowel disease (IBD). It most often affects the ileum, or the lower part of the small intestine, and the beginning of the colon, but it can affect any part of the digestive tract. The inflammation can extend deep into the intestinal lining, creating painful swelling and irritation and frequent diarrhea. The inflammation can also produce scar tissue that can cause cramps as the movement of food is slowed through the intestine.

As many as 700,000 people in the United States may be affected by this disease, which occurs equally in men and women, most often between the ages of 20 and 29, and particularly among those who smoke cigarettes or have a parent or sibling with IBD. A chronic disorder that cannot be cured, Crohn's symptoms can be managed by medications and diet, although most people eventually require surgery.

History

Burrill B. Crohn was among the first to describe the disease in medical literature in 1932. A gastroenterologist at Mount Sinai Medical Center in New York, Crohn treated patients whose similar symptoms did not fit a known disease. His work advanced scientific understanding of the disease that came to bear his name as well as many other gastrointestinal conditions.

Symptoms

The symptoms depend on where in the digestive tract they are, and they can vary from mild to severe and flare up suddenly before a period of remission. The most common symptoms are diarrhea, which may be watery or bloody; cramping abdominal pain; and weight loss. Other symptoms include anemia, fatigue, nausea, loss of appetite, fever, the need to empty already-empty bowels, and rectal bleeding, as well as pus, mucus, or stools draining from around the rectum. Symptoms that Crohn's disease may cause outside of the intestines are mouth ulcers, swollen gums, eye inflammation, joint pain and swelling, tender red skin bumps, and inflammation in the liver or bile ducts. Children with Crohn's disease may experience developmental and growth-related delays.

Causes and Risk Factors

The body's immune system mistakenly attacks and destroys healthy body tissue in Crohn's disease, although the precise cause for this remains unknown. A virus or bacterium may trigger the disease when the immune system, working to fight a foreign substance in the digestive tract, has an abnormal response and also attacks healthy cells.

Emotional stress and certain foods do not cause Crohn's disease, although stress may worsen the symptoms, and some people find that certain foods can trigger symptoms.

Most men and women are diagnosed with Crohn's disease before they reach 30 years of age. Other risk factors that increase the likelihood of a diagnosis include having a sibling or parent with the disease; being of Eastern European Ashkenazi Jewish descent; smoking cigarettes; taking nonsteroidal anti-inflammatory medications that can lead to bowel inflammation; living in an urban area or industrialized country, especially in a northern climate; and eating a diet high in fat or processed foods.

Diagnosis

A doctor will take a family history and may perform a physical exam, including ordering medical tests to rule out inflammatory bowel diseases with similar symptoms. Abdominal tenderness or a mass, skin rash, swollen joints, or mouth ulcers may show evidence in a physical examination.

The most accurate method of diagnosing Crohn's disease and ruling out other conditions are intestinal endoscopies, such as upper GI endoscopy and enteroscopy; capsule endoscopy; and colonoscopy. Other diagnostic tools include barium enema or upper gastrointestinal series examination; CT scans; magnetic resonance imaging (MRI) of the abdomen; and lab tests, including blood tests and stool culture to rule out other possible causes of the disorder.

Treatments

Treatment for Crohn's disease depends on the location of the problem, the severity of the disease, and its response to treatment. The goals of treatments are to control inflammation and limit complications, relieve symptoms, correct or prevent nutritional deficiencies, and improve long-term prognosis.

Treatment includes medications, changes in diet, and if necessary, surgery. The drugs usually prescribed work to suppress the immune system's abnormal response that causes inflammation and control or reduce symptoms, including the frequency of flare-ups. Common Crohn's medications include anti-inflammatories, immunosuppressants, and biologic therapy for severe cases that do not respond to medications, as well as antibiotics and pain relievers.

To treat severe symptoms, bowel rest may be prescribed to allow the intestines to heal. This involves drinking only clear liquids or taking nothing by mouth. Nutrients are given by an intravenous catheter in the arm. It is vital that those with Crohn's disease maintain good nutrition because the disease causes appetite loss and increases the body's need for energy. Diarrhea and other common symptoms may reduce the ability to absorb water and vital nutrients such as fat, carbohydrates, protein, minerals, and vitamins.

People who find that spicy or high-fiber foods trigger flare-ups rely on soft, bland foods to reduce discomfort.

Surgery does not cure the disorder, and it is rarely performed. But up to 70 percent of people will need surgical treatment to remove diseased portions of the intestine and join healthy sections together.

Prognosis and Outcomes

Crohn's disease has no cure, and symptoms may flare up suddenly and then lessen or disappear temporarily. Symptoms can be managed with appropriate medication and careful attention to diet, which usually significantly improves the quality of life. Most women with Crohn's disease deliver babies successfully, but they should not become pregnant during a flare-up, while beginning a new treatment, or while on steroid medications.

Ray Marks

See also: Abdominal Diseases; Digestive Diseases; Inflammatory Bowel Disease; Ulcerative Colitis

Further Reading

Crohn's & Colitis Foundation of America. (2015). What is Crohn's disease? Retrieved from http://www.ccfa.org/what-are-crohns-and-colitis/what-is-crohns-disease/.

Mayo Clinic. (2014, August 13) Crohn's disease. Retrieved from http://www.mayoclinic.org/diseases-conditions/crohns-disease/basics/definition/con-20032061.

National Institute of Diabetes and Digestive and Kidney Diseases. (2014, September 3). Crohn's disease. Retrieved from http://www.niddk.nih.gov/health-information/health-topics/digestive-diseases/crohns-disease/Pages/facts.aspx.

Sklar, J., & Sklar, M. (2007). *The First Year: Crohn's Disease and Ulcerative Colitis: An Essential Guide for the Newly Diagnosed*. Boston: Da Capo Press.

CUTTING AND SELF-HARM

Cutting and other forms of self-harm are seemingly bizarre behaviors in which individuals—typically adolescents or other young people—purposefully make small cuts, burns, or other relatively minor injuries to their own bodies. These acts of self-harm are frightening and difficult to understand for parents, other family members, and friends. Although commonly thought to be failed suicide attempts or actions to get attention, these acts are actually attempts by mentally troubled individuals to control their emotional pain, according to psychologists. Mental health experts classify the acts as nonsuicidal self-injuries (NSSIs).

Acts of Self-Harm

In a typical case of cutting, knives, razor blades, scissors, paper clips, or other sharp tools are used to make a series of short straight lines, often parallel to each other. The cuts are usually made on the forearms, though other parts of the body may also be cut, such as the upper arms, upper thighs, and chest. Some people form letters or words out of the cuts to describe how they're feeling about themselves, such as "loser," "stupid," "failure," or "fat."

Burning may be done with any type of hot object, including lit cigarettes, matches, stovetop flames, plugged-in irons, or radiators. Other types of self-harm include punching oneself, banging one's head against the wall, biting one's skin, pulling out one's hair, picking at wounds to prevent healing, intentionally falling down the stairs, self-suffocation, and self-poisoning.

The cutting, burning, or other acts of self-harm are typically done in private, so other people may not immediately be aware that it is happening. One common sign of this behavior is the constant wearing of long sleeves, even in hot summer weather, to cover cuts or burns on the arms. Another sign that often coincides with self-harming behaviors is a noticeably altered mood, in which the individual suddenly becomes quiet, withdrawn, and depressed. When asked about the mood change, the individual is likely to deny it or to make excuses for it, rather than admit to struggling with a serious problem. When asked about cuts, excuses might include blaming the cat, an itchy rash, or some accident.

Over time, the adolescent's cutting or burning tends to become more frequent and harder to hide.

Reasons for Self-Harm

According to psychologists, self-injury is basically a coping strategy for people who are experiencing deep unhappiness, emotional troubles, stress, and a lack of control in their lives. It is not usually done for attention, as is commonly believed, but as a way to try to relieve these troubles. It sometimes starts after a particularly challenging event, such as the breakup of a relationship. Sometimes it starts as a matter of impulse or curiosity.

The cuts, burns, and other injuries may cause physical pain—though the pain is usually limited, and the injuries usually heal eventually. The sharp sensations may let the practitioners know that they are living, feeling beings—serving to jolt them out of their emotional deadness—or the physical pain may lift them out of the psychological pain they feel. In some cases, self-harmers want to feel the pain as a way of punishing themselves for not being good enough in some area (such as not being smart or attractive enough).

Evidence indicates that, for many people struggling with emotional problems, self-injury produces biochemical effects similar to cocaine and other drugs that cause the release of endorphins in the brain. Those chemicals produce feelings of pleasure and can lead to addiction. However, self-harm causes these feelings only in people who become addicted to the behavior. Other, psychologically healthy people will not get such pleasurable feelings from self-harm. Addiction is the reason that cutting becomes more frequent—and with larger cuts—over time. As in other addictions, such as cocaine addiction, it takes more and more of the behavior to yield the same "high" over time.

In many cases, teenagers who self-harm have additional mental health issues with which they are struggling. They may have eating disorders. They may be unusually sensitive to negative personal experiences. They may have a history of sexual abuse, physical abuse, and/or emotional abuse within their families. Some—though not all—self-injurers have serious mental disorders, such as schizophrenia, bipolar disorder, or personality disorders. Acts of self-harm often occur while the practitioner is under the influence of drugs or alcohol.

Prevalence

Self-harm typically begins at about the age of 14 or 15, and the behavior may continue for years. Some people continue the practice well into adulthood. For other people, the practice is a "phase" that they eventually outgrow, similar to drug use and other "experimental" behaviors that many teens try out.

Cutting and other kinds of self-harm tend to be most common in teenage girls, though many boys also engage in the practice. Although often associated with the "Goth" subculture, cutting is not practiced by all Goths, and many people who cut themselves are not Goths.

A study by researchers at King's College London, published in 2011, followed more than 1,000 teenagers in Australia for several years to track their self-injurious behaviors. According to the study's findings, 1 in 12 teens (but 1 in 10 girls) self-harmed, mainly by cutting or burning. In about 90 percent of the cases, the acts of self-harm stopped by the time the individuals turned 20.

Other studies have placed the prevalence of cutting in teen girls as high as one in five. Part of the reason for the greater prevalence of self-harm in girls, according to researchers, is that girls are generally under more social stress than boys. Girls tend to feel that their peers expect them to be very attractive, very intelligent, and very popular. The phenomenon of a high cutting prevalence among popular, pretty teen girls was described in the book *Girls on the Edge*, by physician and psychologist Leonard Sax. No matter how popular and pretty the girls might be, according to Sax, their feelings of insecurity and the pressure from peers could lead to illogical self-harming attempts to cope. In contract to these popular girls, wrote Sax, most boys who self-harm tend to be unpopular.

Treatment

Treatment is necessary not only to bring relief to the troubled mental state of the self-injuring individual, but also to prevent further harm to the individual's physical health. Some people who self-harm—especially when they're drinking or using drugs—accidentally cause permanent disfigurement or even fatal wounds.

The first step in getting treatment usually happens after the behavior is discovered by a parent or other relative. Many parents mistakenly believe that the cuts or other wounds mean that the person is trying to commit suicide. Psychologists advise that parents try to have an open, honest discussion with the self-injurer—without becoming overly angry or hostile. The person should know that the parent cares, wants to understand, and wants to help.

One common problem among self-injuring teens is that many live in families in which open communication does not come easily. In their families, the honest expression of emotions may be discouraged. Psychologists note that the repression of emotional expression can be unhealthy. Young people who have other outlets for emotional expression—such as a temper tantrum or a crying fit every now and then—are less likely to engage in acts of self-injury. Thus, an important aspect of treatment for self-harmers is the acceptance of honest emotional expression within the family.

Ultimately, it may be necessary for the self-harmer to get professional psychotherapy. Such help can be found with psychiatrists, clinical psychologists, or licensed mental health therapists, especially those who specialize in adolescent conditions. In addition, some medical centers offer special therapy programs for self-harmers.

An example of such a program is the SAFE (Self-Abuse Finally Ends) Alternatives program at Linden Oak Hospital in Naperville, Illinois. This 30-day inpatient program was started by certified addictions counselor Karen Conterio, who also wrote a book on the subject titled *Bodily Harm* (1999). This and similar programs seek to address the problems underlying the self-harming acts, such as depression, anxiety, repressed anger, low self-esteem, and ineffective mechanisms to cope with stress. Depending on the particular case, the program may incorporate the use of psychiatric medications, such as antidepressants and antianxiety drugs.

A. J. Smuskiewicz

See also: Bipolar Disorder; Depression; Mental Disorders; Social Health

Further Reading

Cleveland Clinic. (2015). Self-injury/cutting overview. Retrieved from https://my
     .clevelandclinic.org/childrens-hospital/health-info/diseases-conditions/hic-pediatric
     -congenital-heart-defects.

Conterio, K. (1999). *Bodily Harm: The Breakthrough Healing Program for Self-Injurers*. New
     York, NY: Hachette.

Cornell University College of Human Ecology. (2015). What is self-injury? The Cornell Re-
     search Program on Self-Injury and Recovery. Retrieved from http://www.selfinjury
     .bctr.cornell.edu/about-self-injury.html.

Levenkron, S. (1998). *Cutting: Understanding and Overcoming Self-Mutilation*. New York, NY:
     W. W. Norton.

Moran, P., Coffey, C., Romaniuk, H., Olsson, C., Borschmann, R., Carlin, J. B., & Patton,
     G. C. (2011). The natural history of self-harm from adolescence to young adulthood:
     A population-based cohort study. *Lancet*, 379, 236–43.

Sax, L. (2011). *Girls on the Edge: The Four Factors Driving the New Crisis for Girls—Sexual
     Identity, the Cyber bubble, Obsessions, Environmental Toxins*. New York, NY: Basic Books.

Strong, M. (1999). *A Bright Red Scream: Self-Mutilation and the Language of Pain*. New York,
     NY: Penguin.

CYCLIC VOMITING SYNDROME

Cyclic vomiting syndrome (CVS) is a debilitating disorder characterized by intense, repeated episodes of vomiting and severe nausea that can last for hours or days. CVS, while originally thought to be a pediatric disease, affects individuals of all ages. The disorder affects about 0.04 to 2 percent of children, and the incidence of new cases is approximately 3 per 100,000 children yearly. For adults, the true prevalence of CVS is unknown. Moreover, there are limited data on the race of CVS patients. With regard to gender, CVS is found in both men and women and has been more predominant in men.

The symptoms of CVS include (1) having vomiting episodes that begin with severe vomiting that lasts less than a week, (2) experiencing three or more different episodes of vomiting in the past year, and (3) exhibiting no symptoms (vomiting and nausea) between episodes. During an episode, a person may suffer from fever, dizziness, nausea, sensitivity to light, abdominal pain, diarrhea, headache, and dehydration. Individuals who have experienced CVS symptoms for at least three months, with the first onset having occurred at least six months prior, may have CVS. There is currently no cure for CVS, and the treatment of CVS varies. Generally, people who have CVS are told to get plenty of rest and sleep and to take medications to prevent or to abort episodes. The recurrent, severe vomiting that happens during CVS episodes is a determinant of several health complications, including dehydration, electrolyte imbalance, peptic esophagitis, hematemesis, Mallory-Weiss tear, and tooth decay.

Dr. Samuel Gee (1882) first described CVS of childhood in his paper, "On fitful and recurrent vomiting," where he reported the condition in nine children. Over the past century, there has been periodic evidence of CVS in pediatric literature and very few reports of adult CVS. However, in the last decade, reports of CVS in adults have been more dominant in the medical literature than pediatric CVS has been. Dr. B U.K. Li at Northwestern University and Children's Memorial Hospital (Li et al. 2008) and Dr. David Fleisher of University of California, Los Angeles (UCLA) and University of Missouri (Fleisher et al. 2005) are responsible for major advances in describing and understanding pediatric CVS. Dr. Fleisher and his colleagues, recognized as the early "discoverers" of adult CVS, have laid the foundation in the pathophysiology and treatment of CVS.

Despite the fact that CVS was discovered more than a century ago, the etiology, origin, and development of CVS remain relatively unknown. CVS thus continues to be a misunderstood disease by medical practitioners. Yet, medical researchers have posited that there is a strong link between migraines and CVS, although the relationship is unclear. For one, migraine headaches, abdominal migraines, and CVS are all associated with severe symptoms and pain, have similar triggers, and affect children who either have a family history of migraines or will develop migraine into their adulthood. Based on the similarities between migraines and CVS, doctors prescribe drugs often used to treat migraines to CVS patients. Additionally, a study involving 28 patients treated at two London teaching hospitals found a relationship between anxiety/depression and headaches (Lee et al. 2012).

Diagnosing CVS has been difficult for doctors, as no test (x-rays, CT scans, blood tests) can be performed to detect CVS. Making a diagnosis requires a thorough examination of a person's symptoms and medical history as a way to eliminate other disorders or diseases that may cause vomiting and nausea. Diagnosis is often a long process because the doctor has to investigate whether there is a pattern or cycle to the patient's vomiting. Besides the fact that there are no tests that can detect CVS, many doctors know little or nothing about the rare disorder, further making diagnosis difficult.

CVS has four phases: (1) the symptom-free interval phase, which is when the individual experiences no symptoms; (2) the prodrome phase, which is characterized by nausea that may or may not be accompanied with abdominal pain; (3) the vomiting phase, which consists of nausea and vomiting and difficulty eating, drinking, and taking medications without vomiting; and (4) the recovery phase, when the nausea and vomiting stops and the appetite and energy return. Treatment may vary during each phase.

Generally, treating CVS involves identifying and avoiding triggering factors, taking prophylactic drug therapy (such as tricyclic antidepressants [TCAs], which are shown to be effective in several studies) to prevent recurrent episodes, abortive treatments to improve acute episodes, and supporting patients and their families psychologically. People with CVS could prevent episodes by avoiding and working through triggers. Some common triggers in children are excitement and emotional stress. For adults, anxiety and panic attacks are triggers. Infections, allergies, colds, sinus problems, and the flu can trigger an episode. Additionally, eating too much or eating just before bed has been found to be a trigger just as certain foods like chocolate and cheese can be triggers. Some other symptoms include physical exhaustion, menstruation, motion sickness, and hot weather.

At the onset of a CVS episode, staying in bed and sleeping in a dark, quiet place is recommended. Once the nausea and vomiting become severe, treatment may require hospitalization and intravenous fluids to prevent dehydration and to receive drugs for the nausea and pain. During the prodrome phase, people can take abortive measures by taking medication for nausea and pain. Some medications used to treat nausea in CVS patients are Zofran and Ativan. For the pain, some patients can take ibuprofen. However, some individuals with CVS who suffer from intense pain during episodes are given stronger painkillers such as Dilaudid or morphine, which are stronger and can be habit-forming. Some patients are prescribed medications such as Zantac or Prilosec to calm the stomach by reducing the amount of acid it makes. During the vomiting phase of CVS, the goal is to prevent dehydration and to end the cycles of nausea, vomiting, and abdominal pain. Thus, rehydrating the patient and antiemetic, antianxiety, and/or analgesic medications are recommended. Last, when CVS individuals are in the recovery phase, they should drink plenty of water and replace electrolytes, necessary salts in our bodies that keep us healthy.

CVS disrupts the personal and professional lives of patients and reduces their quality of life. For instance, CVS sufferers are often absent from school and employment, which affects their life options, finances, and reliability. CVS has an emotional and physical toll on patients, stressing the need for support from family, friends, and medical professionals. There is a need for further research to understand the natural history of the disorder and possible treatments that allow CVS sufferers to lead a life free of symptoms. Current research includes investigating whether tapering TCAs can return the patient to an asymptomatic state. Finally, while CVS has deleterious effects on individuals, it is now accepted as well-defined problem and is being researched more frequently, which will hopefully lead to greater understanding and effective treatment of CVS.

Dena Simmons

See also: Abdominal Disease

Further Reading

Fleisher, D., Gornowicz, B., Adams, K., & Feldman, E. (2005). Cyclic vomiting syndrome in 41 adults: The illness, the patients and the problems of management. *BioMed Central Medicine, 3,* 20–28.

Gee, S. (1882). On fitful or recurrent vomiting. *St. Bartholomew Hospital Report, 18,* 1–6.

Hejazi, R. A., & McCallum, R. W. (2011). Review article: Cyclic vomiting syndrome in adults—rediscovering and redefining an old entity. *Alimentary Pharmacology & Therapeutics, 34,* 263–273.

Lee, L., Abbott, L., Moodie, S., & Anderson, S. (2012). Cyclic vomiting syndrome in 28 patients: Demographics, features, and outcomes, *European Journal of Gastroenterology and Hepatology, 24*(8), 939–943.

Li, B., Lefevre, F., Chelimsky, G., Boles, R., Nelson, S., Lewis, D., Linder, S., Issenman, R., & Rudolph, C. (2008). North American Society for pediatric gastroenterology, hepatology, and nutrition consensus statement on the diagnosis and management of cyclic vomiting syndrome. *Journal of Pediatric Gastroenterology and Nutrition, 47,* 379–393.

National Digestive Diseases Information Clearinghouse (NDDIC). (2014). Cyclic vomiting syndrome. Retrieved from http://digestive.niddk.nih.gov/ddiseases/pubs/cvs/#four.

Withers, G. D., Silburn, S. R., & Forbes, D. A. (1998). Precipitants and aetiology of cyclic vomiting syndrome. *Acta Paediatrica*, 87(3), 272, 277.

CYSTIC FIBROSIS

Overview

The normal mucus that lines the lungs, nose, other organs, and body cavities is slippery and watery. Its purpose is to prevent them from getting too dry or infected. The mucus of those who have cystic fibrosis is thick and sticky, and it clogs the lungs, blocks the airways, causes breathing problems, and makes it easy for bacteria growth that can lead to lung infections and damage. The mucus can also block ducts in the pancreas, leading to a deficiency in digestive enzymes, as well as produce very salty sweat.

Cystic fibrosis, or CF, is a genetic disease of the secretory glands, which produce mucus and sweat. In addition to the lungs, it affects the pancreas, liver, intestines, sinuses, and sex organs. It is inherited from parents who each carry a faulty CFTR gene (a mutation) that makes a protein that controls the movement of salt and water through the body's cells. A child who inherits this mutation from only one parent usually has no symptoms but, as a carrier, can pass the defective CFTR gene to offspring.

In the United States, about 30,000 people live with CF (nearly half are adults). About 1,000 new cases are diagnosed each year, usually by age two. CF affects males and females; although it is most common among Caucasians of Northern European descent, it is also prevalent among Latinos and American Indians. There is no cure, but recent improvements in treatments to remove mucus from the lungs, control infections, and treat intestinal complications have contributed to longer lifespans and improved quality of life.

Symptoms

A noticeable symptom of CF in babies is a salty-tasting skin. Other symptoms vary depending on the age of onset; in the very young, they may include poor growth or poor weight gain. Those who have a milder version of the disease may not experience symptoms until they become teens or young adults. Many other symptoms may occur later or worsen over time as the disease affects the respiratory, digestive, or reproductive systems. The thick mucus blocks enzymes from the pancreas that aid in digestion. The salty sweat results in the loss of salt and an imbalance of minerals in the blood, which can cause dehydration; other results include decreased blood pressure, heat stroke, increased heart rate, and increased risk of diabetes and osteoporosis.

The most common symptoms include a persistent cough that produces thick mucus, repeated lung infections, shortness of breath, coughing, wheezing, breathlessness, sinus infections, nasal polyps, fatigue, inflammation of the pancreas, gallstones, frequent greasy stools, intestinal gas, constipation, rectal prolapse, club-shaped or enlarged fingertips and toes, and male infertility and difficulty becoming pregnant.

Causes and Risk Factors

The disease is genetically transmitted when both parents carry at least one copy of a defective gene, although not every child will have CF. Carriers are those who inherit only one copy of the defective gene and do not have CF. Each time two carriers have a child, the chances for their offspring having the disease are 25 percent the child will have CF, 50 percent the child will be a carrier and not have CF, and 25 percent the child will not be a carrier or have the disease.

Diagnosis

A genetics test is the only way to detect who is at risk for CF; it can detect faulty CF genes in 9 of 10 cases. A complete diagnostic evaluation for CF includes a sweat test, genetic test, family history, and clinical evaluation. Most children are diagnosed by age two, although some receive a diagnosis as adults if symptoms appear later.

Additional diagnostic tests may include chest and sinus x-rays; lung-function tests; and a sputum (spit) culture, which studies bacteria growth. Screening newborns is a routine practice in all 50 states and the District of Columbia.

Treatments

Cystic fibrosis cannot be cured, but the goals of treatments are preventing or controlling lung infections, loosening and removing mucus from the lungs to clear airways, preventing and treating intestinal blockages, maintaining good nutrition, and avoiding dehydration.

Treatment is individualized, depending on the symptoms and severity. Medications that include antibiotics to fight infections, enzymes to thin the mucus, and bronchodilators to keep airways may be administered by inhalers. Oxygen therapy may be recommended for severe lung disease, and some cases may require a lung transplant. Chest physical therapy involves pounding the chest and back to loosen the mucus from the lungs so that it can be coughed up. Pulmonary rehabilitation to maintain or improve the illness includes exercise and nutritional counseling, breathing techniques, and counseling or group support.

To aid in digestion, pancreatic enzyme pills may be prescribed, as well as vitamin supplements, high-calorie nutritional shakes, and a high-salt diet or supplements, If necessary, surgical and other procedures may be indicated, including a feeding tube at night, lung transplantation, bowel-blockage removal, and mucus suctioning by an endoscopy.

Prevention

Although CF cannot be prevented, measures to reduce its effects and complications include avoiding smoke, dust, and other allergens; drinking plenty of fluids; carefully managing nutritional requirements; getting immunized for preventable diseases; exercising; and washing hands often to lower the risk of infection.

Prognosis and Outcomes

Cystic fibrosis remains a life-limiting disease without a cure. Early treatment, as well as improved treatments and care for CF, make it possible for most young people who have CF live to age 40 or older in the United States. Depending on the severity of symptoms, early and regular medical care along with a carefully managed treatment regimen can improve quality of life. Most often, those who develop lung problems do not respond to treatment are at higher risk for premature death.

Future

Studies of gene therapy are under way, as are test of many new medicines. One is ivacaftor, approved in 2012, for people age six and older with a specific gene mutation of cystic fibrosis. This drug repairs protein to better allow water and salt to reach the lungs. Also under research is an inhaled spray containing normal copies of the CF gene that delivers it to the lungs of those with the disease.

Ray Marks

See also: Digestive Diseases; Lung Diseases

Further Reading

Cystic Fibrosis Foundation. (2015). About cystic fibrosis. Retrieved from http://www.cff.org/.

KidsHealth. (2015). Cystic fibrosis. Retrieved from http://kidshealth.org/parent/medical/lungs/cf.html.

Mayo Clinic. (2015, July 7). Cystic fibrosis. Retrieved from http://www.mayoclinic.com/health/cystic-fibrosis/DS00287.

National Heart, Lung, and Blood Institute. (2013, December 26). What is cystic fibrosis? Retrieved from http://www.nhlbi.nih.gov/health/health-topics/topics/cf/.

Orenstein, D. M., & Spahr, J. E. 2012. *Cystic Fibrosis: A Guide for Patient and Family.* Philadelphia: Lippincott/Williams & Wilkins.

DEEP VEIN THROMBOSIS

Deep vein thrombosis is a condition in which a thrombus, or blood clot, forms in a vein deep in the body, usually the lower legs, thighs, or pelvis. It may cause pain, but it can occur without any symptoms. Often called DVT, it can develop as a result of being confined to a hospital or nursing home bed, medical conditions that affect blood clotting, or after sitting still while traveling for a long time.

Deep vein thrombosis becomes a very serious condition when a blood clot breaks loose from the vein; travels through the bloodstream; and becomes lodged in the lung, where it blocks blood flow and causes a pulmonary embolism, which can cause permanent lung damage, low blood-oxygen levels, and damage to other organs not receiving enough oxygen, as well as sudden death. Common symptoms include warmth and tenderness, pain or swelling, and skin redness. Treatment aims to break up blood clots and prevent new ones from forming, as well as easing the symptoms of pain and inflammation. Once a diagnosis is made, DVT can be treated effectively.

Although age is a risk factor, DVT can occur at any age. As many as 900,000 people in the United States may be affected each year, and it's estimated that 60,000 to 100,000 cases are fatal, with up to 30 percent of those within one month of receiving a diagnosis; sudden death takes place in about 25 percent of those who have a pulmonary embolism.

Symptoms

Although about half of those with DVT experience no symptoms, the most common ones include swelling, pain, or tenderness along a vein in the leg, often starting as cramping or soreness in the calf while walking or standing; increased warmth or enlarged superficial veins in the affected leg; and discolored or red skin. Occasionally, the symptoms of a pulmonary embolism are also the initial symptoms of DVT, and these may include shortness of breath, pain when breathing deeply, coughing up blood, rapid breathing, and an increased heart rate.

Causes and Risk Factors

Blood clots that may lead to DVT are caused by blood that is prevented from circulating or clotting properly. Risk factors include immobilization following surgery or an injury; a fractured hip or leg; inherited blood clotting disorder; and, rarely, prolonged periods of sitting on an airplane flight or in a car. Other risk factors include pregnancy, birth control pills or hormone replacement therapy; obesity, cancer, heart failure, or inflammatory bowel disease; smoking tobacco; age older than 60; and a personal or family history of DVT or pulmonary embolism.

Diagnosis

The most common diagnostic test for DVT is duplex ultrasound, which uses high-frequency waves to measure the speed of blood flow, see the structure of the veins, and detect any blood clots. Without a clear diagnosis from an ultrasound, a veno-gram may be used to examine the deep veins and clots inside them; it is an x-ray made visible by the injection of contrast dye into the veins. A CT scan or an MRI may also be used to detect blood clots. Blood tests are taken to check for the pres-ence of elevated level of D dimer, a clot-dissolving substance found in most people with DVT, or an inherited blood-clotting disorder that can cause DVT.

Treatments

The treatment goals for DVT include stopping a blood clot from growing, prevent-ing a clot from breaking off and traveling to the lungs, and reducing the chance of a recurrence. Medications include anticoagulants, or blood thinners; thrombin in-hibitors, which interfere with the process of blood clotting; and thrombolytics, which dissolve large blood clots quickly. Compression stockings may be prescribed to prevent swelling because the pressure they exert reduces the chances that the blood will clot. Surgery may be necessary when medication is not an option or if medications have not been effective—a filter is inserted into the vena cava, a large vein in the stomach, to prevent any clots that break loose from lodging in the lungs.

Prevention

Common preventive measures include reducing risk factors that can be controlled, such as maintaining a healthy body weight, stopping smoking, and getting regular exercise. For those who face an increased risk of DVT, exercise and movement fol-lowing surgery or illness are key, as are following medical advice for medications and other treatments.

   Although the risk of DVT during long travels is low, it increases with four hours or more of travel time or in the presence of other risk factors. Walking the aisles of a plane, train, or other conveyance is recommended, as is stopping the car every hour and moving, stretching, and flexing the feet to increase blood flow to the calves. Wearing loose clothing and drinking nonalcoholic fluids also helps to minimize the risk of travel-related DVT. Wearing compression stockings and taking blood thin-ners may also be prescribed for traveling.

Prognosis and Outcomes

One-half of those who have had DVT will have long-term complications such as swelling, pain, discoloration, and scaling in the affected leg. About one-third of those with DVT and a pulmonary embolism will experience a recurrence within 10 years.

Jean Kaplan Teichroew

See also: Physical Activity; Thrombophlebitis; Venous Disorders

Further Reading

Centers for Disease Control and Prevention. (2015, June 22). Deep vein thrombosis (DVT)/pulmonary embolism (PE)—Blood clot forming in a vein, data & statistics. Retrieved from http://www.cdc.gov/ncbddd/dvt/data.html.

Cleveland Clinic. (2014, April 25). Deep vein thrombosis (DVT). Retrieved from http://my.clevelandclinic.org/services/heart/disorders/hypercoagstate/hic_Deep_Vein_Thrombosis_DVT.

Mayo Clinic. (2015). Deep vein thrombosis (DVT). Retrieved from http://www.mayoclinic.com/health/deep-vein-thrombosis/DS01005.

National Heart Lung and Blood Institute. (2011, October 28). What is deep vein thrombosis? Retrieved from http://www.nhlbi.nih.gov/health/health-topics/topics/dvt/.

Society for Vascular Surgery. (2010, December) Deep vein thrombosis (DVT). Retrieved from http://www.vascularweb.org/vascularhealth/pages/deep-vein-thrombosis-%28-dvt-%29-.aspx.

DEMENTIA

Current use of the term *dementia* [taken from the Latin for *de* (privation) and *mens* (mind)] reflects progressive loss of cognitive and intellectual functions associated with structural brain disease.

Lock (2013), in *The Alzheimer Conundrum*, contends that operational definitions of dementia used over time reflect our history, politics, and medical research. Dementia is not a specific disease: It is a categorical term describing a wide range of symptoms associated with a decline in memory, or other thinking skills, severe enough to reduce a person's ability to perform everyday activities.

The Centers for Disease Control and Prevention (CDC 2015) reports the two most common forms of dementia are Alzheimer's disease and vascular dementia. Dementia is often incorrectly referred to as "senility" or "senile dementia," which reflects the formerly widespread—but incorrect—belief that serious mental decline is a normal part of aging.

History

Berchtold and Cotman (1998) chart the evolution the concept of *de mens* (without mind) before the 1700s—described as the *clinical scope*—and the 1800s and beyond—identified as the *cognitive paradigm*. Before the 1700s, popular terminology included amentia (absence of [a] mind), dotage, senility, and stupidity—each suggesting defective intellectual judgment. Confirming this notion, the *Oxford English Dictionary* (1644) defined dementia as *without mind*. In the 1800s and beyond, society incorporated the [then] popular vernacular of without mind to evolve as a *cognitive paradigm*. Our current legal definition is informed by [the] *incapability of informed consent*, that is, without mind. Early Western medical and social histories describe behaviors, illnesses (madness and shaking disease), and deaths that were most probably caused by dementia. Berchtold and Cotman reference Shakespeare's *Hamlet* and *King Lear*, wherein the author made numerous and keen descriptions of dementia (140).

In 1801, French physician Philippe Pinel first used the term *demence* (incoherent) to describe his work with a 34-year-old woman suffering from an unusual disease process. Over a period of just a few years, this young woman lost her memory, speech, and ability to walk or use common objects like a fork or a hairbrush. The medical-political-social history of the term *dementia* incorrectly suggested that serious mental decline is a normal part of aging and evoked images of extreme disability and dependence, questions of competence in employment, legal transactions, and the conduct or ordinary activities of living.

Nearly 100 years later, the German physician, Alois Alzheimer, treated a 50-year-old patient identified as Auguste D. Following her death in 1906, Dr. Alzheimer published his findings on the clinical postmortem studies of the patient. First described as a distinctive disease, Alzheimer's disease was included in a textbook in 1910. The description was of a brain that was shrunken, full of fluid, evidenced structural damage in the form of neurofibrilary tangles, and had bone structures growing in the brain tissues.

Agronin (2004), author of *Alzheimer's Disease and Other Dementias*, reports that Alzheimer's disease (AD) is the most common type of dementia, accounting for 60 to 80 percent of cases. Vascular dementia, the second most common cause of dementia, is associated with stroke. Less common types of dementia include alcohol dementia (sustained use/abuse of alcohol), trauma dementia (brain and spinal injury), and the rare form called front-temporal dementia.

Types, Causes, and Symptoms

Dementia, a general term describing a group of symptoms such as losses of memory, judgment, language, complex motor skills, and other intellectual function, is caused by permanent damage or death of the brain's nerve cells, or neurons. The most common forms of dementia include Alzheimer's disease (AD), vascular dementia (multi-infract), dementia with Lewy bodies, Parkinson's disease, frontotemporal disease, Creutzfeldt-Jacob disease, Huntington's disease, and Wernicke-Korsakoff syndrome. The National Institute of Aging (NIA) reports that AD represents 60 to 70 percent of all cases of dementia. For more in depth descriptions of dementia, see the information available at the Alzheimer's Association website, at http://www.alz.org/dementia/types-of-dementia.asp.

Agronin (2004) asserts that dementia, in all forms, results from the dysfunction or death of large numbers of neurons and posits that dementia types are associated with protein deposits.

Other causes of dementia include the effects of stroke, toxic reactions (excessive alcohol or drug use), severe nutritional deficiencies (e.g., B12, folate), infections of the brain and spinal column, AIDS, Creutzfeldt-Jakob disease, prion diseases, and brain injury. Recent studies of the long-term effects of brain trauma injury report that lacking proper treatment, brain trauma injuries can lead to Parkinson's disease, Alzheimer's disease, and/or dementia.

The Mayo Clinic (2015) states the symptoms of dementia vary based on the cause. Common signs and symptoms include memory loss (typically short-term memory impairment) and difficulty communicating (an inability to express one's self). The dementia patient exhibits increasing difficulty with more complex tasks (lack planning and judgment skills), motor coordination (dressing, walking, feeding one's self), and changes in personality (hostility, inappropriate behavior, distrust). Severe symptomology includes paranoia, agitation, and hallucinations.

The Global Deteriorate Scale (GDS) (also known as the Reisberg scale) is used by health care professionals to describe stages of dementia; the GDS is most often used to delineate the trajectory of Alzheimer's disease, which is responsible for nearly 70 percent of all dementia cases. The GDS describes seven stages of ability: stage 1, no cognitive decline; stage 2, mild cognitive decline (forgets names, locations, trouble finding words); stage 3, mild cognitive decline (difficulty traveling to new locations or handling problems at work); stage 4, moderate cognitive decline (difficulty with complex tasks of finances, shopping, and planning); stage 5, moderately severe cognitive decline (needs help to choose clothes, and needs prompting to bath); stage 6, severe cognitive decline (loss of awareness or recent events and experiences, needs assistance going to the toilet and bathing); and stage 7, very severe cognitive decline (limited vocabulary, eventually becoming nonverbal, and loses ability to walk, sit, and eat).

Available dementia drug treatments are limited to slowing or minimizing the development of the symptoms. These pharmaceutical compounds are known as cholinesterase inhibitors (donepezil, or Aricept; rivastigmine, or Exelon; galatamine, or Razadyne), which may boost boosting levels of cholinesterase a chemical messenger involved with memory and judgment. Memantine, or Namenda, which regulates glutamate another chemical messenger is involved in learning and memory. Cholinesterase inhibitors are primarily used to treat Alzheimer's disease, vascular dementia, Parkinson's disease dementia, and Lewy body dementia.

Nonmedical approaches may be used in concert with medications; these include environmental and behavioral modifications: Modify the environment by reducing clutter and noise. Less distraction may help the patient to focus and function. Modify your responses by focusing on reassuring and validating the person; be in their world—they no longer have skills and abilities to function in your world. Modify tasks by breaking the task into easier steps; celebrate each success. Other nonmedical basics include enhancing communication, using eye contact, and speaking slowly. Encourage physical exercise, word and thinking games; establish a nighttime ritual; keep a calendar (use words and pictures); and plan for the future. Reach out to support groups and therapists.

Agronin (2004), Greutzner (2001), and the CDC (2015) recommend positive lifestyle behaviors to reduce the risk of developing the chronic diseases that are statistically linked to AD, the most common form of dementia. These conditions include hypercholesterolemia, hypertension, obesity, and Type 2 diabetes mellitus. In the simplest of terms, eat well and exercise.

Linda R. Barley

See also: Aging, Healthy; AIDS; Alzheimer's Disease; Brain Diseases; Creutzfeldt-Jakob Disease; Diet and Nutrition; Mental Disorders; Parkinson's Disease

Further Reading

Agronin, M. (2004). *Alzheimer Disease and Other Dementias*, 4th ed. New York: Wolters Kluwer, Lippincott, Williams & Wilkins.

Alzheimer's Association. (2016). Retrieved from http://www.alz.org/.

Berchtold, N., & Cotman, C. (1998). Evolution in the conceptualization of dementia and Alzheimer's disease: Greco-Roman period to the 1960s. *Neurobiology of Aging, 19*(3), 173–189.

Centers for Disease Control and Prevention (CDC). (2015). Alzheimer's disease. Retrieved from http://www.cdc.gov/aging/aginginfo/alzheimers.htm.

Dunne, R. (2002). *Dementia Care Programming: An Identity Focused Approach*. State College, PA: Venture Publishing.

Gruetzner, H. (2001). *Alzheimer's: A Caregiver's Guide and Sourcebook,* 3rd ed. New York: John Wiley & Sons.

Lock, M. (2013). *The Alzheimer Conundrum*. Princeton, NJ: Princeton University Press.

Mayo Clinic. (2015). Alzheimer's disease. Retrieved from http://www.mayoclinic.org/diseases-conditions/alzheimers-disease/home/ovc-20167098.

DEPRESSION

Depression is a mood disorder that affects almost 20 million people in the United States, from children to older adults. It affects the way a person thinks, feels, behaves, and functions; it is diagnosed when a person feels sad, hopeless, discouraged, unmotivated, or disinterested in life for two weeks or longer and when these feelings interfere with daily activities. The exact cause of depression is not known, but chemical changes in the brain, hormones, inherited traits, and stressful life events are some of the many factors that are involved.

Depression often starts between the ages of 15 and 30, with the average age of onset at 32, and it is much more common in women. Older adults are often at high risk, and a small percentage of teens experience debilitating depressive disorder. Depression is a high risk for suicide, and in addition to affecting mental health, it can also affect physical health. Depression is treatable with medication, psychotherapy, or a combination of both.

Types of Depression

One of the most common mental disorders in the United States, depression is classified with three main types: major depression, persistent depressive disorder, and bipolar disorder.

Major depression is at least five symptoms for a two-week period that interfere with the ability to work, study, eat, and sleep. Major depressive episodes may occur once or twice in a lifetime or reoccur frequently. Persistent depressive disorder (formerly known as dysthymia) is a form of depression that usually continues for two years or longer; it is not as severe as major depression, but it has the same symptoms. Bipolar disorder, once called manic-depression, is a mood cycle from severe or mild highs to severe depression. During bipolar depression, a person experiences the symptoms of major depression.

Symptoms

Common symptoms of depression include a persistent sad or anxious mood; feelings of hopelessness, anger, frustration, pessimism, guilt, worthlessness, or helplessness; a loss of interest or pleasure in activities once enjoyed, including sex; less energy or fatigue; difficulty concentrating, remembering, or making decisions; insomnia and other sleep problems; poor appetite and weight loss, or overeating and weight gain; thoughts of death or suicide, suicide attempts; restlessness and irritability; as well as headaches, digestive disorders and pain, and other persistent physical symptoms that don't respond to treatment and for which no other cause can be diagnosed.

Causes and Risk Factors

Depression is caused by a combination of genetic, biological, environmental, and psychological factors. Those at increased risk include women, people 45 to 64 years old, veterans returning from combat, Hispanics and non-Hispanics of other or multiple races, as well as those without a high school education, those previously married or unemployed, and older adults.

Other identified risk factors include people who have low self-esteem or are too dependent, self-critical, or pessimistic; physical or sexual abuse, the death or loss of loved ones, relationship or financial problems; childhood trauma or depression; family history of depression, suicide, bipolar disorder, or alcoholism; an unsupportive environment for those who are lesbian, gay, bisexual, or transgender; having an anxiety or eating disorder or posttraumatic stress disorder; alcohol or substance use disorder; heart disease, cancer, or other serious illness or chronic pain; and some medications for high blood pressure or sleeping.

Diagnosis

Depression is diagnosed when a person has a depressed mood or loss of interest in activities once enjoyed for most of the day daily or nearly daily for at least two weeks and when at least five symptoms are present at the same time. The symptoms are listed in the *Diagnostic and Statistical Manual of Mental Disorders (DSM-5)*, which is the standard classification of mental disorders used by mental health providers in the United States. Therapists, psychiatrists, and other mental health providers make a diagnosis of depression based on these specific criteria.

A health care provider may also conduct a physical examination and order lab tests to rule out medical causes for depression symptoms, as well as check for signs of substance abuse. If no medical condition is found to cause depression, a psychological evaluation of depression symptoms and other mental illnesses is next. Depression often occurs along with anxiety and eating disorders and obsessive-compulsive disorder (OCD).

Treatments

Effective treatments for reducing the symptoms of depression include medications and forms of talk therapy. Antidepressant medications work to lift mood and ease the feelings of sadness and hopelessness. A variety of antidepressants known as selective serotonin reuptake inhibitors (SSRIs) and serotonin norepinephrine reuptake inhibitors (SNRIs) are available; some people experience benefits after a few weeks. These medications may also pose significant side effects, including weight gain, headaches, nausea, sexual problems, agitation, and sleep problems. Other similar medications, or a combination of mood stabilizers, antipsychotics, or anti-anxiety medications may be prescribed, depending on individual mental and physical needs.

The combination of medication and forms of psychotherapy have been shown to be most effective in treating depression symptoms; both cognitive-behavioral therapy (CBT) and interpersonal therapy (IPT) teach people with depression to identify, work through relationship problems, and change problematic thinking and behaviors to regain a sense of control and pleasure, as well as to learn how to cope with daily stresses.

For those with treatment-resistant depression, which doesn't respond to antidepressant medication or therapy, electroconvulsive therapy (ECT) and transcranial magnetic stimulation (TMS) may be prescribed. Other steps to manage symptoms include joining a support group; regular exercise; relaxation, meditation, and breathing techniques; self-help materials; and family or marriage counseling.

Prognosis and Outcomes

Undiagnosed and untreated depression usually worsens and can last for many years, which contributes to an increased risk of suicide as well as negatively affecting personal relationships at home, work, and school. Depression usually responds well to treatment with antidepressant drugs, psychotherapy, or a combination of both, and most people receiving treatment experience a significant improvement in their symptoms. It may take some time to find the correct medication for an individual, and inadvisable sudden quitting can cause depression to worsen.

Future

Researchers conduct clinical trials to identify new and more effective treatments for depression and related disorders, including what behavior and brain function might reveal about treatment success in depression using cognitive-behavioral therapy; the effectiveness of combining therapies and certain medications; and how a computer-based treatment program affects emotions, behaviors, and brain systems, which may lead to procedures that can reduce symptoms of depression and improve positive emotions, relationships, and well-being.

Karen Jeanne Coleman

See also: Anxiety Disorders; Bipolar Disorder; Mental Disorders; PTSD (Posttraumatic Stress Disorder); Women's Health

Further Reading

Anxiety and Depression Association of America. (2015). Depression. Retrieved from http://www.adaa.org/understanding-anxiety/depression.

Depression and Bipolar Support Alliance. (2015). Depression. Retrieved from http://www.dbsalliance.org/site/PageServer?pagename=education_depression.

Diagnostic and Statistical Manual of Mental Disorders, 5th ed. (DSM-5). (2013). Washington, DC: American Psychiatric Association.

Mayo Clinic. (2015, July 22). Depression (major depressive disorder). Retrieved from http://www.mayoclinic.org/diseases-conditions/depression/basics/definition/con-20032977.

National Institute of Mental Health. (2015). What is depression? Retrieved from https://www.nimh.nih.gov/health/topics/depression/index.shtml.

Solomon, A. (2001). *The Noonday Demon: An Atlas of Depression.* New York: Scribner.

DERMATITIS

Dermatitis refers to skin inflammation, or rashes, caused by infections and exposure to allergens and irritating substances. Rashes can range from mild to severe, and they can create a variety of skin conditions, including itching, swelling, reddening, and blisters. The rashes are not contagious or life-threatening, although they can cause great discomfort and self-consciousness.

The most common types of dermatitis are contact dermatitis; atopic dermatitis, which is often called eczema; and seborrheic dermatitis, or cradle cap in infants and dandruff in adults. Dermatitis can affect anyone, but age, occupation, family history, and underlying health conditions may increase the risk of development. Nearly everyone gets contact dermatitis at least once in a lifetime. Worldwide, around 10 to 20 percent of children and up to 3 percent of adults of all skin colors have atopic dermatitis; most people develop it by the time they reach five years old. People younger than three months old and adults between 30 and 60 years old are those most susceptible to seborrheic dermatitis.

Of the many other forms are neurodermatitis, nummular dermatitis, statis dermatitis, perioral dermatitis, pompholyx, and dermatitis herpetiformis, an autoimmune blistering disorder associated with a sensitivity to gluten. Depending on the cause, treatment may include creams, lotions, or moisturizers to sooth itching or dry skin; antihistamine medications; topical corticosteroid ointments; and occasionally, corticosteroid pills or shots.

Symptoms

Itching and inflamed skin are often the first symptoms of dermatitis. Depending on the cause and the type of dermatitis, the skin may appear stiff or mildly swollen and have lesions, scabs, flaking, or small red bumps and pimples that may form weeping blisters. It may feel warm, tender, or burning and grow scaly, raw, or thick. More severe cases may have crusty scales, painful cracks, oozing blisters, or swelling in eyes, face, and genital areas.

Causes and Risk Factors

The exact causes of dermatitis are unknown due to the wide spectrum of the disorders, but in general, allergies, irritants, genetic factors, and health conditions cause different types of dermatitis. Factors that may increase the risk of developing certain types of dermatitis include age (atopic dermatitis usually starts in infancy); family or personal history of eczema, allergies, and asthma (atopic dermatitis); an occupation with exposure to some metals, solvents, and cleaning supplies (contact dermatitis); and congestive heart failure, Parkinson's disease, HIV, and other health conditions (seborrheic dermatitis). Each form of dermatitis has some specific or unique causes.

Contact dermatitis can result from contact with common irritants, including dust, sand, wool, and synthetic fabrics; detergents and soaps; personal hygiene products; hair dyes, fragrances, and perfumes; chlorine and other chemicals; adhesives; or allergy-provoking substances such as poison ivy, pollen, fish, eggs, and peanuts. Atopic dermatitis commonly runs in families with a genetic tendency for allergic conditions such as asthma, hay fever, or eczema, while possible underlying factors include a combination of dry, irritable skin and an immune system malfunction. Seborrheic dermatitis is common in people with oily skin or hair, and it may appear or disappear on its own depending on the time of year. Hereditary, physical stress, or neurological factors contribute to this condition, which is caused by overproduction in the sebaceous glands.

Neurodermatitis, most common among women between 30 and 50 and those who have a family history of dermatitis or obsessive-compulsive disorder, may be triggered by nerve injury, stress or emotional trauma, bug bites, tight wool or synthetic clothing, and dry skin, as well as traffic exhaust, allergens, sweat, heat, and poor blood circulation. Nummular dermatitis—coin-shaped red plaques on the legs, hands, arms, and torso—may be due primarily to family history as well as irritating weather conditions; skin injuries and infections; tight clothing; and sensitivities to rubber, nickel (found in earrings and zippers), formaldehyde, and other materials. Stasis dermatitis—the accumulation of blood and fluid buildup in the tissues that leads to skin irritation near the ankles—is caused by poor circulation in the legs, most likely caused by varicose veins, extreme obesity, congestive heart failure, or other conditions affecting leg circulation. Perioral dermatitis—red blisters and scaling near the mouth and chin—may be caused by exposure to topical steroids, makeup, or moisturizers. Pompholyx—itchy blisters on the sides of the fingers, palms of the hands, and soles of the feet—may be due to emotional tension, heat and sweat, or sensitivity to nickel, cobalt or chromate metals; a family history of atopic eczema is also a risk factor. Dermatitis herpetiformis—lesions usually seen on the elbows, knees, buttocks, and back—is the result of an immunologic response to gluten in the diet.

Diagnosis

To determine the type of dermatitis and make a diagnosis, a dermatologist may perform patch testing to test sensitivity to particular substances or examine the location and appearance of the rash. Lab tests may be conducted to rule out other skin problems; testing typically includes a culture for bacteria or other infection and, possibly, a biopsy or blood tests. Family and personal medical histories are reviewed regarding relevant health issues, and answers to specific questions may lead to determining the cause of the rash.

Treatments

Treatment is determined by the cause of the dermatitis. Atopic dermatitis, for example, cannot be cured, but treatment effectively reduces the symptoms of itchy, dry skin. Most treatment plans for dermatitis include the application of topical corticosteroid creams; creams or lotions that affect the immune system; and phototherapy, or controlled exposure to light. Oral antihistamine medications and oral or topical antibiotics may be prescribed as well.

Relief from itchy dry skin may be helped by taking warm oatmeal or bleach baths, frequent skin moisturizing, and avoiding temperature extremes. Wet compresses and over-the-counter anti-inflammation and anti-itch products, such as hydrocortisone cream and calamine lotion, can temporarily relieve symptoms.

Prevention

For contact and other types of dermatitis not caused by risk factors beyond control, people should identify and avoid substances that cause it. Allergens should be avoided as much as possible, and proper care should be taken to remove irritants immediately from the skin. Wearing cotton clothing, changing laundry detergent, and managing stress can also reduce the risk of a flare-up.

Prognosis and Outcomes

Treatment can stop the dermatitis from getting worse, as well as relieve the uncomfortable symptoms. Ongoing or recurring treatment is necessary for dermatitis that flares up over a lifetime. With appropriate treatment, contact dermatitis usually clears up in several weeks or sooner. If exposure to irritants or allergens cannot be avoided, dermatitis is likely to recur. The immune system, which has been sensitized to a substance, may react to future exposure and cause a flare-up. Most people who have dermatitis due to exposure to workplace irritants are successful in managing their symptoms, and they recover without problem.

Ray Marks

See also: Allergies; Asthma; Autoimmune Disease; Celiac Disease; Eczema; Immune System Disorders; Psoriasis; Skin Conditions

Further Reading

American Academy of Dermatology. (2011, July). Contact dermatitis. Retrieved from https://www.aad.org/dermatology-a-to-z/diseases-and-treatments/a—d/contact-dermatitis.
Cleveland Clinic. (2015, May 25). Dermatitis. Retrieved from http://my.clevelandclinic.org/disorders/Dermatitis-Atopic_Eczema/hic_Dermatitis.aspx.
Dermaharmony. (2011, June 7). Dermatitis—causes and treatment. Retrieved from http://www.dermaharmony.com/dermatitis/default.aspx.
Mayo Clinic. (2015). Dermatitis. Retrieved from http://www.mayoclinic.org/diseases-conditions/dermatitis-eczema/basics/definition/con-20032183.

DIABETES, TYPE 1

Type 1 diabetes is a chronic condition in which the pancreas loses its ability to make insulin, a hormone needed to convert sugar (glucose), starches, and other food into energy needed for daily life. In this form of diabetes—formerly called insulin-dependent diabetes or juvenile diabetes—the immune system attacks and destroys the cells in the pancreas that produce insulin. The result is a buildup of glucose in the blood, which can lead to serious problems. Long-term complications can develop gradually over time; they may be disabling or even life-threatening, affecting the heart, blood vessels, nerves in the feet and elsewhere, eyes, kidneys, skin, gums, and teeth. Osteoporosis, pregnancy complications, and hearing impairment are also possible results of the disease. Stress, hormonal changes, periods of growth, physical activity, medications, illness or infection, and fatigue can adversely affect efforts to tightly control blood sugar levels

Type 1 diabetes usually strikes children and young adults; although onset can occur at any age, most people are diagnosed before the age of 30. More than 1.25 million people in the United States live with Type 1 diabetes, including about 200,000 children and young adults. Some 40,000 people are diagnosed every year. Type 1 diabetes is not preventable, and it can result in a reduction in quality of life and shorten the average life span by about 15 years. But people can live a healthy life by keeping their blood glucose levels in the target range set by their doctor.

Symptoms

Diabetes often goes undiagnosed because the symptoms are not always obvious and may take a long time to develop. Type 1 diabetes may come on gradually or suddenly. Symptoms may include unusual thirst and frequent urination; extreme hunger; unusual weight loss; extreme fatigue and irritability; blurred vision; sores that heal slowly; dry, itchy skin; and loss of feeling or tingling in the feet.

Causes and Risk Factors

The exact cause of Type 1 diabetes is unknown, but it develops when the body's immune system destroys pancreatic beta cells that make the hormone insulin that regulates blood glucose. Once those cells are destroyed, they cannot produce insulin, so sugar builds up in the bloodstream instead of being used for energy.

Some known risk factors include a genetic susceptibility, or a family history of Type 1 diabetes, which is associated with a slightly increased risk of developing the disease; trigger due to viral infection from German measles, mumps, or certain other viruses, which may cause the immune system to turn against the body instead of helping it fight infection and sickness; and race and ethnic background. In the United States, the prevalence is higher among Caucasians than among black or Hispanic people.

Diagnosis

Most people are diagnosed within a short period of time once the pancreas shuts down its production of insulin. A variety of diagnostic tests may be used.

- Fasting blood glucose test takes a blood sample to check blood glucose levels after an overnight fast of at least eight hours. Usually conducted first thing in the morning, it is the most commonly used test for diagnosing diabetes.
- Random blood glucose takes a blood sample to check blood glucose levels at a random time of the day. It is the preferred test in medical emergencies when people have severe diabetes symptoms.
- Oral glucose test checks blood glucose levels before and two hours after drinking a sugary beverage, indicating how the body processes glucose. People with Type 1 diabetes will see a sharp rise and a sustained high level of glucose.
- Hemoglobin (A1C) test measures average blood sugar levels for the previous few months. Diabetes is diagnosed when A1C is 6.5 percent or higher. This test takes less time than the oral glucose test and does not require fasting.

These tests help distinguish between Type 1 and Type 2 diabetes. The doctor takes blood tests to check for autoantibodies that are common in Type 1 diabetes once a diagnosis has been made. The presence of ketones, or by-products from the breakdown of fat, in urine also suggests Type 1 diabetes rather than Type 2.

Treatments

Treatment of Type 1 diabetes involves management; the disease has no cure. Proper management of Type 1 diabetes is a lifelong commitment that can help people live long, healthy lives; it involves the following measures.

Insulin: People with Type 1 diabetes must take multiple insulin injections daily or continually infuse insulin through a pump. Following the insulin regimen prescribed by a doctor plays a vital role in diabetes care. Insulin does not cure the disease, but it does allow a person with Type 1 diabetes to stay alive, and it does not necessarily prevent the possibility of complications, including kidney failure, blindness, nerve damage, heart attack, stroke, and pregnancy complications.

Regular exercise and healthy body weight: Activity blood sugar, which results in more stable blood glucose levels, can help avoid some of the long-term health problems.

Healthful foods and carbohydrate counts: Paying particular attention daily to the amounts of sugars and starches in food and the timing of meals is a crucial, as is counting carbohydrates in foods, which is necessary to take enough insulin to properly metabolize them.

Blood sugar monitoring: People with Type 1 diabetes must test their blood sugar six or more times a day to make sure blood sugar level remains within target range to delay or prevent complications. When blood sugar level drops below target range, ingesting fruit juice, glucose tablets, hard candy, or regular soda can stabilize the blood sugar. When blood sugar rises above target range, adjusting meal plans or medications or taking an additional insulin can return blood sugar back to the normal range.

Support: Talking to a counselor or joining a support group can provide encouragement and understanding and be good sources of information.

Prevention

Type 1 diabetes cannot be prevented, and there is no practical way to predict who will get it. Once a diagnosis has been made, it requires lifelong treatment and management. Scientists do not know exactly what causes the body's immune system to attack the beta cells, but they believe that both genetic factors and viruses are involved.

Prognosis and Outcomes

Diabetes is a lifelong disease and there is no cure. But people can lead full, active lives with Type 1 diabetes. Careful management of blood glucose can prevent or delay the many possible complications of diabetes, although they can occur, even in people with good diabetes control.

Future

Researchers are making progress in identifying the genetics and triggers that predispose some people to develop Type 1 diabetes. Researchers continue to develop new methods to develop preventive immunotherapies and to cure the disease by transplanting insulin-producing cells into the body. They are also working on improvements with devices that make blood glucose testing and insulin injections easier, less painful, and more effective.

Leah Sultan-Khan

See also: Addison's Disease; Autoimmune Disease; Celiac Disease; Charcot-Marie-Tooth Disorder; Cholesterol; Diabetes, Type 2; Prediabetes; Rheumatoid Arthritis; Sjögren's Syndrome

Further Reading

American Diabetes Association (2011). *Complete Guide to Diabetes: The Ultimate Home Reference from the Diabetes Experts.* Alexandria, VA: American Diabetes Association.
American Diabetes Association. (2015). Type 1 diabetes. Retrieved from http://www.diabetes.org/.
Centers for Disease Control and Prevention. (2015, March 31). National diabetes fact sheet. Retrieved from http://www.cdc.gov/diabetes/basics/diabetes.html.
JDRF. (2015). Type 1 diabetes facts. Retrieved from http://jdrf.org/about-jdrf/fact-sheets/type-1-diabetes-facts/.
Mayo Clinic. (2014, August 2). Type 1 diabetes. Retrieved from http://www.mayoclinic.com/health/type-1-diabetes/DS00329.
Mayo Clinic. (2014). *The Essential Diabetes Book.* New York: Time Home Entertainment Inc., 2014.
The Nemours Foundation (2015). Type 1 diabetes: What is it? Retrieved from http://kidshealth.org/parent/diabetes_center/diabetes_basics/type1.html.

DIABETES, TYPE 2

Type 2 diabetes is a lifelong chronic disease in which the pancreas does not produce enough insulin, or the body does not properly use the insulin it makes. The result is that glucose builds up in the blood stream instead of being used for energy. If untreated, Type 2 diabetes can be life-threatening, especially over time, when it can lead to serious problems. Potential complications associated with Type 2 diabetes are cardiovascular diseases, including heart attack and stroke; nerve damage in the feet and legs; kidney damage; eye damage that can increase the risk of cataracts and glaucoma; bacterial and fungal infections affecting the skin and mouth; osteoporosis; pregnancy complications; and hearing impairment.

Once known as called adult-onset diabetes or noninsulin-dependent diabetes mellitus, Type 2 diabetes is the most common form of diabetes; about 27 million people in the United States have it.

This type of diabetes is usually associated with excess body weight, age, physical inactivity, family history of diabetes, and other factors. Childhood obesity contributes to the increase in cases of Type 2 diabetes among children and teens. Complications associated with Type 2 diabetes can reduce life expectancy by about 5 to 10 years among middle-age adults with Type 2 diabetes. Most people can prevent the onset of Type 2 diabetes with healthful meals, regular exercise, healthy body weight, and taking medications.

Symptoms

Type 2 diabetes usually occurs slowly over time, and symptoms may not show up for many years. Symptoms typical of Type 2 diabetes include increased thirst and frequent urination, increased hunger, weight loss, fatigue, blurred vision, sores or frequent infections that heal slowly, areas of darkened skin, and pain or numbness in the feet or hands.

Causes and Risk Factors

Type 2 diabetes develops when the body becomes resistant to insulin or when the pancreas stops producing enough insulin, which is needed to move blood sugar, or glucose, into cells where it is used for energy. This process causes sugar to build up in the bloodstream.

It is not known why some people develop Type 2 diabetes and others don't. Common risk factors include being overweight (especially with abdominal obesity); prediabetes (higher-than-normal levels of blood glucose); age 40 or over; physical inactivity; high blood pressure or high cholesterol; a family history of diabetes; belonging to certain high-risk ethnic groups (African Americans, Hispanics, American Indians, and Asian Americans); and a personal history of gestational diabetes or having a baby weighing nine pounds or more at birth.

Diagnosis

A diagnosis of Type 2 diabetes is based on tests.

- Fasting blood glucose test takes a blood sample to check blood glucose levels after an overnight fast of at least eight hours.
- Hemoglobin (A1C) test measures average blood sugar levels for the previous few months. Diabetes is diagnosed when A1C measures 6.5 percent or higher; prediabetes measures 5.7 to 6.4 percent.
- Oral glucose test checks blood glucose levels before and two hours after drinking a sugary beverage, indicating how the body processes glucose.

Treatments

Treatment of Type 2 diabetes requires a lifelong commitment to managing blood sugar regularly. Because there is no cure, checking and recording blood sugar level once a day or several times a week is the only way to control blood sugar levels within target range and prevent or delay further complications. Recommended management measures include maintaining a healthy body weight and eating a well-balanced diet with plenty of fruits, vegetables, and whole grains; regular physical activity to help reduce blood sugar levels; moderate alcohol consumption; and taking medications and possibly insulin to lower blood sugar.

Prognosis and Outcomes

Type 2 diabetes can be prevented or delayed by making lifestyle changes if necessary, including maintaining a healthy weight with regular physical activity and a healthful diet; avoiding smoking tobacco; getting adequate sleep; and managing blood pressure, cholesterol, and glucose.

Diabetes is a lifelong disease that has no cure. Some people with Type 2 diabetes no longer need medication when they lose weight and become more active because their body's insulin and an appropriate diet help control their blood sugar level.

Leah Sultan-Khan

See also: Cholesterol; Diabetes, Type 1; Diet and Nutrition; Food Guides from the USDA; Heart Diseases; Obesity; Physical Activity; Prediabetes; Stroke

Further Reading

American Diabetes Association. (2015). Type 2. Retrieved from http://www.diabetes.org /diabetes-basics/type-2/?loc=util-header_type2.

American Diabetes Association (2011). *Complete Guide to Diabetes: The Ultimate Home Reference from the Diabetes Experts*. Alexandria, VA: American Diabetes Assn.

Centers for Disease Control and Prevention. (2015, February 9). Prevent Type 2 diabetes. Retrieved from http://www.cdc.gov/Features/DiabetesPrevention/index.html.

Mayo Clinic. (2014, July 24). Type 2 diabetes. Retrieved from http://www.mayoclinic.org /diseases-conditions/type-2-diabetes/basics/definition/con-20031902.

Mayo Clinic. (2014). *The Essential Diabetes Book*. New York: Time Home Entertainment Inc., 2014.

DIET AND NUTRITION

Nutrition, as a science discipline, refers to the study of nutrients, which are contained in foods, beverages, and supplements. Nutrients are chemical substances the body uses in order to perform vital functions. Antoine Lavoisier was the first to discover, in 1775, that energy could be released from food, and, thus, he is known as the father of nutrition. There are six categories of nutrients: water, carbohydrates, proteins, fats, vitamins, and minerals. Without these essential nutrients, one's health would be compromised and prolonged deprivation could result in death. Thus, it is estimated that one could not live beyond a week without water nor could one live beyond two months without a food source.

Within the body, water helps to dissolve chemical substances and transports them to all tissues, where vital reactions occur. Furthermore, these cellular reactions must take place in a water solution; afterward, the by-products are carried away by water. The body also utilizes water to produce sweat and regulate one's temperature. This explains why approximately 60 percent of the body's weight is made up of water.

Carbohydrates serve as the body's primary energy source. Each gram of carbohydrates provides the body with four calories. A calorie is commonly known as the unit of measurement that quantifies the amount of energy supplied by food. Carbohydrates are composed of sugar molecules. Simple carbohydrates contain one or two sugar molecules. Examples of naturally occurring simple sugars include fructose, found in fruit, and lactose, found in dairy items. Sucrose and high fructose corn syrup are processed simple sugars that are added to foods and beverages for the purpose of sweetening. Complex carbohydrates, such as starch and fiber, contain many interlocking sugar molecules. Fiber is the nondigestible form of carbohydrates; its presence in the diet helps to prevent intestinal disorders like constipation, diverticulitis, and cancer. All the other carbohydrates are digestible and travel through the blood as glucose.

Proteins can also supply four calories of energy per gram, but, more importantly, proteins serve as raw material for building and preserving body muscle and tissues. In addition, proteins function as antibodies, enzymes, and hormones within the body. Proteins are made up of smaller units called amino acids, of which there are 20 types. The body is capable of synthesizing 11 of the amino acids; however, it is essential that the other nine be obtained from one's diet. Proteins that contain all nine of the essential amino acids are referred to as complete, and those lacking one or more are referred to as incomplete. It is possible, through menu planning, to combine incomplete proteins to ensure that one consumes daily the essential nine amino acids.

Fats are nutrients that, in addition to supplying energy, function within the body as insulation to help regulate body temperatures and as padding to protect organs from external injury. Calories consumed in excess of the body's needs are stored as fat, which can later be metabolized for energy as needed. One gram of fat will yield nine calories of energy. There are several types of fat molecules. Fats of a solid consistency, like those found in the marbling of red meats, butter and cream, primarily contain *saturated* fatty acids. Fats of a liquid consistency, such as vegetable oil, contain *unsaturated* fatty acids. This category includes *mono-unsaturated* fats, such as canola, olive and peanut oil, and *poly-unsaturated* fats. This latter group is further delineated as linoleic (omega-6) fatty acids, found in the other vegetable oils, and alpha-linolenic (omega-3) fatty acids, found in fish oil. When liquid oil is converted to a solid fat through the process of hydrogenation, the product is referred to as a *trans fat*; shortening and stick margarine are examples of trans fats. With regard to health, diets high in saturated fats and trans fats are known to negatively affect cholesterol levels in the blood, while diets high in unsaturated fats are associated with improved cholesterol levels.

Vitamins are divided into two groups: fat-soluble (A, D, E, and K) and water-soluble (B and C). All of the B vitamins, which include B_1 (thiamin), B_2 (niacin), B_3 (riboflavin), B_6 (pyridoxine), B_{12} (cobalamin), folate, biotin, and pantothenic acid, are involved, as coenzymes, in the metabolism of carbohydrates, proteins and fats to release energy. Furthermore, vitamins C, D, and K help with bone formation, while vitamins B_6, B_{12}, folate, and K are involved in blood cell development. Neurological activities are maintained by vitamins A, B_1, B_6, and B_{12}, and the integrity of cell membranes are maintained by vitamin E. Lastly, vitamins A, C, and E protect the body against oxidative damage.

Minerals are also involved in energy metabolism, specifically iodine, chromium, manganese, and molybdenum. Bone formation occurs through the actions of calcium, phosphorus, magnesium, and fluoride, while blood cell development is influenced by iron, zinc, and copper. Furthermore, the regulation of fluid and electrolyte balance occurs through the body's use of sodium, potassium, chloride, and phosphorus. And lastly, selenium performs antioxidant functions.

The term *diet* refers to the food and beverages one consumes regularly. Thus, a healthful diet is one that is diverse, in which items from all the food groups are represented. The *MyPlate* icon, released by the U.S. Department of Agriculture (USDA) in 2011, visually conveys the food groups required for a nutritious diet.

The *vegetable group* includes starches, such as corn and potatoes, as well as dark green, red, and orange vegetables. These items are rich in vitamins, minerals, and complex carbohydrates. The *fruit group* includes apples, mangoes, melons, bananas, berries, and grapes, to name a few. These items are rich in vitamins, minerals, and simple carbohydrates. The *grain group* includes foods, such as cereals, breads, crackers, pasta, and rice, made from grains. If the whole grain is used, then the food item will naturally be rich in fiber, iron, and B vitamins, with the exception of B_{12}. Levels of folate will be more than adequate because, beginning in 1998, all grain products were fortified with synthetic folate. Refined grains, in which iron and B vitamins were removed during milling, must be nutrient enriched, as mandated by law since 1930. However, there is no mandate for manufacturers to replace the fiber that was lost during milling; thus, refined grains tend to be low in fiber. To this end, grains are typically rich in complex carbohydrates, vitamins, and minerals, with varying amounts of fiber. The protein food group includes meat, poultry, seafood, and eggs, which represent *complete proteins*, as well as legumes, nuts and seeds, which represent *incomplete proteins*. The fats found in animal proteins tend to be saturated and solid with the propensity to clog arteries once entering the bloodstream, while the oil extracted from plant proteins and fish tend to be unsaturated and liquid. Animal proteins contain vitamin B_{12}, and plant oils contain vitamin E. In general, proteins are rich sources of minerals. The *Dairy* group includes low-fat milk, yogurt, cheese, and fortified soy beverages. These items contain simple carbohydrates, proteins, fats, vitamins, and minerals, such as calcium. The type of fat in dairy items is mostly saturated, which, following digestion and metabolism, has an adverse effect on the amount of cholesterol circulating in the blood, potentially leading to heart disease; thus it is important to choose dairy items in which most of the fat has been removed or skimmed, such as skim or 1 percent milk.

In addition to its emphasis on variety, a healthful diet should be balanced. The Institute of Medicine has established for the general population amounts deemed appropriate for the essential nutrients; these amounts are listed in the Dietary Reference Intakes table. Furthermore, the USDA has recommended daily food patterns, with specific amounts for each food group, based on age and gender. Additionally, the Institute of Medicine has specified that the daily caloric intake of adults should be comprised of 45–65 percent carbohydrates, 10–35 percent protein, and 20–35 percent fat. Adhering to these guidelines should enable one to manage his or her body weight.

When there is an imbalance, malnutrition can occur. More than two-thirds of the adult American population is either overweight or obese, a condition characterized by excess body fat.

This condition results from calories being consumed or eaten beyond the metabolic needs of the individual; excess calories are then stored as body fat. In the American diet, foods that contribute to the excess calorie load include items prepared with additional fat and sugar, such as sweetened beverages (soda), desserts (cookies and cakes), and snacks (chips and candy) as well as foods that are deep fried. Fat is stored in adipose tissue and tends to accumulate slowly over time; however, deposits can reach harmful levels that impede physiological functioning and place the individual at risk for other chronic diseases. Thus, overweight and obese persons are more likely to suffer from osteoarthritis, heart disease, stroke, hypertension, Type 2 diabetes, and cancers, such as breast, endometrial, and colorectal malignancies. Experts believe it is the cellular reactions that occur within adipose tissue that lead to oxidative damage and inflammation; this in turn restricts blood circulation, leads to insulin resistance, and disrupts hormonal balance. Furthermore, excess consumption of saturated fats, found in red meat and full-fat dairy products (such as cream, cheese and butter), as well as trans-fats (found in stick margarine, shortening, and hydrogenated vegetable oils), have been found to be directly associated with plaque formation in the arteries of the heart and brain. As the arterial walls thicken with the cholesterol deposits that make up plaque, the passage of blood is impaired; often, to compensate, the heart will pump harder and exert a greater force of blood pressure inside the vessels, a condition known as hypertension. Evidence indicates that in a majority of cases, hypertension coexists with heart disease, stroke, and diabetes. Another dietary factor, excess sodium (found in salted and preserved foods that have been dried, canned, or frozen) is known to contribute to high blood pressure among certain individuals.

Malnutrition can also occur when there are deficits in the diet. The American diet tends to be lacking in fruits, vegetables, and whole grains that are replete with vitamins and minerals. These plant-based foods also contain fiber, antioxidants, and phytochemicals, which are partly responsible for the crop's color; all of these substances are thought to play a role in chronic disease prevention, specifically of cardiovascular disease, stroke, hypertension, Type 2 diabetes, and some cancers. Furthermore, fish, which contains the unsaturated fat known as omega-3, is minimally consumed by Americans; this fatty acid is known to play a beneficial role in the regulation of blood pressure and blood clotting. Alternative sources of omega-3 fatty acids may be found in walnuts, flax seeds, dark leafy greens, or fish oil supplements. Another chronic disease, known as osteoporosis, affects a significant number of postmenopausal women (10 percent). This condition occurs with the demineralization of bone that is part of the aging process; adequate calcium consumption must occur early and be maintained throughout the years in order to achieve peak bone mass by adulthood. Although calcium is naturally found in dairy products, the mean intake of dairy foods by Americans, 12 years or older, is only half of the amount recommended for bone health. For nondairy consumers, alternative sources should include calcium-fortified foods, such as orange juice and soy beverages, or calcium supplements to prevent osteoporosis.

In summary, the *2010 Dietary Guidelines for Americans* suggest the following strategies: (1) Fill half one's plate with fruits and vegetables. (2) Drink water instead of sugary drinks. (3) Switch to fat-free or low-fat (1 percent) milk or fortified soy beverages. (4) Make at least half of one's grain selections whole instead of refined. (5) Avoid oversized portions. (6) Reduce sodium by limiting canned, dried, and processed foods. (7) Vary protein sources; include plant-based proteins more often and seafood twice a week. (8) Cut back on foods high in solid fats, added sugars, and salt. Implementing these behavior changes may significantly reduce one's risk of obesity, cardiovascular disease, stroke, hypertension, Type 2 diabetes, and osteoporosis.

Public health experts believe nutrients should come primarily from foods. Often, nutrients are present in food in a form that has greater bioavailability than when presented in supplement form. However, in certain situations, fortified foods or dietary supplements may be beneficial; these include cases in which one's diet is inadequate or one has an increased need due to a medical condition.

Gloria Shine McNamara

See also: Aging, Healthy; Brain Diseases; Cardiovascular Disease; Cholesterol; Dementia; Diabetes, Type 2; Food Guides from the USDA; Heart Diseases; Mental Disorders; Obesity; Stroke; Wellness

Further Reading

Brown, J. (2011). *Nutrition Now*. Belmont, CA: Wadsworth, Cengage Learning.

Centers for Disease Control and Prevention. (2011). Calcium and bone health. Retrieved from www.cdc.gov/nutrition/everyone/basics/vitamins/calcium.html/.

Centers for Disease Control and Prevention. (2012). Osteoporosis. Retrieved from www.cdc.gov/nchs/fastats/osteoporosis.htm.

Centers for Disease Control and Prevention. (2012). Obesity. Retrieved from http://www.cdc.gov/nchs/fastats/overwt.htm.

Thompson, J., & Manore, M. (2009). *Nutrition: An Applied Approach*. San Francisco, CA: Pearson Benjamin Cummings.

U.S. Department of Agriculture, Agricultural Research Service, Food Surveys Research Group. (2010). *Fluid Milk Consumption in the United State: What We Eat in America, NHANES 2005-2006*. Washington, DC: USDA. Retrieved from http://www.ars.usda.gov/Services/docs.htm?docid=19476.

U.S. Department of Agriculture, Center for Nutrition Policy and Promotion. (2012). *MyPlate*. Retrieved from http://www.choosemyplate.gov/food-groups/.

U.S. Department of Agriculture and U.S. Department of Health and Human Services. (2010). *Dietary Guidelines for Americans*. Retrieved from http://www.dietaryguidelines.gov.

U.S. Department of Health and Human Services, Office of Disease Prevention and Health Promotion. (2011). About Healthy People. Retrieved from http://www.healthypeople.gov/2020/about/default.aspx.

DIGESTIVE DISEASES

Digestive diseases affect the digestive, or gastrointestinal, system. This system includes the esophagus, stomach, large and small intestines, liver, pancreas, and the gallbladder. Disorders range from mild to very serious conditions, and they are very common, affecting more than 100 million people in the United States.

The incidence and prevalence of most digestive diseases increase with age. Notable exceptions are gastroenteritis and appendicitis, intestinal infections that peak among infants and children. Other exceptions include hemorrhoids, inflammatory bowel disease, and chronic liver disease, which occur more commonly among young and middle-aged adults.

Women are more likely than men to report a digestive condition. Whether they experience more troubles with their digestive systems than men is difficult to determine, but they visit doctors more often than men and have a greater opportunity to discuss their digestive symptoms.

Chronic digestive disorders include cancer, celiac disease, Crohn's disease, gallstones, incontinence, inflammatory bowel disease, irritable bowel syndrome (IBS), lactose intolerance, pancreatitis, swallowing problems, ulcerative colitis, ulcers, and unintended weight gain or loss.

Symptoms

Commonly reported symptoms are abdominal pain, bleeding, bloating, constipation, diarrhea, nausea, and vomiting.

Causes

While the causes of many digestive diseases remain unknown, a digestive disease may develop congenitally or from numerous factors such as stress, fatigue, diet, or smoking. Abusing alcohol imposes the greatest risk for digestive diseases, particularly increasing the risk of esophageal, colorectal, and liver cancers.

Physical, mental, and emotional stresses are key causes of poor digestion. When the body experiences stress as a survival mechanism, it diverts energy, blood, enzymes, and oxygen from the digestive organs. In addition to fear, anger, worry, and other mental and emotional stresses, physical stresses caused by infections, trauma from injuries, surgery, and environmental toxins can have a major effect on the efficiency of the digestive system.

Antibiotics can kill a high percentage of the naturally occurring beneficial bacteria that are needed for digestion. Once antibiotic treatment stops, pathogenic bacteria, opportunistic yeasts, fungi, and parasites can move in to fill an opening in the gut area (because there are now very few bacteria). Once they become dominant and multiply, they can damage the gut wall and create toxic substances that can affect the immune system detrimentally.

A poor diet of processed food, or refined carbohydrates (sugar and flour stripped of essential nutrients and fiber) and junk foods almost completely devoid of nutritional value (and high in calories fat, refined carbohydrates, and sugar), forces the body to rob itself of chromium, manganese, cobalt, copper, zinc, and magnesium. Once these minerals are depleted, the body finds it harder to digest any carbohydrates. Those not fully digested ferment into simple sugars and alcohols, providing fuels for yeast and bacteria and leading to indigestion, gas, and bloating. A low-fiber diet results in a slow transit time of food through the digestive tract, which means greater risk of constipation and the absorption of some of the toxins from not-yet-eliminated food waste into the bloodstream. Eating enough raw food supplies enzymes that help digestion. Food allergies, including those to dairy, wheat, and fruits, often lead to digestive disorders.

Drugs directly affect the digestive organs. Over-the-counter, prescription, and recreational drugs that can affect digestion include antacids, antihistamines, NSAIDs, birth control pills, laxatives, steroids, alcohol, caffeine, tobacco, marijuana, cocaine, and many others. The anti-inflammatory drugs aspirin, acetaminophen, and ibuprofen can irritate the lining of the stomach, leading to impaired digestion and infection.

When exposed to environmental toxins (chemicals, radiation, solvents, food additives, air and water pollution, and mercury and other metals), the body naturally reacts to detoxify them, a process that requires a great amount of energy that leaves little for proper digestive function.

Genetics also play an important role in digestive functioning and the ability to withstand stress and resist digestive problems.

Diagnosis

In addition to a complete medical history of symptoms and physical examination, testing for digestive disorders is often necessary. Lab tests look for hidden blood in the stool and abnormal bacteria in the digestive organs.

Numerous imaging tests are available for more detailed diagnosis, including barium beefsteak meal, colorectal transit study, computed tomography scan (CT scan), defecography, lower GI (gastrointestinal) series (or barium enema), magnetic resonance imaging (MRI) and magnetic resonance cholangiopancreatography (MRCP), oropharyngeal motility (swallowing) study, radioisotope gastric-emptying scan, ultrasound, and upper GI (gastrointestinal) series (or barium swallow).

When necessary, more invasive endoscopic procedures are performed, including colonoscopy, endoscopic retrograde cholangiopancreatography (ERCP), esophagogastroduodenoscopy (EGD, or upper endoscopy), and sigmoidoscopy.

Treatments

Depending on the diagnosis and its severity, treatment options include prescription and nonprescription medications, dietary changes, increased exercise, chemotherapy for cancer, and home remedies such as castor oil for constipation. A variety of surgical procedures performed with endoscopy and laparoscopy are available, as is open surgery, including organ transplantation of the liver, pancreas, and small intestine.

Prevention

Eating a healthful diet, controlling stress, exercising, reducing alcohol, and avoiding smoking and drugs are standard health practices that may offset the onset of digestive disorders.

Prognosis

The prognosis for living with a digestive disorder depends on the specific condition, its duration and severity, as well as an individual's general health and age.

Ray Marks

See also: Abdominal Disease; Celiac Disease; Crohn's Disease; Inflammatory Bowel Disease; Irritable Bowel Syndrome; Lactose Intolerance; Pancreatitis; Ulcerative Colitis; Ulcers

Further Reading

Johns Hopkins Medicine Health Library. (2015). Digestive diagnostic procedures. Retrieved from http://www.hopkinsmedicine.org/healthlibrary/conditions/digestive_disorders /digestive_diagnostic_procedures_85,P00364/.
National Digestive Diseases Information Clearinghouse (NDDIC). (2014). Digestive diseases A–Z. Retrieved from www.digestive.niddk.nih.gov/.
National Digestive Disease Information Clearinghouse (NDDIC). (2014, December). Facts and fallacies about digestive diseases. Retrieved from http://crextras.com/lib/distress /chronic/irritable-bowel/digestive-diseases/.

DIVERTICULAR DISEASE

Overview

Diverticular disease is made up of three different conditions including diverticulosis; diverticular bleeding; and diverticulitis, which results in the development of small pockets or sacs in the wall of the colon or large intestine, which is a long, tube-like structure that stores and eliminates waste products.

Diverticulosis, or *diverticula,* refers to the formation of tiny pockets or diverticula in the lining of the bowel that range in size from very small to very large. These form in response to pressure placed on weak areas of the walls of the intestine by gases, waste products, or liquid. They occur most commonly in the region of the large intestine called the sigmoid colon and can rupture to produce diverticulitis.

The condition is very common, occurring in 10 percent of people over age 40 and half of those over age 60. This may not be a problem because the condition may not produce symptoms. Symptoms can, however, occur due to complications and are mostly due to bleeding, or diverticular infection, known as diverticulitis.

Diverticular bleeding occurs with chronic injury to the small blood vessels located near to diverticula, when a small artery located in the diverticulum breaks through the skin into the colon.

Diverticulitis is a painful condition that occurs when one or more diverticula become infected or inflamed, and complications of diverticulitis include tearing of the intestinal wall, with leakage of intestinal contents into surrounding abdominal cavity, and possible peritonitis, abscesses, or intestinal obstruction.

There are two forms of diverticulitis, the simple and complicated forms.

Simple diverticulitis accounts for 75 percent of cases, is not associated with complications, and usually responds to medical treatment.

Complicated diverticulitis occurs in 25 percent of cases and usually requires surgery due to complications such as abscesses; fistulas or abnormal links between two areas of the body not normally connected, such as the bladder and bowel; blockage of the colon; peritonitis or infection around the abdominal organ; or sepsis, which is an overwhelming body-wide infection that can lead to multiple organ failures.

Types of Symptoms

Diverticuli, infection, and inflammation of diverticula can occur suddenly and without warning and get worse after that. Inflammation of a diverticulum can occur when there is thinning of the diverticular wall and increased pressure in the colon or the presence of particles lodged in diverticula. Both events may decrease the blood flow to the diverticulum.

In diverticulitis, diarrhea may fluctuate with constipation, and there may be painful tenderness or cramping in the lower left abdominal area, accompanied by fever and chills. Nausea, bloating, vomiting, weight loss, and bleeding may also occur.

There may be a frequent need to urinate, changes to bowel movement, lessening desire to eat, and/or loss of appetite.

Causes and Risk Factors

Genetics, lower fiber diets, and age are chief risk factors for diverticular disease.

Other risk factors are lack of exercise, obesity, and smoking.

Diagnosis

Because the disease is often asymptomatic, it is often discovered by chance during tests for other conditions.

Usually, a medical history, including a physical examination, may be conducted along with diagnostic barium enema x-rays to outline the lower intestinal tract, CT scanning, ultrasound testing, and colonoscopy—a test that allows the doctor to look inside the large bowel, in a hospital setting, using a narrow, flexible, tube-like telescopic camera called a colonoscope. This test can confirm the presence of diverticula and rule out other reasons for a change in bowel movements, such as polyps or bowel cancer.

Flexible sigmoidoscopy, which examines the sigmoid colon with a thin flexible tube that contains a camera, and blood tests may be conducted to affirm the diagnosis or rule out competing diagnoses. Angiography may be used to establish the status of the circulatory system in the event of severe bleeding, and to locate the source of the bleeding.

Treatments

Treatments usually include these recommendations:

- Adoption of a liquid or high-fiber diet, including vegetables, whole grains, fruits.
- Antibiotics and use of laxatives, as required, may be recommended.
- Antispasmodic drugs to reduce mild symptoms of abdominal pain.
- Surgery may be used for any perforation, abscess, fistula, or recurring cases of diverticulitis. There are three types of surgery: primary bowel resection, bowel resection with colostomy, and abscess drainage. In primary bowel resection, the diseased bowel area is removed, and the rest of the digestive tract is then reconnected to this area. The bowel resection with colostomy procedure is used when the rectal area is damaged. Here, a surgical opening is made in the abdominal wall, where waste will pass through into an attached plastic bag in the future. Abscess drainage procedures may be used to simply drain and clean any present abscess.

Prevention and Future Directions

Eating appropriate amounts of food, including fiber, and drinking plenty of water and exercising regularly are likely to be helpful, as are getting enough rest and sleep. Keep a healthy weight.

Patients with diverticular disease who experience unexplained fever, chills, or abdominal pain should notify their health provider.

It is hoped that, in the future, better ways of understanding the way diverticula develop and become infected will yield better ways of preventing and managing the condition. Studies in nutrition may be especially helpful.

Prognosis

About 15 to 25 percent of cases with diverticulosis will develop diverticulitis, while 5 percent will experience diverticular bleeding.

About 85 percent of cases with simple diverticulitis will respond to medical treatment, while 15 percent will require surgery. After successful treatment for a first diverticulitis attack, one-third will continue to have episodic cramps, and another third will experience a second attack. The outcome is worse after a second bout of diverticulitis, and complications occur at high rates in this group, and only 10 percent remain symptom free.

Repeated diverticulitis attacks can produce scar tissue that leads to narrowing and obstruction of the colon region.

Ray Marks

See also: Abdominal Diseases; Bleeding Disorders; Digestive Diseases

Further Reading

American College of Gastroenterology. (2015). Diverticulosis and diverticulitis. Retrieved from http://patients.gi.org/topics/diverticulosis-and-diverticulitis/.

Mayo Clinic. (2014, April 7). Diverticulitis. Retrieved from http://www.mayoclinic.org/diseases-conditions/diverticulitis/basics/definition/con-20033495.

National Institute of Diabetes and Digestive and Kidney Diseases. (2013, September). Diverticular disease. Retrieved from http://digestive.niddk.nih.gov/ddiseases/pubs/diverticulosis/index.aspx.

UpToDate. (2015, September 16). Patient information: Diverticular disease (beyond the basics). Retrieved from http://www.uptodate.com/contents/diverticular-disease-beyond-the-basics.

DYSMENORRHEA

Dysmenorrhea is painful cramping during menstruation. It is a common problem, affecting around 50 percent of postpubescent women. The condition is most regularly seen in women between the ages of 20 and 24, and symptoms often decrease with age. In the United States, about 10 to 20 percent of those affected by dysmenorrhea have severe pain that leaves them unable to participate in everyday functions like work and school for several days each month. Women who smoke or who entered puberty at a young age (under 11) are at greater risk for dysmenorrhea, as are those who have irregular menstrual cycles or heavy bleeding during their period.

There are two types of dysmenorrhea: primary dysmenorrhea and secondary dysmenorrhea. The first occurs in otherwise healthy women and is usually seen in younger adults. The menstrual pain felt as a result of primary dysmenorrhea is not related to uterine or other issues. While the cause is not entirely known, the increased level of hormone-like substances (prostaglandins) during menstruation is thought to play a role in the condition. Prostaglandins are the natural substances that trigger the uterus to contract and expel menstrual blood. So far, research has shown that the higher the level of prostaglandins, the greater the chance of dysmenorrhea.

Secondary dysmenorrhea is a condition that typically develops in women older than 25 as a result of problems associated with the uterus or pelvic organs. These women have usually had normal, relatively pain-free menstruation until the onset of their uterine or pelvic disorders. Such issues that may trigger secondary dysmenorrhea include uterine fibroids, which are noncancerous growths in the uterus; pelvic inflammatory disease, a bacterial infection in the pelvic organs; and endometriosis, a condition in which uterine lining tissues mistakenly implant and grow on the fallopian tubes, ovaries, or elsewhere outside of the uterus. Stress and anxiety are also factors that may trigger secondary dysmenorrhea.

The symptoms of dysmenorrhea include an intense throbbing or aching in the lower abdomen, sharp pains that come and go, and a persistent ache that radiates through the lower back and legs. Some women also experience diarrhea, nausea, headaches, and/or dizziness during menstruation as a result of dysmenorrhea. Although dysmenorrhea itself does not lead to other medical conditions, the underlying issues that cause secondary dysmenorrhea might if left untreated. For example, endometriosis can lead to fertility issues, and pelvic inflammatory disease may increase the risk of ectopic pregnancy, a sometimes life-threatening problem that occurs when a fertilized egg implants outside of the uterus.

A pelvic exam should be able to show whether a woman has primary dysmenorrhea or secondary dysmenorrhea. If the exam reveals no irregularities or abnormalities, the problem is most likely primary dysmenorrhea. Primary dysmenorrhea is often treatable with such home remedies as a low-sugar, low-sodium, and no-caffeine diet or increased stress-reducing activity such as yoga and meditation. Warm showers and baths and over-the-counter anti-inflammatory medication is also often recommended. If the pain is severe, a medical practitioner may recommend such treatment as prescription anti-inflammatory medication and pain relievers or birth control pills. If secondary dysmenorrhea is suspected, a doctor may recommend such tests as an ultrasound, a CT scan, or other imaging tests. Additionally, a complete blood count test can be used to pinpoint infections and other such problems. Laparoscopic outpatient surgery can also be used to explore the pelvic region and reproductive organs for signs of fibroids, endometriosis, cysts, and other issues that may be creating the painful menstrual cramps. This is usually only recommended for a small percentage of women who have not responded to other tests and treatments.

Evidence shows that dysmenorrhea was a known problem in ancient civilizations such as Egypt and Greece. Early practitioners applied aromatic oils and ointments to treat inflammation and pain associated with the problem. Roman physicians wrote extensively about their use of asparagus root to relieve menstrual pain. By the 19th century, dysmenorrhea was seen as a common but serious problem, though the suspected causes were wide and varied. In 1938, a connection between ovulation and dysmenorrhea was made, followed by the discovery of increased prostaglandins creating menstrual pain in 1965. Over time, different courses of treatment were prescribed and studied. Newer research has shown that calcium channel blocking agents are helpful in decreasing pain associated with dysmenorrhea. Experimentation has also revealed that transcutaneous electrical nerve stimulation, a noninvasive procedure in which electrical impulses are used to block pain in the pelvis, may also be effective for some women.

Tamar Burris

See also: Abdominal Diseases; Women's Health

Further Reading

Centers for Disease Control and Prevention. (2015). Heavy menstrual bleeding. Retrieved from http://www.cdc.gov/ncbddd/blooddisorders/women/menorrhagia.html.

Cleveland Clinic. (2015). Diseases & conditions: Dysmenorrhea. Retrieved from https://my.clevelandclinic.org/health/diseases_conditions/hic_Dysmenorrhea.

Ehrenthal, D. B., Hoffman, M. K., & Adams-Hillard, P. J. (2006). *Women's Health: Menstrual Disorders*. Philadelphia, PA: The American College of Physicians.

Marshburn, P., & Hurst, B. (2011). *Gynecology in Practice: Disorders of Menstruation*. Burlington, MA: Wiley-Blackwell.

Mayo Clinic. (2015). Menorrhagia. Retrieved from http://www.mayoclinic.org/diseases-conditions/menorrhagia/basics/definition/con-20021959.

Mayo Clinic. (2015). Menstrual cramps. Retrieved from http://www.mayoclinic.org/diseases-conditions/menstrual-cramps/basics/definition/con-20025447.

E

EAR DISEASES

The ear is a sensory organ with three main components—the outer, middle, and inner ear—all necessary for hearing to occur. For hearing to occur, sound waves in the air travel through the outer ear to the middle ear, where they cause the eardrum to vibrate. The vibrations are then conveyed by three small bones called ossicles in the middle ear to the inner ear. The inner ear sends messages it receives via the auditory nerves to the brain, and this will result in the ability to hear or interpret the sound. The inner ear also controls balance.

There are many types of diseases that affect the ears. Two categories produce hearing loss: conductive problems and sensorimotor problems. In conductive problems, the sound cannot pass through the outer or middle ear. This may be caused by a blockage in the ear canal or tube known as the external ear canal. In sensorineural problems, the cause lies either in the cochlea of the inner ear or in the auditory or hearing nerve.

Ear disease causes significant discomfort and hearing loss, as well as work loss, decreased productivity, and decreased ability to communicate effectively. In children, this can cause developmental delays, and academic failure.

Types of Ear Conditions

Cholesteatoma is a condition in which skin cells grow in the wrong place in the middle ear and mastoid bone of the ear region. They may also invade the inner ear, brain, or any other structure of the ear area and brain. They can severely damage the ear, and can be removed surgically.

Herpes zoster otitis causes a viral infection related to the facial nerves and the nerves of the inner ear. The symptoms include intense ear pain; a rash located to the ear and face regions; and, on occasion, paralysis of the facial muscles. The affected individual may experience abnormal sounds, difficulty hearing, nausea and vertigo, or lack of balance and dizziness.

Meniere's disease involves fluid buildup in the ear and defective functioning of the inner chamber that can affect hearing. The condition can cause vertigo or dizziness and nausea, due to disruption of fluid balance in the sacs in the inner ear, and a reduced ability to detect movement. Possible causes are trauma to the head or ear, autoimmune health conditions, allergies, or syphilis. The disease may occur episodically and is erratic in its progression. If the condition progresses to total deafness, the episodes of vertigo and ringing in the ears may spontaneously subside.

Otitis media is a middle ear infection caused by a virus or bacterium. Some symptoms of this include earache, headache, mild deafness, fever, loss of appetite. *Chronic suppurative otitis media* is the term given to a situation in which the middle ear infection persists and is draining the whole time.

Otosclerosis is a metabolic condition that causes new bone to grow and reduces the function of the bones in the middle ear, which reduces the ability of the bones in this area to vibrate, thus eliminating the transfer of sound to the inner ear and causing permanent hearing loss. It can also affect the inner ear directly and can occur in both ears at the same time.

Perforated eardrums can be caused by serious infections and head injuries. Most can heal within three months.

Swimmer's ear involves an infection of the ear canal, which links the inner ear to the ear lobe or pinna, resulting in an inflamed ear canal. This is commonly said to be due to an infection of the skin lining the ear canal—for example, a fungal infection from swimming. Excess water in the ear can make one more prone to infections. Internal damage to the ear can also promote opportunities for infection. It can also occur in people with eczema.

Vestibular neuritis refers to an inflammation of the vestibular nerve located in the inner ear. It produces symptoms similar to Meniere's diseases and can develop suddenly. Its distinct cause is unknown, but it is said it is possibly related to an infection, even though more than half of those with the condition do not appear to have an infection.

Types of Symptoms

The symptoms experienced by those with an ear condition will depend on the cause of the problem. A common symptom however is pain, discomfort, or hearing loss.

Other symptoms can include irritability, tinnitus or ringing in the ear, sleep problems, changes in balance, and fever.

Causes and Risk Factors

Trauma, injury, and infections are common causes of ear dysfunction.

Benign tumors such as acoustic neuromas can cause vertigo, hearing loss, and loss of facial nerve functions.

Otosclerosis may have an inherited component and is often worse in pregnancy.

Diagnostic Tools

The physician can conduct an overall medical history examination and a physical examination.

They can examine the ear with an instrument called an otoscope to see if there is any infection.

Treatments

If infection is present, it will usually be treated with antibiotics. Painkillers may be given to reduce any pain. Using ear drops and keeping the ear dry may help in conditions such as swimmer's ear.

Sodium fluoride tablets may be recommended for those with otosclerosis of the inner ear.

If a perforated eardrum does not heal, a surgical intervention known as typmanoplasty to repair the eardrum might be needed. It can also be treated by a procedure called a myringoplasty, which involves a tissue graft procedure.

Mastoid surgery is done on occasion to relieve pressure in ear from infected tissue and mastoid in the middle ear bone, which may require cleaning.

A stapedectomy or stapedotomy—where a pistin is introduced surgically to replace an affected stapes bone so sound can travel to the inner ear—has been shown to work well.

A hearing aid may be recommended in cases of hearing impairments.

A cochlear implant is a small electronic device or connecting system that is implanted surgically into the ear. It is wired so that its electronic impulses send sound waves to the auditory nerves for transmission to the brain for processing, and it can help in cases where the hearing problem does not respond to a hearing aid. Children born deaf may also benefit from this form of surgery, especially if done sooner rather than later.

Prevention

Preventing infections, careful cleaning of the ears, and avoiding trauma and excessive noise are important for ensuring ear health.

Ray Marks

See also: Meniere's Disease; Tinnitus; Vestibular Diseases

Further Reading

American Academy of Otolaryngology—Head and Neck Surgery. (2015). Better ear health. Retrieved from http://www.entnet.org/?q=node/1250.

Mayo Clinic. (2013, April 20). Ear infection (middle ear). Retrieved from http://www.mayo clinic.org/diseases-conditions/ear-infections/basics/definition/con-20014260.

National Institute on Deafness and Other Communication Disorders. (2015, September 30). Hearing, ear infections, and deafness. Retrieved from http://www.nidcd.nih.gov/health /hearing/Pages/Default.aspx.

National Institutes of Health. (2012). Ear disorders. Retrieved from http://health.nih.gov /topic/Ear Disorders.

EATING DISORDERS

A group of serious psychiatric conditions, eating disorders are characterized by an unhealthy relationship with food, causing overeating or not eating enough to stay healthy, as well as extreme concerns about body shape or weight. They have a negative impact on physical and mental health and, often, the ability to function, and they have the highest mortality rate of any mental disorder. The precise causes of eating disorders are not known, but they are most likely a combination of genetics, emotional and psychological health, and social pressures to be thin.

The most common types of eating disorders are anorexia nervosa, bulimia nervosa, and binge-eating disorder. A fourth type, OSFED, for "other specified feeding or eating disorder," also causes significant distress or impairment, but it does not meet strict diagnostic criteria for another eating disorder. Up to 30 million men and women of all ages suffer from an eating disorder in the United States; about 95 percent are between 12 and 26 years old, and although most are women, an estimated 10 to 15 percent are men. More rare eating disorders, often found in infants or people with an intellectual disability, are pica, the persistent eating of nonfood items for at least one month; rumination disorder, which involves repeatedly and persistently regurgitating food after eating; and avoidant/restrictive food intake disorder, characterized by the failure to meet minimum daily nutrition requirements due to a lack of interest in eating.

Each eating disorder causes specific symptoms, and people with an eating disorder also often experience depression, anxiety disorders, obsessive-compulsive disorder, substance abuse problems, and other psychiatric disorders. Eating disorders may lead to heart and kidney problems and be life-threatening; early intervention is important. The goals of treatment are to restore healthier eating habits and, if possible, reverse complications caused by the disorder. Treatment options can include medical monitoring, psychotherapy, nutritional counseling, and if needed, medication or hospitalization.

Symptoms

Anorexia nervosa, often called anorexia, is recognized abnormally low body weight, caused by the refusal to eat or highly restrictive eating, sometimes to the point of starvation, as well as an intense fear of weight gain and a distorted perception of weight or body shape, sometimes leading to compulsive exercise. This disorder can cause osteoporosis or thinning bones, brittle hair and nails or hair loss, dry skin, mild anemia, muscles wasting away, severe constipation, drop in blood pressure and body temperature, sensitivity to cold, excessive facial or body hair due to inadequate protein, lethargy, organ failure, and the absence of menstrual periods or infertility in women.

Bulimia nervosa, more commonly called bulimia, is the feeling of not being able to control the amount of food eaten. It is characterized by frequently eating unusually large amounts of food and then feeling a lack of control that results in purging by way of vomiting, excessive use of laxatives or diuretics, fasting, or excessively exercising. People with bulimia also fear weight gain and want to lose weight because they have negative feelings about their size and shape; they can actually be within the normal range for their age and weight. The symptoms of bulimia nervosa that come from purging include chronic sore throat, swollen salivary glands, worn tooth enamel, gastroesophageal reflux disorder (GERD) from repeated vomiting, electrolyte imbalance (salt concentrations in the blood), intestinal problems from abusing laxatives, kidney problems from diuretics, and severe dehydration.

Like people with bulimia, those with *binge-eating disorder* feel a lack of control regarding eating, often due to insatiable cravings and often tied to dysfunctional thoughts. Because they do not purge food, people with this disorder may have normal weight but are more often overweight or obese. They experience shame and guilt about their overeating, which can lead to further overeating and contribute to heart disease, high blood pressure, high cholesterol, Type II diabetes, gallbladder disease, join pain, and sleep apnea.

Causes and Risk Factors

While the exact causes of eating disorders are unknown, a variety of conditions may contribute to their development. Family history and genetics play a role for some: Those who have siblings or parents with an eating disorder have an increased risk. Psychological and personal factors that place some people at higher risk include low self-esteem, perfectionism, feeling a lack of control, anxiety, depression, troubled relationships, history of abuse, and having been bullied about body size. Social factors may also contribute to risk, such as peer and media pressures to have the "perfect" body, as well as cultural values based on physical appearance. Still being researched are biological causes of eating disorders, specifically an imbalance of brain chemicals that control hunger, appetite, and digestion that have been found in some people.

Diagnosis

Each eating disorder has a specific set of diagnostic criteria listed in *The Diagnostic and Statistical Manual of Mental Disorders (DSM-5),* the publication mental health providers use to diagnose mental conditions.

Because no single test can diagnose an eating disorder, health professionals look at how a disorder affects overall health and ask screening questions about medical history, physical and emotional health, and eating habits. A physical exam checks for outward manifestations of the disorder. Blood and urine tests check for signs of malnutrition, changes in liver functioning, or electrolytes and other consequences of an eating disorder or rule out other causes of weight loss; x-rays can show weakened bones. A person suspected of having an eating disorder may also be referred to a mental health professional who will conduct an assessment for depression and anxiety.

Treatment

No single treatment plan exists for an individual with an eating disorder. But people with eating disorders have responded well to treatments tailored to their own needs. Treatment often includes medical and mental health professionals along with nutritional counseling and management.

Treatment for anorexia focuses on restoring a healthy weight, treating the related psychological issues, and maintaining the positive changes to prevent relapse. Treating bulimia nervosa involves interrupting the binge-purge cycle, identifying and managing unhealthy feelings, and maintaining positive behavioral changes. For binge-eating, the treatment goal is to interrupt and stop binges. Psychotherapy addresses the thoughts, emotions, and behaviors that trigger each of the disorders, which is vital to restoring physical well-being and healthy eating practices, as well as ending binge-purge cycles or binge eating.

Medications do not cure eating disorders, but some antidepressants may help manage symptoms of depression or anxiety as well as help reduce binge-eating and purging, decrease the chance of relapse, and improve attitudes about eating. Hospitalization may be needed for those with malnutrition or other serious health problems such as severe depression or suicidal thoughts.

Prevention

Targeting people who may show early signs of an eating disorder, prevention programs aim to change attitudes, perceptions, and behaviors associated with eating disorders and halt the development of a serious problem. The programs work to reduce dissatisfaction about body size and shape, depression, and self-esteem based on appearance and focus on healthy eating habits and appreciation for the body and its functions.

Prognosis and Outcomes

Eating disorders can be life-threatening, and getting professional treatment is key, particularly early on in the course of a disorder. Recovery from an eating disorder is possible, but it takes place over time with mindful application of the treatment. Sustaining recovery requires careful planning and the help of a treatment team.

Future

Scientists are conducting brain imaging and genetic studies to better understand risk factors, identify biological markers, and develop specific medications to target areas in the brain that control behaviors associated with eating. Efforts are ongoing to develop new treatments, including the research showing that outcomes improve when parents are included in family-based treatment approaches for their children; it is not clear if this will work for adults with anorexia, but research is under way to incorporate families.

Susana Leong

See also: Anxiety; Depression; Gastroesophageal Reflux Disease (GERD); Heart Diseases; Kidney Diseases; Osteoporosis; Social Health; Women's Health

Further Reading

Costin, C. (2012). *8 Keys to Recovery from an Eating Disorder: Effective Strategies from Thera-peutic Practice and Personal Experience.* New York: W. W. Norton & Co.

Diagnostic and Statistical Manual of Mental Disorders, 5th ed. (DSM-5). (2013). Washington, DC: American Psychiatric Association.

Mayo Clinic. (2015, April 29). Eating disorders. Retrieved from http://www.mayoclinic.org /diseases-conditions/eating-disorders/basics/definition/con-20033575.

National Association of Anorexia Nervosa and Associated Disorders. (2015). Binge-eating disorder. Retrieved from http://www.anad.org/get-information/get-informationb inge-eating-disorder/.

National Eating Disorders Association (NEDA). (2015). Types and symptoms of eating dis-orders. Retrieved from https://www.nationaleatingdisorders.org/types-symptoms-eating -disorders.

National Institute of Mental Health. (2014). Eating disorders: About more than food. Re-trieved from http://www.nimh.nih.gov/health/publications/eating-disorders-new-trifold /index.shtml#pub1.

ECZEMA

Eczema is a generic term used to describe many types of skin inflammation or forms of skin irritation or swelling. It is derived from the Greek, and aptly means "to boil out." The condition occurs most commonly in infants and children, but it can af-fect people of all ages. If the onset occurs early on in life, children commonly can be rid of the problem after their third year. In other cases, the condition may occur without any cure across the lifespan. All races can be affected, and a family history of allergies is not uncommon. Eczema may also predict the onset of other allergic diseases later on in life. As much as 20 percent of children and 1 to 2 percent of adults may suffer from eczema, with girls generally being more affected than boys. Worldwide and depending upon the region, up to 10 percent of adults and 30 percent of children may be affected, and the presence of the condition is increasing. Al-though all races are affected, studies of health care office visits show Asians and blacks appear to visit health care offices more frequently for problems with eczema than whites. If both parents have eczema, there is an 80 percent chance their children will have this condition.

While all body regions may be affected by eczema, in children and adults, the condition typically occurs on the face, neck, elbows, knees, and ankles. In infants, eczema typically occurs on the forehead, cheeks, forearms, legs, scalp, and neck. The condition can sometimes occur as a brief reaction that only leads to symptoms for a few hours or days, but in other cases, the symptoms persist over a longer time and the condition is then referred to as chronic dermatitis.

There are different categories of eczema that have been described.

1. *Atopic dermatitis*

This condition is the most common form of eczema and is often long lasting. The individual with this condition commonly suffers from itchy, inflamed skin that can come and go, depending on exposure to triggers or allergens factors.

2. *Contact eczema*

This condition, also called *contact dermatitis*, is a local reaction that includes redness, itching, and burning in areas where the skin has come into contact with an allergen or irritant. The condition is sometimes referred to as *allergic contact eczema* (allergic contact dermatitis) if the trigger is an allergen and *irritant contact eczema* (irritant contact dermatitis) if the trigger is an irritant. Skin reactions to poison ivy and poison sumac are examples of allergic contact eczema.

3. *Seborrheic eczema*

This condition is an inflammation of unknown cause, where yellowish, oily, scaly patches of skin on the scalp, face, and occasionally other parts of the body are evident. Dandruff and "cradle cap" in infants are examples of seborrheic eczema. It is commonplace for seborrheic dermatitis to inflame the face at the creases of the cheeks and/or the nasal folds.

4. *Nummular eczema*

This condition is characterized by coin-shaped patches of irritated skin—most commonly located on the arms, back, buttocks, and lower legs. These may appear crusted and scaly and can be extremely itchy.

5. *Neurodermatitis*

This condition, known as *lichen simplex chronicus*, is a form of chronic skin inflammation caused by a scratch-itch cycle that becomes intensely irritated.

6. *Stasis dermatitis*

This condition is a skin irritation on the lower legs, generally related to the circulatory problem known as venous insufficiency, in which the function of the valves within the veins has been compromised.

7. *Dyshidrotic eczema*

This condition is an irritation of the skin on the palms of hands and soles of the feet characterized by clear, deep blisters that itch and burn.

The most common type is atopic eczema.

Symptoms

Typical symptoms of eczema include itchiness of the skin, redness of the skin, roughness of the skin, swelling, or a leathery thickening of the skin. There may also be cracking and "weeping" of the skin, the presence of open sores that can become infected may be seen, and the skin may feel like it has been burned. Affected areas can also appear very dry, thickened, and scaly.

Causes and Risk Factors

A chief cause of this health condition is thought to be genetic, and the defective gene(s) produce abnormalities of the skin. There may also be a related immune system problem.

Eczema can also be triggered by environmental irritants or allergens—which are substances that cause allergies, including soaps, perfumes, and chemicals—as well as foods such as nuts, eggs, seafood, and food additives; preservatives; and colorings.

Stress or changes in temperature or humidity may pose a risk for outbreaks of eczema.

Diagnosis

There is no specific test to diagnose eczema definitively. Your health provider can reach a diagnosis by:

A physical examination, as well as a skin biopsy may be helpful in arriving at a diagnosis.

The medical history, especially any exposure to an irritant or allergen will be important to identify.

Allergy tests, or patch tests that can help test allergies may be helpful as well.

Other tests may be done to rule out competing diagnoses that cause skin inflammation.

Treatments

Treatments may include oral or topical corticosteroid creams, immune-suppressing drugs, antihistamines, oral or topical antibiotics, and various self-care activities, including frequent skin hydration and avoiding extremes of temperature.

It is important to reduce exposure to allergens or irritants if these have been identified, and moisturize the area frequently.

Natural supplements, diets, and herbal medicines are possible areas of intervention a sufferer can explore as well.

Parents can help their children as indicated and teach their preteen or teenage children how to carry out skin care and effective precautions against flare-ups, especially recognizing stressful situations and how to manage them.

General prevention strategies might include:

- Avoidance of over-bathing.
- Keeping skin hydrated.
- Making appropriate lifestyle modifications to reduce stress and exposure to irritants, such as hard soaps, detergents, or solvents.
- Wearing loose-fitting clothing, especially cotton clothing, that may be less irritating than wool or synthetic fibers.
- Using protective clothing, humidifiers in summer and winter, and paying attention to hygiene.
- Using cool compresses to help control itching.
- Exercising to reduce stress, but avoiding activities that make one too hot or too cold.
- Avoiding sudden changes in temperature or humidity.
- Being aware of foods that may cause an outbreak and trying to avoid these.

Prognosis and Complications

On rare occasions, eczema can prove fatal. More often than not, it is a cause of considerable disability to the individual and family members. Some cases with eczema develop other allergic reactions later on. Other may suffer from infections, and most can effectively manage their disease with medical treatments and by avoiding irritants. In many cases, eczema goes into remission or ceases altogether for months or even years. For many kids, it begins to improve round age five to six, but others may experience flare-ups in the teenage and early adult years.

Research and Future Directions

Some research suggests eczema results from an overly acidic body and skin, which creates an overactive immune system response. This is why some recommend an eczema sufferer minimize his or her intake of acidic foods and drinks, such as coffee, alcohol, and pizza and take in more alkaline foods and drinks.

In another area, the U.S. Food and Drug Administration (FDA) has approved two drugs known as topical immunomodulators for the treatment of mild-to-moderate eczema: Elidel and Protopic. These are skin creams that work by altering the immune system response to prevent flare-ups.

The FDA has warned doctors to prescribe Elidel and Protopic with caution, however, due to concerns over a possible cancer risk associated with their use. The warning advises doctors to prescribe short-term use of Elidel and Protopic only after other available eczema treatments have failed in adults and children over the age of two. It is not to be used in children under two years of age.

Behavior modification, emotional support, probiotics-dietary supplements, or immunity-boosting products have been recommended by some but need to be investigated further, and the latter should be used with caution.

Ray Marks

See also: Cellulitis; Dermatitis; Meningitis; Obesity, Morbid; Psoriasis; Skin Conditions; Thrombophlebitis

Further Resources

American Academy of Dermatology. (2012). Proper treatment helps ease burden of eczema. Retrieved from http://www.skincarephysicians.com/eczemanet/proper_treatment.html.

Eczema. (2012). Retrieved from http://eczemablog.blogspot.com/2008/11/eczema-ltd-for-treatment-of-eczema.html.

Eczema causes. (2012). Retrieved from http://www.healthy-skin-guide.com/excema-causes.html.

Eczema rash treatment. (2012). Retrieved from http://www.healthy-skin-guide.com/eczema-rash-treatment.html.

Eczema treatment. (2012). Retrieved from http://www.eczematreatment.blogspot.com/.

KidsHealth. (2012). Eczema. Retrieved from http://kidshealth.org/parent/infections/skin/eczema_atopic_dermatitis.html.

National Eczema Association. (2012). Retrieved from http://www.nationaleczema.org/.

Stoppler, M. C. (2012). Eczema. MedicineNet.com. Retrieved from http://www.medicinenet
.com/eczema/article.htm1.

EHLERS-DANLOS SYNDROME

Ehlers-Danlos syndrome is a group of inherited disorders characterized by defects in the connective tissues, which are proteins and other substances that provide strength and elasticity to the skin, joints, blood vessel walls, and other organs. People with this syndrome usually have overly flexible joints; stretchy, fragile skin; small fragile blood vessels; and abnormal scar formation and wound healing.

The six major types of Ehlers-Danlos syndrome, or EDS, are classified according to their signs and symptoms. They share common symptoms, but each type involves a unique defect in the connective tissue and is considered a distinct hereditary disorder, meaning that someone with one type will not have a child with another type. The types are known as arthrochalasia type, classic type, dermatosparaxis type, hypermobility type, kyphoscoliosis type, and vascular type.

Symptoms are often recognizable in early childhood, and most people are diagnosed as young adults. It affects men and women equally of all racial and ethnic backgrounds. Worldwide, the hypermobility type affects about 1 in 10,000 to 15,000 people, and the classic type about in 1 in 20,000 to 40,000 people. The other types are very rare. Although incurable, EDS symptoms can be treated and managed with medications, physical therapy, and surgery, if necessary.

History

The syndrome was first recognized in 1901 by Edvard Ehlers, a Danish dermatologist, and in 1908 by the French physician Henri-Alexandre Danlos. They recognized characteristic features of the inherited disorders, and the Ehlers-Danlos syndrome was named in 1936. In the 1980s, Ehlers-Danlos syndrome was classified as having more than 10 types, but researchers devised a simpler classification in 1997 and reduced the number of major types to six.

Symptoms

The symptoms of Ehlers-Danlos syndrome (EDS) may vary in range and severity depending on the type and the individual. But key symptoms typically include abnormal looseness and excessive extension of the joints, which may be unstable and prone to injury; hip dislocation; chronic joint pain; the tendency to develop early onset of osteoarthritis, or degenerative joint disease; unusually loose, thin, stretchy skin that may bruise easily; paper-like scars that often become discolored and wide; poor wound healing; and very fragile skin, blood vessels, and other tissues and membranes.

Some symptoms of the vascular and kyphoscoliosis types may be serious and life-threatening, including blood vessels rupturing unpredictably that cause internal bleeding, stroke, and shock; an increased risk of organ rupture, including tearing of the intestine and rupture of the uterus during pregnancy; and severe curvature of the spine that worsens and can interfere with breathing.

Causes and Risk Factors

Family history is the greatest risk factor because all types of Ehlers-Danlos syndrome are caused by genetic defects, some of which are inherited and passed from parents to their offspring. Those with the most common types of Ehlers-Danlos syndrome have a 50 percent chance of passing on the gene to each child.

Diagnosis

A diagnosis of Ehlers-Danlos syndrome is based on a physical exam and the appearance of loose joints or hypermobility, fragile and stretchy skin, and family history. Genetic tests may confirm the diagnosis for most types of EDS and may rule out other problems. A skin biopsy that determines the chemistry of the connective tissue also may aid in diagnosis. To check for heart or vascular problems, an exam might include an echocardiogram, and specialized x-rays may help detect movable lumps under the skin determine the extent of spinal curvature.

Treatments

No cures exist for Ehlers-Danlos syndrome, and treatments are based on symptoms; foremost are protecting the skin from injury and sun damage and treating wounds and infections with great care. Because the skin is so fragile, surgical suturing can be difficult. Special braces may help to stabilize affected joints and help maintain their stability, while physical therapy and exercising strengthen the muscles supporting them to reduce or prevent joint injury. Any activities involving joint impact are to be avoided, including contact sports. Children must be extremely careful to avoid falling or hurting themselves.

Medications that help control pain and keep blood pressure low may be recommended. The best form of treatment is monitoring to prevent injuries, dangerous aneurisms, and cardiac trouble. Rarely, surgery is used to repair joints, although the connective tissue may not heal properly due to its inherent weakness.

Prevention

Genetic counseling is important to gain detailed information about the pattern of inheriting EDS, the risks of recurrence, and identifying other family members who may be at risk, including future offspring. Vigilant screening and lifestyle alterations can help reduce symptoms and complications.

Prognosis and Outcomes

There is currently no cure for any types of the syndrome, and prognosis depends on the type, but most people can manage their symptoms and lead a normal life. Severe cases are rare, but they can be fatal.

Most women can have successful pregnancies, although with increased risk of miscarriage, premature rupture of membranes, premature births, cervical incompetence, and premature labor, in addition to the 50 percent chance of passing on EDS on to her child and a 50 percent chance that the child will be affected.

Ray Marks

See also: Genetics and Genomics

Further Reading

Ehlers-Danlos Syndrome National Foundation. (2015). What is EDS? Retrieved from http://www.ednf.org/index.php?option=com_content&task=view&id=2202&Itemic.

Ehlers-Danlos Syndrome Network C.A.R.E.S., Inc. (2015, August 2). What is Ehlers-Danlos syndrome? Retrieved from http://www.ehlersdanlosnetwork.org/.

Mayo Clinic. (2015). Ehlers-Danlos syndrome. Retrieved from http://www.mayoclinic.org/diseases-conditions/ehlers-danlos-syndrome/basics/definition/con-20033656.

National Organization for Rare Disorders. (2015). Ehlers Danlos syndrome. Retrieved from https://rarediseases.org/rare-diseases/ehlers-danlos-syndrome/.

U.S. National Library of Medicine. (2015). Ehlers-Danlos syndrome. Retrieved from http://ghr.nlm.nih.gov/condition/ehlers-danlos-syndrome.

EMPHYSEMA

Emphysema is a chronic irreversible health condition affecting the lungs. It specifically involves the air spaces in the lungs, along with changes in the small air sacs or alveoli as well as air passages known as bronchioles. These air spaces may become permanently enlarged, while alveoli walls as well as numbers of *alveoli*—which promote oxygen exchange between the air and bloodstream—may be destroyed, and as a result, their mechanical function becomes impaired. This can cause the *bronchioles*, which allow air to leave the lungs to collapse. Although the person with this condition can breathe in effectively, they cannot breathe out effectively because the elastic function of the lung is gradually lost or impaired, and air is trapped in the lungs. Also affected are small blood vessels of the lungs and airways, so oxygen flow through the lungs is further reduced. The disease often occurs in combination with chronic bronchitis, and if so, this is termed chronic obstructive airways or pulmonary disease (COPD).

Emphysema, along with COPD, is a major cause of disability, hospital usage and costs, as well as premature death, especially among men. The disease—both alone or in combination with COPD—is common and has a strong relationship with smoking.

Symptoms

Key symptoms of emphysema include shortness of breath on activity or at rest as well as coughing and possibly wheezing.

Fatigue and recurrent infections of the lungs, plus weight loss may occur as the disease progresses.

The shortness of breath reduces the oxygen needed by the brain and other vital organs. This reduces the person's energy levels and ability to perform tasks of daily living.

Key Causes

Smoking, as well as an inherited predisposition due to a gene abnormality related to an enzyme found in the lung that prevents the destruction of alveoli walls, have been cited as possible causes.

People who have bronchial asthma and those exposed to indoor or outdoor air pollution, secondhand smoke, or manufacturing or worksite fumes or dust may also be prone to developing emphysema.

Diagnosis

The diagnosis of emphysema involves a detailed examination of the respiratory system, such as listening to breath sounds. There may be signs of heart failure in the advanced stages of the disease. Specific tests may include blood tests, chest x-rays, electrocardiograms, lung function tests, tests of blood gases, and CAT scans of the lungs.

Treatments

The goal of treatment for emphysema is to improve life quality by controlling the symptoms and preventing disease flare-ups. Quitting smoking, drug therapy, pulmonary rehabilitation, oxygen therapy or taking in pure oxygen from an oxygen concentrator, and surgery may be employed depending on the status of the condition and age of individual.

Supplemental treatments include vaccinations against flu; diuretics to reduce fluid in cases of heart failure; bronchodilators; exercises to help drainage of lung fluid or mucus buildup, as well as to build strength of respiratory muscles; and counseling and antidepressant medication if patient feels depressed. Weight control and nutrition are also important health-promoting aspects in this condition.

Prognosis

If the disease goes unchecked, it steadily worsens over time, and people with this condition usually have a lower life expectancy than those who do not. Complications involve right-sided heart failure; the production of an excess number of red blood cells that causes an increased risk of blood clots; the presence of air in the lung or pleural cavity, called a pneumothorax; large holes in the lungs, or bullae; and respiratory failure with collapse of the lungs due to infection. The outlook is worse for those with heart failure and respiratory failure.

If precautions against factors that heighten the problem are taken, people can lead reasonably normal lives, although they may have to curtail some aspects of this.

Prevention

Smoking cessation in the course of the disease may slow the rate of disease progression, if smoking is the cause of the condition, as may avoidance of air pollution, dust; and inhalants.

Avoiding the flu and exposure to extremes of temperature may be helpful.

Ray Marks

See also: COPD (Chronic Obstructive Pulmonary Disease); Cor Pulmonale; Lung Cancer; Lung Diseases; Pneumonia; Secondhand Smoke

Further Reading

Mayo Clinic. (2014, April 5). Emphysema. Retrieved from http://www.mayoclinic.org/diseases
-conditions/emphysema/basics/definition/con-20014218.

Virtual Medical Centre. (2015, September 29). Emphysema. Retrieved from http://www
.myvmc.com/diseases/emphysema/.

ENDOCARDITIS

Endocarditis, also called *bacterial endocarditis* or *infective endocarditis*, is a health condition in which an infectious agent, most commonly a bacterium, traveling in the bloodstream settles in the lining of the heart (or endocardium), a heart valve, or a blood vessel and causes inflammation.

It is not that common, but it may arise more frequently in those who already have a heart condition or as a congenital condition present at birth, especially in association with heart defects. In addition to being caused by a bacterium, it can be caused by a fungus. The condition can cause an abnormal heartbeat, stroke, or kidney failure, and if not treated, it can be fatal.

The condition can occur rapidly or in a subacute form over time, is more common in people over age 50, and is more common in men than women.

Symptoms

Abnormal color urine
Chills and fever
Vague, flu-like symptoms
Low-grade fever
Fatigue
Muscle aches
Night sweats
Paleness
Painful joints
Persistent cough
Swelling of feet, legs, or abdomen
Tiny pinpoint-sized areas of bleeding on the chest and back
Weakness
Weight loss

Causes

Autoimmune disease
Bacteria
Congenital heart defects
Fungi
Heart damage
Infection during surgery

Key Risk Factors

Atrial septal defects
Dental surgery or cleaning
Endoscopic surgery of the gastrointestinal, respiratory, or urinary tracts
Kidney failure patients who are on dialysis
Presence of an artificial heart valve
Presence of a congenital heart defect
Exposure to illegal drugs using dirty needles or not cleaning the skin
History of endocarditis
History of coronary artery bypass surgery
History of rheumatic fever
Presence of a cardiac pacemaker or implanted defibrillator
Heart attack
Mitral valve prolapse
Tonsillectomy
Ventricular defects

Diagnosis

A diagnosis of endocarditis is reached via a medical history and physical exam, as well as through blood cultures and echocardiograms. Other tests include chest x-rays, electrocardiograms, and assessments of C-reactive protein.

Treatments

Use of antibiotics, both in response to an infection as well as to prevent infections in susceptible people, is often given intravenously over a four- to six-week period in the case of the condition. Surgery may be conducted if the condition is caused by a fungus or if there is a need to repair or replace a damaged heart valve.

Complications should be treated as indicated.

Prognosis

Early treatment yields the best result. Possible complications include heart valve damage, jaundice, shortness of breath, blood in urine, stroke, and brain abscesses and headaches, especially if the infection damages the heart valves.

Prevention

Preventive antibiotics are recommended for those at risk, especially before any form of surgery. As well, continued medical follow-up is recommended for those with a prior endocarditis history. Intravenous drug users should seek appropriate help to diminish their risk. Good oral health care is also recommended.

Ray Marks

See also: Autoimmune Disease; Congenital Heart Disease; Heart Diseases; Inflammation

Further Reading

American Heart Association. (2015, April 24). Infective endocarditis. Retrieved from http://www.heart.org/HEARTORG/Conditions/CongenitalHeartDefects/TheImpactofCongenitalHeartDefects/Infective-Endocarditis_UCM_307108_Article.jsp#.Vjz4-GtKjwo.
Mayo Clinic. (2014, June 14). Endocarditis. Retrieved from http://www.mayoclinic.org/diseases-conditions/endocarditis/basics/definition/con-20022403.
National Heart, Lung, and Blood Institute. (2010, October 1). What is endocarditis? Retrieved from http://www.webmd.com/heart-disease/tc/endocarditis-topic-overview.

ENVIRONMENT

While the term *environment* has several accepted definitions, when referring to the health-related aspects of environment, one commonly accepted description refers to all things that are external to the human being, including air, water, soil, and the agents and organisms that exist within. This meaning of environment is commonly known as the "physical" or "natural" environment. The natural environment is recognized as an important factor influencing health status, and the World Health Organization lists the natural environment as a major determinant of health. Environment, as it relates to human health, may also refer to the "built environment" (the human-made structures and settings in which humans exist and operate) or the "social environment" (comprising transportation systems, housing, industry, and the interactions, or social networks, that humans share with other humans). Both the built environment and social environment have also been linked to health outcomes among humans.

The environment can be viewed as both a protective factor and risk factor for human health, disease, and disability. There are many ways in which the environment determines disease and disease-related risk factors. The natural environment in its unaltered state, for example, plays host to myriad biological agents of disease, most notably pathogens such as viruses, bacteria, and parasites, and well as wild animals. The unaltered natural environment also poses threats to human health in the form of hazardous weather conditions, temperature extremes, radiation, dangerous topography, and nutrient deficiencies in the soil, among others. Further, the natural environment may be altered, posing additional hazards to humans, such as through the addition of toxic chemicals (including fertilizers, pesticides, nuclear radiation, and lead) leading to hazardous conditions. The built environment also creates health threats to humans, from industrial air pollution to hazards on the roads. Conversely, alterations to the environment can act as protective factors in relation to human health. Examples include signage on highways, baby-proofing homes, water treatment facilities, vector-control programs, and waste management facilities.

While humans have been aware of the connections between some environmental hazards and human health for centuries, the rigorous study of environmental health is a relatively recent phenomenon in human history. One of the most influential historical figures in the field of modern public health is British physician John Snow, considered by many to be the father of modern epidemiology. In 1854, Snow accurately identified the source of a serious cholera outbreak in London, England, to be a public well built just a few feet from a disused and polluted cesspit. Dr. Snow's discovery demonstrated a direct link between water contamination and disease and represented some of the earliest work in the movement toward understanding the importance of environmental hygiene and sanitation. In subsequent years, both in Europe and the United States, environmental health became a concern of many physicians, politicians, and social activists.

In 20th-century United States, noted author and biologist Rachel Carson published what many consider to be the defining treatise of the modern environmental movement. Published in 1962, Carson's book *Silent Spring* raised considerable concern about the rapid industrialization of the United States' agricultural system by exposing the hazardous nature of the pesticide DDT. *Silent Spring* garnered widespread notoriety, and in the years following its publication, regulations on chemical pesticides were evaluated and strengthened. During 1960s and 1970s and directly following Carson's exposé, the environmental movement in the United States gained considerable momentum. The first Earth Day, organized to raise awareness about environmental concerns in the midst of the antiwar protest movement, was held in April 1970. In December of that same year, President Richard Nixon created the U.S. Environmental Protection Agency, a new agency within the federal government tasked with the protection of both human health and the environment. Today, the EPA continues to function and has evolved into a comprehensive environmental protection and conservation agency operating through 10 regional centers and more than 12 offices, including the Offices of Water (OW), Air and Radiation (OAR), Solid Waste and Emergency Response (OSWER), and Chemical Safety and Pollution Prevention (OCSPP).

As a subfield of public health, *environmental health* refers to the study of the health-related outcomes of the interactions between the environment and human beings. The field of environmental health involves identifying and examining health-related risk factors in the environment with the goal of minimizing those risks to improve health outcomes. Environmental health specialists are specially trained individuals who work to minimize these environmental risks and study the complex social and genetic factors that are frequently related to the risks posed by hazardous environmental conditions.

While the complex interplay of environment, genetic endowment, and individual behavioral capacities often make it quite difficult to measure the true extent of the impact of environmental risk factors on human health, it is clear that the environment, in myriad ways, contributes to the burden of many of the chronic diseases that plague the human population today.

In the latter half of the 20th century, several noteworthy environmental disasters punctuated the importance of the need for further study of the health impacts of hazardous environmental toxins. In the mid-1970s, at the height of the first major environmental movement in the United States, international attention focused on Love Canal, a small neighborhood in western New York State, where residents were reporting an unusually large number of birth defects, physical abnormalities, and other serious health issues. Love Canal, home to a large tract of single-family residences and two public schools, was a 36-square-block neighborhood that, unbeknownst to its residents, was built on a toxic waste site used by Hooker Chemical decades earlier. Love Canal was declared a federal health emergency site in 1978, eventually resulting in the relocation of 800 families.

Love Canal was one of a number of environmental disasters that illustrated the serious health effects of environmental hazards. Two years before the Love Canal incident, just outside of Seveso, Italy, an industrial accident exposed several local communities to dangerous levels of chemicals, resulting in contaminated water and food supplies. In 1984 in Bhopal, Madhya Pradesh, India, a methyl isocyanate gas leak from a Union Carbide pesticide plant resulted in thousands of gas-related deaths and more than 500,000 related injuries. Just two years later, the explosion and release of radioactive contaminants into the atmosphere in Chernobyl, Soviet Union (today Ukraine), caused acute radiation sickness among those most proximal to the nuclear reactor. Several other related long-term health effects are reported due to the Chernobyl disaster, including thyroid cancer, which is frequently cited as the main health impact of the disaster.

Today, the relation between many environmental risk factors and chronic disease is well known. In particular, much research has been done on the links between environmental factors and cancer, cardiovascular disease, and chronic respiratory infections, the leading causes of morbidity and mortality in most developed nations today.

Cancer. Perhaps the most widely studied chronic disease related to environmental risk factors is cancer. According to the U.S. Department of Health and Human Services (2003) at least two-thirds of all cancer cases can be linked to exposure to factors outside of the body. Carcinogenic substances in the environment—including chemicals, gases, radiation, and pathogens—comprise a sizable proportion of these cancer risk factors. It is well established, for example, that prolonged exposure to ultraviolet radiation from the sun increases the risk of developing skin cancers, especially among lighter-skinned individuals. It is also known that exposure to some naturally occurring compounds—such as benzene, radon, and asbestos—increases the risk of cancer in some individuals. Benzene, a liquid that is widely used as a solvent and chemical reagent, is known to cause blood cell cancers. Exposure to radon, a gas that is naturally released during the decay of radioactive elements, increases the risk of lung cancer. Asbestos fibers have been shown to increase the risk of lung cancer and the much rarer cancer, mesothelioma, among workers exposed to asbestos.

The products of combustion are also implicated in the development of cancer with exposure to secondhand smoke (e.g., linked to lung cancer), as well as several other cancers, including cancers of the brain and bladder and childhood leukemia. Some agencies, including the International Agency for Research on Cancer (IARC) and the U.S. National Toxicology Program (NTP) classify diesel exhaust as a likely carcinogen. In fact, the IARC lists more than 100 compounds as known carcinogens to humans, including arsenic, coal, formaldehyde, plutonium, soot, and vinyl chloride.

Biological agents in the environment are also implicated in some forms of cancer. Human papillomavirus (HPV) is the primary cause of cervical and anal cancers. Both hepatitis B and hepatitis C are major causes of liver cancer. The Epstein-Barr virus is linked to some forms of lymphoma. Exposure to aflatoxins, dangerous chemicals produced by certain types of fungi, increases the risk of developing liver cancer.

Cardiovascular Disease. The burden of cardiovascular disease is certainly related to the physical environment because access to healthful foods and environments that promote physical activity is critical to developing lifelong cardiorespiratory health and fitness. Further, the American Heart Association reports that risk of heart disease is higher among individuals exposed to air pollution and ambient particulate matter, particularly among the elderly and patients with already weakened respiratory systems. Indoor air pollution, including secondhand smoke, carbon particles from fireplaces and wood-burning stoves, and fumes from household chemicals can be particularly damaging to the cardiovascular health of the elderly. Research suggests that exposure to significant amounts pollutant particles and nitrogen dioxide in traffic fumes could also contribute to heart disease and even trigger a heart attack.

Chronic Respiratory Disease. The lungs are the central boundary between the human body and the environment and are often the site of diseases caused by, or related to, external environmental conditions. Dust, fine particulates, gaseous toxins, and the products of combustion are all environmental risk factors for various chronic, noninfectious respiratory diseases. Asthma and chronic obstructive pulmonary disease (COPD), for example, have been linked to exposure to environmental triggers, including air pollution, secondhand smoke, allergens, and molds.

Other Chronic Health Issues. Several other noteworthy environmental risk factors have been linked to chronic disease conditions. Chen and Goldberg (2009) note that ambient air pollution is associated with acute health events among patients with chronic illnesses such as congestive heart failure and diabetes. Other evidence shows that exposure to lead, even at low doses, results in delayed intellectual development in children. Damage to neurological functioning, including hearing loss and learning disabilities, is linked to exposure to mercury.

Research on the linkages between the environment and chronic disease is ongoing. Scientists are currently studying potential environmental risk factors for diseases such as Parkinson's disease, epilepsy, and Alzheimer's disease, among others.

William D. Kernan

See also: Alzheimer's Disease; Cancer; Cardiovascular Disease; Congestive Heart Failure; Epilepsy; Failure to Thrive; Neoplasms; Parkinson's Disease

Further Reading

Carson, R. (1962). *Silent Spring,* 1st ed. New York, NY: Houghton Mifflin.

Chen, H., & Goldberg, M. S. (2009). The effects of outdoor air pollution on chronic illnesses. *McGill Journal of Medicine*, *12*(1), 58–64.

Crapo, J. D., Broaddus, V. C., Brody, A. R., Malindzak, G., Samet, J., & Wright. J. R. (2003). Workshop on lung disease and the environment: Where do we go from here? *American Journal of Respiratory and Critical Care Medicine*, *168*, 250–254.

Friss, R. H. (2010). *Essentials of Environmental Health.* Sudbury, MA: Jones and Bartlett Learning.

National Toxicology Program. (2011). *The 12th Edition: Report on Carcinogens.* National Institute of Environmental Health Sciences, NIH-HHS.

National Toxicology Program, U.S. Department of Health and Human Services, PO Box 12233, MD K2-05, Research Triangle Park, NC, (919) 541–3419, http://ntp.niehs.nih.gov.

Riegelman, R. (2010). *Public Health 101: Healthy People, Healthy Populations.* Sudbury, MA: Jones and Bartlett Learning.

U.S. Department of Health and Human Services. (2003, August). Cancer and the environment: What you need to know. What you can do. National Cancer Institute and National Institute of Environmental Health Sciences. NIH Publication No. 03-2039.

U.S. Environmental Protection Agency (EPA), Ariel Rios Building, 1200 Pennsylvania Avenue, NW, Washington, DC 20460, (202) 272-0167, http://www.epa.gov.

EPIDEMIOLOGY

Epidemiology is the science behind how disease is spread within populations and factors that influence its spread. The word epidemiology has Greek roots and literally translates to "the study of," *-ology*; "what is upon," *epi*; "the people," *demos* (Carr et al. 2007). The importance of the field of modern epidemiology lies within the five objectives of the field: (1) to identify the cause of a disease, including risk factors (factors that increase an individual's chance for contracting a disease); (2) to determine *prevalence* (the spread of a disease in a community); (3) to document the natural history of a disease, including the *prognosis* (the likely outcome from having the disease); (4) to evaluate current and newly developed practices in administering health care; and (5) to establish evidence for creating public policy to address disease prevention and health promotion (Gordis 2009). To achieve these five objectives, there are two branches of epidemiology: (1) descriptive and (2) analytic. *Descriptive epidemiology* is referred to as the first step in epidemiological studies because it consists of understanding the contextual factors contributing to disease occurrence, which typically involves collecting data on the time, environment, and symptoms of ill individuals (Descriptive epidemiology, n.d.). Hypothesis generation and tentative theory formation are also elements of descriptive epidemiology. *Analytic epidemiology*, referred to as the second step in epidemiological studies, consists of testing the hypotheses generated in the first step to uncover causation or risk factors for disease development (Descriptive epidemiology, n.d.). Moreover, individuals who practice epidemiology are known as epidemiologists.

With the rise of technological innovation and medical understanding, epidemiology is no longer only used to study communicable diseases in the United States and Western context. Now, noncommunicable, chronic diseases are more prevalent and are the leading causes of preventable death in the United States. With this epidemiological shift from acute illness to chronic disease and with the rise of technology, epidemiological studies and foci have changed, and epidemiology has become increasingly complex and statistics-heavy. Many chronic diseases—such as cancer, diabetes, obesity, heart disease, and stroke—have multiple underlying factors that contribute to its manifestation in individuals. Hence, statistical analyses are often used to gain a greater understanding of risk factors for the development and spread of these chronic diseases in populations.

History

Epidemiologic knowledge and advancement throughout history occurred slowly, with periods of great advancement followed by large periods of little to no advancement in the field (Merril & Timmreck 2006). The first documented epidemiologist in the Western world is Hippocrates (ca. 460 BC–ca. 377 BC), an ancient Greek physician who is also considered the father of Western medicine. Hippocrates described a theory of the origin and spread of disease as an imbalance between man and his environment. One book in the Hippocratic collection (*Hippocratic collection* is the term used to refer to texts that are closely associated with Hippocrates' teachings, but with uncertain authorship) titled *Air, Waters, and Places*, published in c. 400 BC, is acclaimed as the first ever endeavor to systematically propose a causal association between environmental influences and disease (Rosen 1958). Indeed it was the books *On Airs, Waters, and Places*; *Epidemic I*; and *Epidemic III* that generated notoriety for Hippocrates and supported the notion that he was the first Epidemiologist in the Western world (Merril & Timmreck 2006). Hippocrates' substantive contribution to epidemiology include basic essentials of the field today: (1) scientific observations on how diseases spread in a population and (2) notes on how diseases affect and manifest in people (Merril & Timmreck 2006). However, before the Hippocratic tradition, little discussed are the practitioners of Chinese medicine and Ayurvedic medicine (from India) who also acknowledged the role that environmental factors and lifestyle factors played in people's health and disease status (Carr et al. 2007).

In the centuries following Hippocrates, epidemiology underwent significant changes with the help of many key people. What follows is a cursory overview of select individuals who contributed to furthering epidemiology: the list and descriptions are nowhere near exhaustive because many people have significantly contributed to the field. Thus, only three individuals who furthered epidemiology in the Western context are featured.

Edward Jenner (1749–1843), a medical doctor from England and now considered the father of immunology, is often credited with pioneering the smallpox vaccination (BBC 2012). During Jenner's time, smallpox was a rampant, lethal disease, especially for children. However, at the time, rumors spread that cow milkmaids who suffered from cowpox, a milder form of smallpox transferrable between cows and humans, never contracted smallpox. To empirically test this observation, Jenner collected some pus from a cowpox pustule, created an incision on the arm of his eight-year-old nephew, and inserted the pus. Later, he exposed his nephew to smallpox, and his nephew demonstrated immunity. Jenner repeated this process with other individuals and achieved similar results. In fact, the word vaccination is derived from the Latin root *vacca*, which means "cow." Although Jenner is credited with the discovery of the smallpox vaccination, smallpox inoculation had been previously discovered and described elsewhere. For instance, Benjamin Jetsy, a British farmer and dairyman, had written about the same procedure of vaccination just 20 years earlier after exposing his wife and children to cowpox based on his personal observation of his milkmaids not contracting smallpox (Merril & Timmreck 2006). Even earlier, Madhav, an 8th-century Indian physician who wrote a book with 79 chapters on diseases and causes of diseases, had written a special chapter on smallpox that detailed a different, yet equally valid method of inoculation (Hopkins 2002). Nevertheless, history often gives sole credit of the smallpox vaccination to Jenner, despite the fact that Jenner may have known of Jetsy's research and that inoculation against smallpox had been around centuries prior (albeit, not in the Western context). To this day, vaccinations are used to protect against serious diseases and are employed as a primary prevention technique in the public health arena. In fact, most schoolchildren in the United States are required to have undergone certain vaccination regimes prior to being allowed to enroll in public school. Such policies reduce the possibility of certain life-threatening communicable diseases being acquired early on in life and quickly spreading through the population via an epidemic because most members of the population possess immunity.

Another individual who greatly furthered the field of epidemiology is the Hungarian physician, Ignaz Philipp Semmelweis (1818–1865) (Semmelweis Society International 2009). Although during his time he was considered a lunatic, Semmelweis is now credited with recognizing the importance of proper hygiene and sanitation, specifically the benefits of handwashing, in reducing the transmission of disease. Puerperal fever, also called childbed fever, killed many patients in the hospitals Semmelweis oversaw. Semmelweis observed that mothers who gave birth at home were significantly less likely to contract puerperal fever than mothers who gave birth in the hospitals (Merril & Timmreck 2006). In addition to observing the higher incidence and prevalence of puerperal fever in hospitals as opposed to homes, he also noted that the problems started with the physician exam. He found out that physicians examining the laboring women often came straight from conducting autopsies; the physicians often still had decaying matter on their hands when they examined their live patients. These observations, and a few others, led Semmelweis to formulate a hypothesis of disease transmission. Semmelweis then conducted an experiment to test if the incidence of puerperal fever could be reduced through good sanitary practices: He provided staff at one hospital with an antiseptic handwashing solution and let the other hospital operate as normal. Results indicated that the incidence of puerperal fever reduced by 90 percent at the hospital in which staff used Semmelweis's antiseptic handwashing solution (Merril & Timmreck 2006). Even with such unmistakable statistical support for his hypothesis, Semmelweis and his theory were disregarded and ridiculed because they went against the then-conventional wisdom. Once germ theory became popularized, lending a plausible, understandable mechanism through which Semmelweis's findings could be explained, did Semmelweis retrospectively receive credit for his contribution to public health and epidemiology. Unfortunately, Semmelweis never lived to see that day; he had died many years earlier, after placement in a mental asylum. Today, good hygienic practices are often cited in preventing and containing communicable diseases, like influenza (the flu), by reducing the likelihood of disease transmission. Furthermore, Semmelweis's careful observations, subsequent hypothesis generation, thoughtful experimental design, and statistical data analyses are characteristic of the process that many epidemiologists currently use today to study disease transmission in a population.

John Snow (1813–1858), considered the father of modern epidemiology, was a well-respected physician who, throughout his career, studied cholera (Merril & Timmreck 2006). His main contribution to the field of epidemiology involves the use of descriptive and analytic epidemiology to successfully study and isolate the cause of a cholera epidemic in London, England, during 1853. Snow tracked cholera death rates in the South District of London, an area equally serviced by two water companies. He noticed that the death rates from cholera in the population serviced by the Lambeth Water Company were significantly lower than the death rates from cholera in the population serviced by Southwark and Vauxhall Water Company (Merril & Timmreck 2006). Upon further research, Snow learned that the Lambeth Water Company had relocated its source supply of water so that it was upstream from the source contaminated with London sewage, whereas the Southwark and Vauxhall Water Company did not. Armed with vital statistics, death rates, and source of water supply data, Snow was able to support his hypothesis that cholera was a waterborne disease that spread throughout the community via sewage-contaminated river water. Snow used rigorous scientific methodology in researching the cholera epidemic of 1853 and, thus, helped lay the foundation for the modern epidemiological paradigm of using observational data to assess possible causes of diseases. Today, many epidemiological studies use observational data and rely on statistical data analysis to understand disease etiology (causes of disease occurrence) and risk factors for spread, including for chronic disease.

Sukhminder Kaur

See also: Etiology; Family Health; Risk Factors

Further Reading

BBC. (2012). Edward Jenner (1749–1823). *Historic Figures.* Retrieved from http://www.bbc.co.uk/history/historic_figures/jenner_edward.shtml.

Carr, S., Unwin, N., & Pless-Mulloli, T. (2007). *An Introduction to Public Health and Epidemiology,* 2nd ed. Buckingham, GB: Open University Press.

Descriptive epidemiology. (n.d.). *Miller-Keane Encyclopedia and Dictionary of Medicine, Nursing, and Allied Health*, 7th ed. Retrieved from http://medical-dictionary.thefreedictionary.com/descriptive+epidemiology.

Gordis, L. (2009). *Epidemiology*, 4th ed. Philadelphia, PA: Saunders Elsevier.

Hopkins, D. R. (2002). *The Greatest Killer: Smallpox in History*. Chicago, IL: University of Chicago Press.

Merril, R. M., & Timmreck, T. C. (2006). *Introduction to Epidemiology*, 4th ed. Sudbury, MA: Jones and Bartlett Publishers.

Rosen, G. (1958). *A History of Public Health*. New York, NY: MD Publications.

Semmelweis Society International. (2009). Dr. Semmelweis's biography. Retrieved from http://semmelweis.org/about/dr-semmelweis-biography/.

EPILEPSY

Epilepsy is a seizure disorder resulting from a sudden burst of abnormal electrical activity in part or the entire brain. Seizures may be an alteration in behavior, consciousness, movement, or sensation depending on how many brain cells misfire and which area of the brain is involved. Epilepsy can develop at any time in a person's life, but it is more common in young children and adults over 65. According to the National Institute of Neurological Disorders and Stroke (2012), about 1 in 100 people in the United States have experienced an unprovoked seizure or been diagnosed with epilepsy.

A single seizure does not constitute epilepsy, which can occur as a result of a temporary medical condition such as a high fever, imbalance in blood glucose, or alcohol or drug withdrawal or immediately following a brain concussion. A person is considered to have epilepsy only when he/she has two or more unprovoked seizures that cannot be attributed to another medical condition.

Symptoms

The form a seizure takes depends on where in the brain the excessive electrical activity occurs. A person may experience just one type of seizure or more than one and will typically return to normal when the seizure is over.

Epilepsy is classified into either *partial* or *generalized* seizures. Partial seizures affect only part of the brain and may alter consciousness or awareness depending on where they start and which parts of the brain are involved. Generalized seizures affect the entire brain, alter consciousness and can be convulsive or nonconvulsive. Below is a list of common partial and generalized seizures.

Simple Partial Seizure. This partial seizure does not alter consciousness and was formerly known as a "focal seizure" because it occurs in a small part of the brain known as the focus. It is also known as an "aura" because it often serves as a warning that a bigger seizure will follow. This seizure lasts 30 to 60 seconds and may involve unusual sensations such as stomach upset or a strange smell, overwhelming feelings of joy or fear, or movements.

Complex Partial Seizure. This form of partial seizure involves a loss or alteration of awareness. It was formerly known as "psychomotor or temporal lobe seizure" because it commonly occurs in the brain's temporal or frontal lobes. This seizure lasts one to two minutes and may involve aimless wandering and confusion, staring blankly, or repeated movements that may progress to a generalized seizure.

Absence Seizure. This is a generalized seizure that occurs most often in children and involves very brief staring spells. It was formerly known as "petit mal seizure" and typically lasts less than 10 seconds. This seizure may involve a sudden blank stare, impaired awareness, rapid blinking, and eyes rolling upward.

Tonic-Clonic Seizure. This is a generalized seizure that involves loss of consciousness. It was formerly known as "grand mal seizure," lasts one to three minutes, and occurs in two phases. The tonic phase includes stiffening of the muscles where the body becomes rigid as it falls to the ground and a person may cry out or groan. The clonic phase includes jerking of the body in convulsions and may involve loss of urinary or bowel control, shallow breathing, bluish skin color, and drooling with an extended period of confusion and fatigue afterward.

Atonic Seizure. This is a generalized seizure that is also known as a "drop attack" and typically lasts only a few seconds. This seizure involves a loss of awareness and sudden loss of muscle tone, often resulting in a person falling down, dropping objects, or nodding the head involuntarily.

Myoclonic Seizure. This is a generalized seizure that typically lasts a few seconds and results in a sudden jerk of a part of the body such as the arm or leg. In this seizure, awareness is retained, and sometimes, a person may fall over when the seizure involves both sides of the body.

First Aid

First aid for seizures involves responding in ways that can keep the person safe until the seizure stops by itself. The Edmonton Epilepsy Association (2011) recommends the following first aid for convulsive and nonconvulsive seizures:

Convulsive seizures

1. Stay calm and let the seizure take its course.
2. Time the seizure.
3. Protect from injury by placing something soft under the head and moving sharp objects out of the way.
4. Loosen anything tight around the neck and check for medical identification.
5. Do not restrain the person.
6. Do not put anything in the mouth.
7. Gently roll the person onto his or her side to allow saliva and other fluids to drain away and keep the airway clear.
8. After the seizure, talk reassuringly to the person until he or she is reoriented.

Nonconvulsive seizures

1. Stay calm and let the seizure take its course.
2. Move dangerous objects out of the way.
3. Do not restrain the person.
4. Gently guide the person away from danger or block access to hazards.
5. After the seizure, talk reassuringly to the person until complete awareness returns.

Causes

According to the Centers for Disease Control and Prevention (2012), a specific underlying cause is not identified in two-thirds of the cases of epilepsy. However, epilepsy can be caused by the following conditions that affect a person's brain:

- Traumatic brain injury or head injury (car accident, sports injury, shaken baby syndrome)
- Oxygen deprivation (e.g., during childbirth).
- Brain infections (e.g., meningitis, encephalitis)
- Brain tumors
- Other neurologic diseases (e.g., Alzheimer's disease)
- Stroke
- Certain genetic disorders

Triggers

Seizures are rarely predictable and may be triggered by a variety of mechanisms. Some common triggers that can provoke seizures include:

- Missed doses of medication (most common)
- Lack of sleep or fatigue
- Stress or excitation
- Fever (febrile seizure)
- Elevated body temperature
- Colds, flu, or some kind of infection
- Menstrual or hormonal cycle
- Flashing or bright lights (photosensitivity)
- Toxicity/drug overdose

Once triggers have been identified, exposure can be limited to maintain seizure control.

Diagnosis

Diagnosing epilepsy is a multi-step process usually based on the following evaluations:

- An investigation of a first seizure (including any witness observations)
- Person's medical history
- Physical examination
- Neurological and behavioral exam (test motor abilities, behavior, and intellectual capacity)
- Supportive tests such as the EEG, CT scan, and MRI

Electroencephalograph (EEG) is an instrument used to measure electrical activity in the brain through small sensors called electrodes attached to the patient's scalp, which is recorded on a printout. It is used to identify the location, severity, and type of seizure disorder. This is the most common test to help diagnose epilepsy and is often used in conjunction with video monitoring to determine the nature of a person's seizures.

Computerized axial tomography (CAT or CT scan) is a safe and noninvasive procedure that uses low-radiation x-rays to create a computer-generated, three-dimensional image of the brain. The scan can reveal abnormalities (bleeding, tumors, and cysts) in the brain that may be causing seizures.

Magnetic resonance imaging (MRI) is a safe and noninvasive scanning technique that uses radio waves and a strong magnetic field to produce detailed images of the brain in three dimensions. The scan can reveal brain abnormalities that may be causing seizures.

Treatments

There is no cure for epilepsy, so children and adults use a variety of treatments to help control or even eliminate their seizures. Epilepsy treatments can be categorized into three main areas: medications, nondrug treatments and complementary therapies. Nondrug treatments include surgery, diet, and vagus nerve stimulation.

Medications. The most common approach to treating epilepsy is to prescribe antiepileptic drugs, which are based on the type of epilepsy, frequency and severity of the seizures, age of patient, and related health conditions. Medications eliminate seizures in 50 percent of cases and reduce the frequency and or intensity of seizures in another 30 percent. The remaining 20 percent of people cannot be brought under control by conventional drug therapy; they may be drug-resistant and require other treatments.

Surgery. Brain surgery for epilepsy is usually performed when other treatments fail to adequately control seizures or if there is an identifiable brain lesion believed to cause seizures that don't interfere with vital functions like speech, language, or hearing. The area of the brain with abnormally discharging neurons has to first be identified and then removed. The success rate of surgery is up to 80 percent in patients with an identified seizure focus.

Diet. The ketogenic diet is a strict high-fat, low-protein and carbohydrate therapeutic diet used in the treatment of difficult to control (intractable) epilepsy in children. The diet causes the body to burn fats rather than carbohydrates for energy, putting it in a state of "ketosis," which reduces the intensity and frequency of seizures. The diet may successfully control epilepsy in 30 to 50 percent of children with intractable epilepsy.

Vagus Nerve Stimulation (VNS). VNS is a type of treatment in which short bursts of electrical energy are directed to the brain via the vagus nerve in the neck by a small, pacemaker-like device surgically implanted near the patient's collarbone. The device can reduce seizures, on average, by 20 to 40 percent and completely control seizures in about 5 percent of people.

Complementary Therapies. Complementary therapies such as relaxation, yoga, acupuncture, aromatherapy, biofeedback, and behavior therapy have helped people with their epilepsy and improved their quality of life by reducing stress and improving seizure control.

Prevention

The possibility of developing epilepsy can be reduced by the following techniques:

- Proper prenatal care during pregnancy and childbirth to prevent brain damage
- Proper immunization against certain diseases of childhood, adolescence, and adulthood, which involve the central nervous system
- Wearing safety gear (seatbelts, bicycle helmets) to prevent head injury and other trauma
- Reducing or treating risk factors such as physical inactivity, obesity, diabetes, high blood pressure, and smoking to lessen the likelihood of stroke and heart disease
- Identifying the genes for many neurological disorders through genetic screening and prenatal diagnosis

Leah Sultan-Khan

See also: Brain Diseases; Environment; Meningitis

Further Reading

American Academy of Neurology. (2012). Epilepsy. Retrieved from http://patients.aan.com/disorders/index.cfm?event=view&disorder_id=918.

American Epilepsy Society. (2012). Retrieved from http://www.aesnet.org.

Centers for Disease Control and Prevention. (2012). Epilepsy. Retrieved from http://www.cdc.gov/Epilepsy/.

Edmonton Epilepsy Association. (2011). Epilepsy: An overview. Retrieved from http://www.edmontonepilepsy.org/documents/Epilepsy%20-%20An%20Overview.pdf.

Epilepsy Action. (2012). Advice and information. Retrieved from http://www.epilepsy.org.uk/info.

Epilepsy Foundation. (2012). About epilepsy. Retrieved from http://www.epilepsyfoundation.org/aboutepilepsy/.

Mayo Clinic. (2012). Epilepsy. Retrieved from http://www.mayoclinic.com/health/epilepsy/DS00342.

National Institute of Neurological Disorders and Stroke. (2012). Epilepsy. Retrieved from http://www.ninds.nih.gov/disorders/epilepsy/detail_epilepsy.htm.

U.S. National Library of Medicine. (2012). Epilepsy. Retrieved from http://www.nlm.nih.gov/medlineplus/epilepsy.html.

Wyllie, E. (2008). *Epilepsy: Information for You and Those Who Care about You.* Cleveland, OH: Cleveland Clinic Press.

ESOPHAGEAL CANCER

Esophageal cancer is the uncontrolled multiplication of cells within the esophagus, the digestive tube that connects the mouth to the stomach. Cancerous cell growth typically begins in the inner layer of this tube. The cancer may then spread to the outer layers, as well as to other tissues and organs of the body.

Esophageal cancer can take one of two main forms. In *squamous cell carcinoma*, cancer develops from the squamous cells that line the inner esophagus. In *adenocarcinoma*, cancer develops from gland cells in the lower esophagus, near the stomach.

Prevalence and Mortality

In 2014, there were some 18,000 newly diagnosed cases of esophageal cancer in the United States, representing about 1 percent of all new cancer cases. Some 15,000 Americans died from esophageal cancer in 2014, representing almost 3 percent of all cancer deaths.

Esophageal cancer has a high mortality rate, and mortality increases as the disease advances. The five-year survival rate is about 38 percent for individuals diagnosed and treated when the cancer was confined to the esophagus. For individuals with cancer that has spread to regions near the esophagus, the five-year survival rate is about 20 percent. In cases in which the cancer has spread to regions distant from the esophagus, the five-year survival rate is only about 3 percent. On average, 18 percent of people with esophageal cancer will be alive five years after diagnosis.

Risk Factors

Some individuals are at an elevated risk for esophageal cancer. People who have gastroesophageal reflux disease (GERD) are at increased risk of adenocarcinoma as a result of acid that backs up into the esophagus from the stomach. The acid causes changes in esophageal cells that can lead to cancer. People with a condition called Barrett's esophagus, which is sometimes associated with GERD, are also at elevated risk of adenocarcinoma. Tobacco use—in the form of cigarette smoking, chewing tobacco, or other products—raises the risk of esophageal cancer. Excessive alcohol use does the same.

The risk of esophageal cancer increases with age, especially after age 45. The disease is most frequently diagnosed between ages 65 and 74. In addition, men are at greater risk than women, and African Americans are at greater risk than other ethnic groups.

Symptoms and Diagnosis

Symptoms are usually slow to develop in individuals with esophageal cancer. As the cancer advances, however, several symptoms may become noticeable. These symptoms include difficulties in swallowing, painful swallowing, hoarseness, frequent coughing, indigestion, heartburn, chest pain, and weight loss.

A diagnosis of esophageal cancer may include a number of evaluations. A patient's symptoms and medical history are evaluated. A physical examination is performed. X-rays are used to look for internal visual evidence of cancer. Blood tests are used to look for biochemical evidence. A tissue biopsy, in which esophageal cells are examined under a microscope, may be performed to verify a diagnosis of esophageal cancer.

The tissue sample is obtained by inserting a thin, flexible tube called an endoscope into the esophagus. Tools at the tip of the endoscope collect the sample. A camera on the endoscope allows the physician to inspect the inside of the esophagus for signs of cancer or other abnormalities. In some cases, ultrasonography may be combined with endoscopy, enabling an analysis of sound waves to reveal more information about the condition of the esophagus.

Additional tests can be used to determine if the cancer has spread to tissues beyond the esophagus. These tests include positron emission tomography, computed tomography (CT), and further endoscopy procedures.

Treatment

Treatment for esophageal cancer is often unsuccessful because of the slow, gradual development of its symptoms. By the time the symptoms are noticed and the cancer is detected, the disease has often progressed to an advanced stage in which much of the esophagus as well as other tissues are affected.

For some patients, surgeons may need to remove part or all of the esophagus. Part of the upper stomach may also need to be removed. People without an esophagus must be fed through a feeding tube inserted into the stomach. In certain cases, the esophagus can be reconstructed using tissue from the small intestine to make a new tubular connection between the mouth and stomach.

In endoscopic mucosal resection, the inner lining of the esophagus is removed. This procedure is effective only for cancer in an early stage of development. Early stages of esophageal cancer may also be treated with radiofrequency ablation (in which high-energy radio waves destroy cancer cells), photodynamic therapy (in which laser beams target cancer cells), and electrocoagulation (in which electric currents kill cancer cells). In many cases, patients with esophageal cancer are treated with a combination of radiation therapy and chemotherapy.

For patients in whom the disease is in advanced stages, only palliative therapy can be offered. In such cases, the cancer cannot be successfully treated. Instead, patients are given drugs to reduce their pain and to help them swallow.

A. J. Smuskiewicz

See also: Cancer; Gastroesophageal Reflux Disease (GERD); Squamous Cell Carcinoma

Further Reading

Ginex, P. K., Jingeleski, M., Frazzitta, B. L., & Baines, M. S. (2009). *100 Questions & Answers About Esophageal Cancer*. Burlington, MA: Jones & Bartlett.

Jobe, B. A., Charles, T. R., & Hunter, J. G. (2009). *Esophageal Cancer: Principles and Practice*. New York: Springer.

Mayo Clinic. (2015). Diseases and conditions: Esophageal cancer. http://www.mayoclinic .org/diseases-conditions/esophageal-cancer/basics/definition/con-20034316.

National Cancer Institute. (2015). Esophageal cancer: Overview. Retrieved from http://www .cancer.gov/types/esophageal.

National Cancer Institute. (2015). SEER stat fact sheets: Esophageal cancer. Retrieved from http://seer.cancer.gov/statfacts/html/esoph.html.

O'Reilly Onconurse. (2016). Esophageal cancer resources. Retrieved from http://www.oreilly .com/onconurse/factsheets/esophageal_resource.html.

ETIOLOGY

Literally, etiology translates to *aitia*, "cause" and *logos*, "the study of": therefore, *etiology* is the study of the causes of disease. Etiology is a critical component of the fields of medicine, public health, and more specifically, epidemiology. The importance of etiology lies within the fundamental understanding that in order to effectively prevent disease onset, provide treatments to people with disease, and prevent the spread of disease, it is paramount to know what causes the disease and the mechanisms of transmission within a population.

Throughout history, many individuals have contemplated the origins of disease and proposed various theories of disease causes and transmission mechanisms. Hippocrates (ca. 460 BC–ca. 377 BC) believed in humorism or humoralism. Humorism states that human beings have four humors, or bodily fluids: black bile, yellow bile, phlegm, and blood. An imbalance of the four humors caused disease (Rosen 1958). For example, Hippocrates declared that fever was caused by an excess of blood. Therefore, Hippocrates (and other physicians at the time) prescribed bloodletting or using bloodsucking leeches to remove "excess blood" as a treatment for feverish patients. Humorism has since been discredited by modern science.

In addition, Hippocrates laid down the initial framework of epidemic constitution that was later expanded on during the 16th and 17th centuries (Rosen 1958). *Epidemic constitution* claimed that certain environmental conditions, specifically atmospheric, give rise to certain diseases and caused them to spread more readily than in the absence of such conditions (Rosen 1958). The notion of epidemic constitution further expanded into miasma theory, which put forth the concept that diseases derive from foul-smelling vapors emitted from decaying organic matter (Miasma Theory, n.d.). In fact, malaria, literally translated to "bad" (*mala*) "air" (*aria*) in Italian, reflects the then-widely held notion of the disease's miasmic origins (Miasma Theory, n.d.).

Although miasma theory was incredibly popular into the early 19th century, a concurrent rival theory also existed: contagion theory. Girolamo Fracastoro (1478–1553), a physician and scholar from Italy, was one of the first people to propose an accurate fundamental tenet of how disease spreads: Tiny particles (he termed them *seminaria*, or "seeds") are responsible for the dissemination of epidemic diseases and can be transmitted via direct and indirect contact (Rosen 1958). Fracastoro was the first scientist to posit that infection was the cause of disease and epidemics were consequences of an infection's spread via contagious particulate matter (Rosen 1958).

Though respected during Fracastoro's time, contagion theory did not garner much support until the 17th century, after Antony van Leeuwenhoek's (1632–1723) technological advancement: the dramatically improved microscope (Rosen 1958). With his newly developed version of the microscope, Leeuwenhoek was able to witness microorganisms. Leeuwenhoek's observation lent credence and provided visible evidence to contagion theory. However, many believed that the miniscule creatures were spontaneously generated, meaning they were borne from inanimate matter. Moreover, some time passed before it dawned on scientists that these tiny animals may actually be the causes of diseases (Rosen 1958).

Francisco Redi (1626–1697), Louis Pasteur (1822–1895), Joseph Lister (1827–1912), and Robert Koch (1843–1910) laid the foundations for and expanded on the now-prevailing paradigm of etiology and contagious disease transmission: germ theory. Germ theory posits that specific microorganisms are responsible for the manifestations of specific diseases and that diseases are contagious (Germ Theory, n.d.). Redi, an Italian physician, hypothesized that maggots did not spontaneously generate from meat (a widely held belief at the time) and conducted an experiment in which he placed meat in jars, covered some jar openings with gauze, and left other jar openings uncovered (Levine & Evers 2009). Redi found that the meat in accessible (open) jars subsequently harbored maggots, whereas meat in inaccessible jars (gauze-covered) contained no maggots. Thus, Redi's findings began to cast doubt on the theory of spontaneous generation. Much later, Pasteur, a French chemist and microbiologist, conducted experiments that generated concrete evidence to finally dismiss the idea of spontaneous generation: Pasteur demonstrated that microbes caused decomposition and that germs were present everywhere, including in the air (Germ Theory, n.d.). After learning of Pasteur's work, Lister, a British surgeon applied the Pasteur's concepts to human medicine (Rosen 1958). Lister developed antiseptic surgical techniques and found that his techniques reduced the rate of infection and death among his patients (Germ Theory, n.d.). Then, Koch, a German physician, gained notoriety for demonstrating that specific germs caused specific diseases, a revolutionary idea at the time (Germ Theory, n.d.).

Thus, the field of etiology dates back centuries, with many theories posited and debunked about the etiology of contagious diseases. Today, with an increased understanding of the origins of communicable diseases and how they spread, coupled with the numerous technological innovations since the 1900s, an epidemiological shift occurred in the United States and other developed countries whereby the incidence and prevalence of life-threatening, contagious illnesses are low and the incidence and prevalence of chronic diseases are on the rise. The shift happened, in part, because of increased etiologic understanding of contagious diseases, the rise of vaccinations, more sophisticated infrastructure and technology, greater hygiene, better food-storage systems, and pasteurization—all are factors that contribute to an average increase in lifespan and major changes in lifestyle.

Nowadays, many people in the United States live sedentary lifestyles and have access to calorie-dense foods. Furthermore, environmental, sociocultural, and biological (genetic) factors are recognized as contributors to chronic diseases such as certain types of cancers, heart disease, high blood pressure, obesity, and Type 2 diabetes. Researchers find that chronic diseases are typically a result of multiple etiologic factors, which is the notion that multiple elements are responsible for the development of chronic diseases. That is, certain components may, in combination, lead to the development of a chronic disease, but the presence of such components does not necessarily guarantee disease manifestation. For example, an individual's body type, current body mass index (BMI), race/ethnicity, diet, and physical activity levels may all be considered risk factors or preventive factors for developing high blood pressure. Therefore, it is becoming increasingly commonplace to employ sophisticated statistical analyses to study chronic disease etiology. Results from such analyses tend to be suggestive instead of definitive as to what "causes" a certain chronic disease to manifest in one individual and not another. Thus, the field of etiology continues to evolve: Chronic disease etiology is much more complex and less definitive than the etiology of contagious diseases, which may only involve certain types of microorganisms. Currently, researchers and practitioners are exploring various risk factors for developing chronic disease because the field of chronic disease etiology is relatively young. In the future, many theories may be proposed and subsequently debunked before a deeper understanding of chronic disease etiology arises.

Sukhminder Kaur

See also: Epidemiology; Family Health; Risk Factors

Further Reading

Germ Theory. (n.d.). In *Contagion: Historical Views of Diseases and Epidemics*. Retrieved from http://ocp.hul.harvard.edu/contagion/germtheory.html.

Kuh, D., & Ben-Shlomo, Y., eds. (2004). *A Life Course Approach to Chronic Disease Epidemiology*, 2nd ed. New York, NY: Oxford University Press.

Levine, R., & Evers, C. (2009). The slow death of spontaneous generation (1668–1859). In *Access Excellence @ The National Health Museum*. Retrieved from http://www.access excellence.org/RC/AB/BC/Spontaneous_Generation.php.

Miasma Theory. (n.d.). In *Brought to Life: Exploring the History of Medicine*. Retrieved from http://www.sciencemuseum.org.uk/broughttolife/techniques/miasmatheory.aspx.

Rosen, G. (1958). *A History of Public Health*. New York: MD Publications.

EYE CANCER

Eye cancer refers to the growth of cancerous cells in the region of the eye. Those that start inside the eye are called *primary intraocular cancers*; the most common types are melanoma and lymphoma in adults. Retinoblastoma is rare, but it is the most common eye cancer in children, usually occurring before the age of five. *Secondary intraocular cancers* begin in the breast or lungs before spreading to the eye; they are more common than primary intraocular cancers. About 90 percent of melanomas start in the skin, and most lymphomas begin in the lymph nodes.

Primary eye cancers most commonly affect people over the age of 50. Caucasians, slightly more men, and those with light-colored eyes are at increased risk. An estimated 1,360 men and 1,220 women in the United States were diagnosed with primary intraocular cancer in 2012. The cause of primary eye melanoma is unknown, but it occurs when changes in DNA cause healthy eye cells to grow and multiply out of control. A weakened immune system is the cause of primary eye lymphoma, which is a rare cancer.

Treatment depends on the type and severity of an eye cancer, but common approaches include surgery, radiation, chemotherapy, laser, or targeted therapy or a combination of options.

Symptoms

Eye cancer may not present any symptoms in its early stages, and each person may experience different symptoms later on, which can include painless blurry, double, or lost vision; flashes of light, spots, squiggly lines, or floating objects (floaters); a sty that doesn't heal; eyelash loss; eyelid tears (ulcerations) or lesions; a bulging eye; change in the position or movement of the eyeball or the shape or size of the pupil; excessive tearing or bloody tears; and pain if a tumor has grown.

Causes and Risk Factors

The causes of eye cancer are unknown, but changes in the DNA of cells contribute to their becoming cancerous. The risk factors for melanomas that start inside the eye include aging, race (Caucasian), having a light eye color, and gender: Men have a very slight higher risk than women. Family history of the disease is rare, but a change in the BAP1 gene may increase the risk. People with mole-like spots associated with their eyes also face a higher risk. Excessive sun exposure is not a proven risk factor for eye melanoma, although it is a risk factor for skin melanoma.

The only known risk factor for primary lymphoma of the eye is a weakened immune system, which includes people who have HIV/AIDS and those who rely on antirejection medications after having an organ or tissue transplant.

Diagnosis

An ophthalmologist, or a specialist in eye diseases, diagnoses melanoma with physical and eye examinations. An ophthalmoscope, which is a lighted instrument and a slit lamp (a microscope with an attached light), often detects eye cancers. Other diagnostic tools are imaging tests, which may include ultrasound; fluorescein angiography, a picture of the eye's blood vessels; a CT scan; or an MRI (magnetic resonance imaging). Occasionally a fine biopsy is needed.

Treatments

Treatment depends on the type, size, and location of an eye cancer. Options or melanoma include observation, also called watchful waiting or close monitoring, of small or slow-growing cancers, particularly if treatment would cause more discomfort than the tumor does itself. Surgery is a standard treatment in which parts or the entire affected eye are removed, depending on the details of the tumor; it is not an option for intraocular lymphoma. A variety of radiation therapies, or the use of high-energy beams to kill cancer cells, are typical treatment for small or medium eye melanomas and may be useful against lymphoma. Laser therapy, or highly focused beams of light that can destroy body tissues, may be used to treat melanoma, but it is not recommended for lymphoma. Chemotherapy, or anticancer medications, has been useful for treating lymphoma, but rarely for melanoma.

Prognosis and Outcomes

With treatment, survival rates for eye melanoma are better when detected in the early stages. When limited to the eye, the five-year relative survival rate is about 80 percent, meaning about three of four people survive for at least five years. The rate drops to about 15 percent if the eye melanoma has spread elsewhere in the body.

Eye lymphomas are rare, but some research suggests that if the cancer remains in the eye and spreads nowhere else, the chance of a five-year survival rate is moderate.

Future

Although medical researchers have developed two new groups of drugs for skin melanomas, it is not known if they will be effective in treating eye melanomas. Immunotherapy drugs help the immune system recognize and attack cancer cells; they are being studied for eye melanomas. Targeted drugs, which target parts of melanoma cells exhibiting gene changes are used treat skin melanomas. Although same gene mutation is not as common in eye melanomas, the drugs may be helpful.

Ray Marks

See also: Eye Diseases, Melanoma

Further Reading

American Cancer Society. (2015, February 2). What is eye cancer? Retrieved from http://www.cancer.org/cancer/eyecancer/detailedguide/eye-cancer-what-is-eye-cancer.

American Society of Clinical Oncology. (2015, May). Eye cancer overview. Retrieved from http://www.cancer.net/cancer-types/eye-cancer/overview?sectionTitle=Overview.

Mayo Clinic. (2015, July 22). Eye melanoma. Retrieved from http://www.mayoclinic.org/diseases-conditions/eye-melanoma/basics/definition/con-20027875.

MD Anderson Cancer Center. (2015). Eye cancer. Retrieved from http://www.mdanderson.org/patient-and-cancer-information/cancer-information/cancer-types/eye-cancer/index.html.

EYE DISEASES

Disorders can affect the eyes either directly or as a secondary symptom of another condition, such as diabetes or migraine. In the United States, about 3.3 million people older than 40 have low vision or are blind, and the number is expected to increase due to the aging U.S. population and the chronic disorders that accompany advanced age. About 14 million people 12 years and older have some visual impairment, and nearly 7 percent of children have a diagnosed eye or vision condition.

Of the many types of eye disorders, these are common: refractive errors, or nearsightedness, farsightedness, astigmatism, and presbyopia; macular degeneration, usually an age-related disease that reduces sharp central vision; cataracts, or clouding of the eye lens; diabetic eye disease; retinal disorders related to the nerves at the back of the eye; amblyopia, often called lazy eye, the most common childhood vision impairment; strabismus, or the imbalance in the positions of the eyes; and glaucoma, or damage to the optic nerve. Bacterial infections and blocked tear glands that cause sties are also common.

Symptoms

The most common symptoms associated with eye disorders include redness, inflammation, and bleeding; changes in vision, including loss and blindness; eye pain; fluid draining from the eye; and seeing double, flashes of light, or "floaters." Some eye disorders may not present early symptoms, they might be painless, or there is no change in vision until a disorder advances.

Causes and Risk Factors

Women are at higher risk for some eye disorders, but key risk factors for one or more eye disorders for both men and women include age; family history; high blood pressure; HIV/AIDS, which makes eyes susceptible to infection; obesity; smoking; and surgical procedures that remove parts of the bones housing the optic nerve or the eye socket to decrease pressure.

Diagnosis

To diagnose an eye disorder, an ophthalmologist performs a complete exam, taking a medical history and discussing vision and related problems, conducting a visual acuity test, and screening for glaucoma. The exam also looks at all parts of the eyes: eyelids, lashes, cornea, iris, lens, and fluid chamber between the cornea and iris, including eye dilation to see the back of the eyes, the retina, optic disk, and the underlying layer of blood vessels.

Treatments

Depending on the disorder, its cause, and severity, treatment approaches may include eye drops, ointments, or gels; prescription eyeglasses; scatter laser or photodynamic therapies; medication injections; treating the underlying illness; and surgery, including vitrectomy to remove blood from the center of the eye if bleeding is severe.

Prevention

Regular checkups by eye specialists help prevent disorders and their consequences, particularly for those who may not exhibit early symptoms. Other recommended strategies include controlling blood sugar levels, cholesterol, and blood pressure; eating green leafy vegetables and fish; maintaining a healthy weight; exercising regularly; avoiding or quitting smoking; and wearing sunglasses and other protective eyewear.

Prognosis and Outcomes

Regular eye examinations and treatment may prevent vision loss. Corrective lenses restore good vision for nearsightedness, farsightedness, and astigmatism. Advanced medical and surgical techniques can improve the disorders glaucoma, macular degeneration, and retinal detachment.

Future

The National Eye Institute is examining better ways to identify and treat vision loss in people with diabetes. The Glaucoma Research Foundation has been studying the best treatment approach for glaucoma. Much progress has been made in eye surgery, allowing many individuals with previously untreatable disorders to experience improved eyesight and quality of life.

Ray Marks

See also: Colorblindness; Diabetes, Type 1; Glaucoma; Hyperopia; Macular Degeneration; Myopia; Sjögren's Syndrome

Further Reading

American Academy of Ophthalmology. (2012). Common eye conditions. Retrieved from http://www.geteyesmart.org/eyesmart/diseases/index.cfm.

Bakri, S. J. (2007). *Mayo Clinic Guide to Better Vision.* Rochester, MN: Mayo Clinic.

National Eye Institute. (2015). Eye health tips. Retrieved from https://nei.nih.gov/healthyeyes/eyehealthtips.

NIH News in Health. (2015, May). Keep your vision healthy. Retrieved from http://newsinhealth.nih.gov/issue/May2015/feature2.

F

FAILURE TO THRIVE

Failure to thrive is the term used to refer to the condition of infants and toddlers characterized by a lack of expected growth or weight gain. Failure to thrive (FTT) occurs because children do not obtain, retain, or use the calories from food required to grow and gain weight appropriately (Dowshen 2011). Therefore, FTT is actually a sign of under-nutrition (Cole & Lanham 2011). However, no precise or medically agreed upon definition exists, because failure to thrive is not classified as a disease; rather, it describes a condition (Dowshen 2011). Underlying medical, social, environmental, or any combination such factors may cause a child to exhibit FTT (Cole & Lanham 2011). Treatment of FTT involves an assessment of the underlying cause and a subsequent, appropriate course of action to address or rectify the cause. If FTT is left untreated, children may not reach—or may be delayed in reaching—developmental milestones, and children may fail to grow normally and fail to appropriately develop mentally, emotionally, and physically. If the underlying cause of FTT is successfully treated soon after the infant or toddler exhibits FTT, children demonstrate normal development or may end up with slightly reduced height, weight, and cognitive abilities (Cole & Lanham 2011). Nevertheless, researchers admit the need to further study potential outcomes of infants and toddlers who present with FTT.

Failure to thrive has been recognized as a condition for at least a century (Dowshen 2011). Prior to its recognition as a condition, it was well known that some infants failed to grow and develop normally: These babies most often died during their infancy. However, with increasing medical knowledge, failure to thrive was identified as a condition stemming from inadequate nutrition. In years past, the medical community classified causes of FTT as "organic" or "nonorganic." Organic causes of FTT included medical or biological complications that impeded or interrupted normal nutritional intake or absorption or that created excess energy expenditure (Cole & Lanham 2011). Examples of organic causes include gastroesophageal reflux, food allergy, malabsorption, thyroid disease, chronic infection, and immunodeficiency. Nonorganic causes of FTT included social or environmental problems that affected an infant's ability to receive or absorb an appropriate number of calories.

Examples of nonorganic causes include problems breastfeeding, incorrect formula preparation, caregiver depression, poor food availability, and poverty. In fact, nonorganic causes of FTT were identified and studied only as of the early 1940s. Dr. René Spitz (1887–1974), an Austrian psychoanalyst, observed orphanages and their effects on infants. He noticed that despite the presence of a relatively germ-free environment, babies confined to hospitals demonstrated a great susceptibility to sickness. Moreover, he observed severe wasting that occurred to infants' minds and bodies and attributed it to the extended period of time spent in institutionalized care: He coined the term "hospitalism" to describe this phenomenon (Spitz 1945). He noted that infants suffering from hospitalism often died within the first year of life or suffered severe, irreversible personality damage and developmental abnormalities (Spitz 1945). He partially ascribed hospitalism to infants' bare environment and to the lack of human touch babies received after babies were weaned from breast milk, which occurred around three to four months of age (Spitz 1945). A short time later, in 1949, Dr. John Bowlby (1907–1990) wrote a report for the World Health Organization (WHO) on the deleterious effects of maternal deprivation that occurred in infants who were institutionalized. He observed infants across many countries—including the United States, United Kingdom, France, Switzerland, Germany, Sweden, and Switzerland—and found similar effects across countries (Bowlby 1952). In the WHO report, Bowlby echoed many of Spitz's findings.

Although causes of failure to thrive were once classified into organic or nonorganic, scientists and practitioners now recognize that causes are often a result of multiple components (Cole & Lanham 2011) and that psychosocial, environmental, and biological factors may be related. Regardless of the underlying elements, the manifestation of atypical weight gain and growth are similar across infants presenting with FTT. Therefore, practitioners use body measurements and growth charts to support the diagnosis of FTT (Cole & Lanham 2011). However, discovering the underlying cause remains paramount to successful treatment because FTT only describes a condition of infants and thus, should not be the sole diagnosis. Nevertheless, an underlying medical cause cannot be identified in 80 percent of the cases, which implies that many cases of FTT may be caused by psychosocial or environmental components. Indeed, the greatest predictor of infant FTT is poverty both in developed and developing areas of the world (Cole & Lanham 2011). Bowlby (1952) observed the same relationship between FTT and poverty more than half a century ago.

Treatment of failure to thrive depends on the underlying condition. If the original condition is medical in nature, then treatment will be dictated by the proper approach for addressing the medical disease or illness. If no medical issue is responsible for the manifestation of FTT, then practitioners must first give nutritional counseling and guidance on the best way for catch-up growth to be achieved by the infant (Cole & Lanham 2011). Additionally, if environmental or psychosocial factors are the underlying issue, a multidisciplinary intervention may be required to promote a healthy home environment and a better relationship between infant and caregiver while simultaneously attending to the infant's cognitive growth and weight gain. Furthermore, practitioners and researchers advise frequent follow-up visits with the infant's physician to evaluate the infant's growth and development.

Expected outcomes of children who endured prolonged FTT are known to have negative long-term physical and cognitive developmental effects (Cole & Lanham

2011). Such children typically are smaller and less cognitively developed, which may translate into poorer academic achievement. However, researchers are less sure if children who temporarily had FTT should expect similar outcomes as their peers who experienced more prolonged FTT. Some evidence suggests that such children experience long-term reductions in height and weight but no discernable cognitive effects (Cole & Lanham 2011).

There have not been rapid developments in the diagnosis, treatment, or expected outcomes associated with failure to thrive. As the fields of medicine and child development advance, greater understanding may help to identify the underlying causes of FTT much quicker than in years past. As stated previously, many of the children suffering from FTT do not have an underlying medical condition, indicating some type of environmental or psychosocial cause. Hence, prevention of most cases of FTT may hinge on educating parents and caregivers about basic infant and child nutrition, psychology, and care.

Sukhminder Kaur

See also: Allergies; Environment; Fetal Alcohol Syndrome; Gastroesophageal Reflux Disease (GERD); Immune System Disorders; Poverty; Thyroid Disease; World Health Organization

Further Reading

Bowlby, J. (1952). *Maternal Care and Mental Health.* Geneva, Switzerland. Retrieved from http://whqlibdoc.who.int/monograph/WHO_MONO_2_(part1).pdf.

Cole, S. Z., & Lanham, J. S. (2011). Failure to thrive: an update. *American Family Physician, 83*(7), 829–834. Retrieved from http://www.ncbi.nlm.nih.gov/pubmed/21524049.

Dowshen, S. (2011). Failure to thrive. Retrieved from http://kidshealth.org/parent/growth/growth/failure_thrive.html#.

Robertson, R. G., & Montagnini, M. (2004). Geriatric failure to thrive. *American Family Physician, 70*(2), 343–350. Retrieved from http://www.ncbi.nlm.nih.gov/pubmed/15291092.

Spitz, R. A. (1945). Hospitalism—An inquiry into the genesis of psychiatric conditions in early childhood. *Psychoanalytic Study of the Child, 1,* 53–74.

FAMILIAL HYPERCHOLESTEROLEMIA

Familial hypercholesterolemia is an inherited disorder that causes high levels of LDL (low-density lipoprotein) "bad" cholesterol levels at birth, which can lead to premature cardiovascular disease. The disorder is caused by a gene mutation on chromosome 19, which is carried by 1 in 500 individuals worldwide. Familial hypercholesterolemia, or FH, is inherited from one parent or, rarely, both; those with two mutated genes face an even higher risk of early heart disease. In the United States, an estimated 1.3 million people have familial hypercholesterolemia. In those with the disorder, the genetic mutation does not allow the liver to remove excess LDL, a cause of cardiovascular disease.

Found in every cell in the body, cholesterol is a waxy substance produced mainly in the liver; it also comes from eating dairy products, eggs, and meat. The body produces the cholesterol it needs to produce vitamin D and some hormones and to insulate nerve fibers and maintain healthy cells. Too much cholesterol can cause heart disease, heart attack, atherosclerosis, and stroke. Cholesterol travels through the blood by attaching to lipoproteins, a type of a protein. Low-density lipoproteins (LDL), often called bad cholesterol, can clog arteries and increase the risk of heart disease.

Anyone with one parent who carries this gene is at risk for the disorder; it is especially common among some ethnic groups, including French Canadians, the Finnish, the Lebanese, the Afrikaners in South Africa, and those of Ashkenazi Jewish descent. Siblings and offspring of those with the disorder face a 50 percent risk of inheriting the defective gene, but children and grandchildren of those without the disorder are not at risk.

In addition to symptoms of heart disease, which may include pain, those with FH may experience cholesterol deposits on their skin or around the eyes. Treatment focuses on minimizing the risk of heart disease, starting with diet, exercise, and usually cholesterol-lowering medications.

History

In 1973, medical researchers Michael Brown and Joseph Goldstein studied people with familial hypercholesterolemia, discovering that the mutated gene and its activities were at the root of the disorder. In 1985, Brown and Goldstein received the Nobel Prize in Physiology or Medicine for their work.

Symptoms

Primary symptoms of familial hypercholesterolemia include having high levels of total cholesterol and LDL cholesterol; xanthomas, which are waxy deposits of cholesterol in the skin or tendons, often visible on the hands, elbows, knees, or ankles; xanthelasmas, or cholesterol deposits in the eyelids; cholesterol deposits around the cornea of the eye known as corneal arcus; and a family history of therapy-resistant high levels of LDL in one or both parents. Chest pain, or angina, may be a symptom of heart disease at a young age.

Causes and Risk Factors

Familial hypercholesterolemia is a genetic disorder caused by a defect on chromosome 19, which makes the body unable to remove low-density lipoprotein (LDL) "bad" cholesterol from the blood. It is inherited from one parent passing the defective gene to a child. Rarely, a person inherits the gene mutation from both parents, which leads to a more severe form of the disorder that may include heart disease and death before reaching age 30. More than 300 forms of gene mutations leading to FH have been identified.

Diagnosis

Diagnosis of familial hypercholesterolemia is based on physical examination to look for the presence of visible symptoms, including xanthomas, xanthelasmas, and corneal arcus, and laboratory blood tests for levels of LDL cholesterol (more than 220 mg/dL in adults with FH; more than 170–200 mg/dL in children with FH), total blood cholesterol (more than 300 mg/dL in adults with FH; more than 250 mg/dL in children with FH), and triglycerides, which are fatty acids, although these are usually in the normal range (below 150 mg/dL) for people with this disorder. Other tests include heart function, genetic testing for the gene mutation, and studies to see how the body absorbs LDL cholesterol. Diagnostic tools also include a personal and family medical history.

Treatments

The first goal of treatment is to reduce the risk of heart disease by lowering the LDL cholesterol levels in the blood. A recommended diet includes limiting beef, pork, and lamb and eliminating butter, whole milk, fatty cheeses and oils, egg yolks, organ meats, and other saturated animal fats. Exercise and weight loss are often recommended to reduce LDL cholesterol levels.

Usually necessary, cholesterol-lowering medications may be prescribed, including statins, bile acid sequestrants, ezetemibe, niacin, gemfibrozil, and fenofibrate.

Those with a severe form of FH may require plasmaphoresis, which removes blood or plasma from the body. Special filters then clear the excess LDL cholesterol before returning the blood to the body; this treatment may be done every three weeks. Those with the gene mutation inherited from both parents may require a liver transplant to provide the missing LDL receptors; this requires long-term follow-up care and continuous immunosuppression medication.

Prevention

Treatment for adults should begin as soon as possible after diagnosis. Early detection and treatment is key for preventing premature heart attacks, including no smoking, regular exercise, eating a healthful diet, and taking medications as prescribed. Children in families with a history of heart attack or heart disease before age 55 for men and 65 for women may benefit by having their cholesterol checked after age 2 and before 10. Genetic counseling can identify those at risk of FH if they have a strong family history of early heart disease

Prognosis and Outcomes

Getting an accurate diagnosis and following treatment recommendations can lead to normal life span. Those with FH face a significantly higher risk of experiencing a fatal heart attack before the age of 40 and a coronary artery blood clot before reaching 60, although about one-third have no symptoms until sudden cardiac death. If untreated, those with FH have 20 times the risk of developing early aggressive heart disease. Risk of death varies, but those who inherit two copies of the defective gene have a poorer outcome because the disorder is commonly resistant to treatment.

Ray Marks

See also: Cholesterol; Diet and Nutrition; Family Health; Food Guides from the USDA; Genetics and Genomics; Physical Activity

Further Reading

FH Foundation. (2015). What is FH? Retrieved from https://thefhfoundation.org/about-fh/what-is-fh/.

National Center for Advancing Translational Sciences. (2015, June 18). Familial hypercholesterolemia. Retrieved from https://rarediseases.info.nih.gov/gard/10416/familial-hypercholesterolemia/resources/1.

National Human Genome Research Institute. (2013, December 26). Learning about familial hypercholesterolemia. Retrieved from http://www.genome.gov/25520184/.

NetDoctor. (2012, June 12). Familial hypercholesterolemia. Retrieved from http://www.netdoctor.co.uk/diseases/facts/familialhypercholesterolaemia.htm.

FAMILY HEALTH

A comprehensive, concise definition describes *family health* as "a family's quality of life, the health of each member, family interactions, spirituality, nutrition, coping, environment, recreation and routines, sleep, and sexuality" (Bomar 2004, 11). The World Health Organization (WHO) defines family health as both the levels of disease in a family and the ability of a family to function as a cohesive unit to promote the health and well-being of the unit (1973). Numerous definitions of family health exist because health is a multidimensional phenomenon and families are complex systems. Even though it is difficult to define, family health is massively important. By understanding how the family system, family members, and health mutually influence each other, treatment regimens as well as public health initiatives and interventions could be more effectively designed to enhance overall health and to promote wellness in families.

During the early 20th century, the dominant health paradigm in the Western context was incredibly narrow and did not incorporate more holistic aspects like social, environmental, and emotional elements. Therefore, the field of family health only emerged in the latter part of the 20th century after the concept of health expanded to include such aspects. When the perception of health shifted from a biomedical model to a biopsychosocial model, the notion of family health developed and become an area of study. Briefly, the biomedical model referred to health and disease as states not influenced by social or emotional conditions. Essentially, the biomedical model defined health as the absence of illness or disease. In other words, under this model, health and wellness promotion are difficult to achieve because one is (1) sick and treatable, (2) sick and untreatable, or (3) "healthy" (i.e., no visible sickness). However, the biomedical model falls short in providing a framework for appropriate prevention and treatment of chronic diseases because many preventable chronic diseases stem from unhealthy behaviors and lifestyles that are tied to social conditions and emotional states. Unhealthy behaviors, lifestyles, social conditions, and emotional states are closely connected to family and family processes.

In the 1970s, scientists began to discover the reciprocal relationship between social, psychological, and environmental factors and health and disease status, which led Engel, an American psychiatrist, to declare the need for a new health paradigm: the biopsychosocial model (Grochowski 2010). The biopsychosocial model acknowledges that biological, social, and psychological elements influence health (Engel 1992), meaning that factors such as socioeconomic status, culture, and family relations are recognized as contributing components to health and disease in individuals. Therefore, under Engel's model, family context, a family member's disease status, mother's education, and a whole host of other factors were acknowledged as contributing to the health of individuals and individuals' families. Consequently, researchers began to study areas like family coping, family-centered medical care, family response to chronically ill children, family psychosocial resilience, and family health promotion to gain greater understanding of family health. Hence, with the advent of the biopsychosocial model, the 1980s and 1990s witnessed a blossoming of the field of family health.

During the 1990s, family systems theory emerged and remains one of the dominant frameworks for understanding family health (Anderson & Tomlinson 1992). In family systems theory, families are considered systems containing subsystems (family members) that wish to sustain balance and harmony. Family members strive for equilibrium within the family by supporting each other in the various spheres of health via developing processes for responding to and adapting to stressors. Stressors are anything that may jeopardize aspects of health or well-being. Specifically, family systems theory states that family health operates within the biopsychosocial model and connects the structure and function of families with the health (illness and wellness) of (1) family members and (2) the family unit (Anderson 2000). In effect, the family systems theory abandoned the old paradigm of cause and effect to lay the framework for the study of multiple causes and reciprocal causation among health-determining aspects.

Operating with the framework of family systems theory, five determinants of family health are identified: (1) biological (genetics), (2) behavioral patterns, (3) cultural and social contexts, (4) environmental circumstances, and (5) health care (access, policy, and services) (Grochowski 2010). Examples of biological determinants include any genetic predisposition to disease resistance or susceptibility, including body size and typical blood pressure levels. Behavioral patterns refer to habitual choices made by individuals and families that affect health. Examples include communication styles, sleep patterns, engagement in physical activity, and diet. Cultural and social contexts indicate the backdrop within which families live and interact, which may include socioeconomic status, religious identity, racial/ethnic group membership, and gender. Environmental circumstances are simply the physical background in which families live that may include air quality; weather conditions; noise level; the presence of parks and recreational centers in the neighborhood; and the layout of families' apartment, house, or other accommodation(s). Health care refers to families' access to quality health services and the policies in place that hinder or facilitate using the services. These five determinants are highly interconnected and work together to influence the health of families. Moreover, the five determinants are not necessarily mutually exclusive. To illustrate, genetic predispositions to disease are influenced by both environmental exposures and behavioral patterns. Additionally, a family's behavioral patterns and environmental context may be the result of a family's social circumstances and health care access (Grochowski 2010).

As of the early 21st century, although much is known about family health in theory, researchers and practitioners are still uncovering the best ways to translate theory into practice. Current family health research in nursing is focused on the development and implementation of best practices drawn from theory. However, lifestyle changes are rapid, and researchers and policymakers are struggling to keep up. Despite that the United States spends more on health care than any other developed nation in the world, Americans and their families do not appear to exhibit greater health and wellness (Grochowski 2010). With declining social and economic conditions in the United States, families may be floundering to achieve optimal family health and wellness. Therefore, it is imperative that practitioners work quickly to identify and implement best practices, drawn from theory, to promote family health in the United States.

Sukhminder Kaur

See also: Diet and Nutrition; Epidemiology; Etiology; Food Guides from the USDA; Genetics and Genomics; Physical Activity; Risk Factors

Further Reading

Anderson, K. H. (2000). The family health system approach to family systems nursing. *Journal of Family Nursing, 6*(2), 103–119. doi:10.1177/107484070000600202.

Anderson, K. H., & Tomlinson, P. S. (1992). The family health system as an emerging paradigmatic view for nursing. *Journal of Nursing Scholarship, 24*(1), 57–63. Retrieved from http://www.ncbi.nlm.nih.gov/pubmed/1541473.

Bomar, P. J. (2004). *Promoting Health in Families: Applying Family Research and Theory to Nursing Practice.* Philadelphia, PA: Saunders.

Engel, G. L. (1992). The need for a new medical model: A challenge for biomedicine. *Family Systems Medicine, 10*(3), 317–331.

Grochowski, J. R. (2010). Introduction: Families and their health. In S. J. Ferguson (Ed.), *Families and Health* (volume III,1–28). Pearson. Retrieved from http://www.pearson highered.com/assets/hip/us/hip_us_pearsonhighered/samplechapter/020562720X.pdf.

World Health Organization. (1973). Pharmacogenetics technical report series, 524. Geneva.

FELTY SYNDROME

Felty syndrome refers to a group of symptoms that occur in people who have long-standing histories of rheumatoid arthritis and are experiencing destruction of their joints, which has caused the development of rheumatoid nodules.

The persons with this rare, potentially serious condition may typically have a low overall blood cell count, a low number of certain white blood cells, an enlarged or swollen spleen, swollen lymph nodes, and occasionally a swollen liver, as well as a high level of circulating rheumatoid factor.

The presence of rheumatoid arthritis, an inflammatory joint disease, causes pain and stiff and swollen joints. Fortunately, only a very small number of these patients will develop Felty syndrome, and the numbers of possible patients, who are more often than not likely to be women who develop the onset of arthritis in their late 30s or early 40s, is declining. It is rare in children and in African Americans, and is most common between the fifth and seventh decades of life. Men who are affected may have an earlier onset than women.

History

The syndrome was first described in 1924 by Dr. Augustus Roi Felty, practicing at Johns Hopkins Hospital in Baltimore; it was later named for him and is also called Felty's syndrome.

Symptoms

Although many patients with Felty syndrome have no symptoms, typical symptoms include fatigue, fever, appetite loss, weight loss, general feeling of discomfort, paleness of the skin and/or brown pigmented patches of skin, and a burning feeling in the eyes or discharge from the eyes.

The condition is commonly accompanied by very severe destruction of the joints, along with deformity, and some patients with Felty syndrome may experience skin or lung infections at higher rates than healthy persons.

Causes

It is not known why people develop Felty syndrome. It is, however, believed to be an autoimmune disorder that may be transmitted genetically and may involve development of antibodies against the type of white blood cell usually affected in this condition.

Diagnosis

Means of diagnosis include physical examination, including examination of the spleen and lymph notes to detect swelling and to examine joints to see of they appear arthritic; blood tests to detect rheumatoid factor, as well as complete blood counts to examine the number of white blood cells; and abdominal ultrasound to help detect any swelling of the spleen.

Treatments

While there is no cure for Felty syndrome, treating the underlying rheumatoid arthritic condition is an option, as well as adding possible injection therapy with a stimulating factor to raise the white cell count where indicated, or possible removal of the spleen, if there is no evident liver disease.

Drugs used to treat the arthritic disease via treatments to suppress the immune system include penicillin and oral gold, methotrexate or azathioprine, which are all standard treatments for this condition.

Prognosis

The most troublesome outcome of Felty syndrome is repeated infections, usually of the skin or respiratory systems. Another is known as portal hypertension, where blood pressure is raised due to blockage or reduced liver blood flow due to scarring or other damage to this tissue. Chronic leg ulcers that are resistant to treatment may also prevail. This condition is serious because rheumatoid arthritis itself is likely to worsen over time.

Prevention

Individuals with rheumatoid arthritis who experience any of the listed symptoms, as well as others who do not have the disease, should see their physician.

Ray Marks

See also: Abdominal Diseases; Autoimmune Disease; Rheumatoid Arthritis

Further Reading

Genetic and Rare Diseases Information Center. (2011, January 6). Felty's syndrome. Retrieved from https://rarediseases.info.nih.gov/gard/8234/feltys-syndrome/resources/1.

Healthline. (2012, July 25). Felty's syndrome. Retrieved from http://www.healthline.com/health/felty-syndrome#Overview1.

National Organization for Rare Disorders. (2015). Felty syndrome. Retrieved from https://rarediseases.org/rare-diseases/felty-syndrome/.

FETAL ALCOHOL SYNDROME

Background

Fetal alcohol syndrome, or fetal alcohol spectrum disorders, refers to a cluster of a varied number of irreversible outcomes that can arise as a result of a mother who drinks alcohol during pregnancy. These outcomes in physical, mental, behavioral, and learning outcomes, along with their individual and collective implications, vary from child to child and cause enormous costs to society. The terms refer to alcohol-related neurodevelopment disorders and/or alcohol-related birth defects or developmental delays that cause adverse fetal, neonatal, and pediatric effects.

Fetal alcohol syndrome is the leading cause of mental retardation and occurs across all races, socioeconomic groups, and ethnicities.

In addition to the costs for the child, each case costs approximately $2 million to the American tax paper over the course of the child's lifetime.

History

The pattern of infant malformation associated with excess alcohol intake during pregnancy was first described in Nantes, France, in 1968 by Lemoine and colleagues. It was first described in the United States in 1973 by Jones and Smith from Seattle in eight children of mothers with chronic alcoholism.

Symptoms and Signs

The most consistent problems observed in children who have fetal alcohol spectrum disorders are growth deficits, performance deficits, and intelligence deficits, plus skeletal and heart problems.

Specific problems include:

Abnormal joints and limbs
Behavioral problems
Developmental delays
Failure to thrive
Smaller than normal heads or head circumference
Deformed facial features
Epilepsy
Organ dysfunction
Learning problems
Poor muscle tone and coordination or fine motor skills
Deficient memory

Causes

The key cause is the use of alcohol by a pregnant mother. Women at high risk may be those who are substance abusers, those who have mental health conditions, women who already have an affected child, recent drug users, smokers, recent abuse victims, and women with multiple sexual partners.

Diagnosis

A person affected by fetal alcohol syndrome may present with characteristic facial deformities; retarded growth patterns; and impairments of cognition, learning, and behavior. However, there is no clear laboratory test for this condition and its diagnosis. The problems tend to become more marked as children become adults.

Treatments

Treatment for women at risk for drug abuse, especially those who need alcohol treatment, includes inpatient and outpatient care, counseling, and other appropriate interventions, including child care.

Treatment for the children requires parents, health professionals, and teachers to work together.

Prognosis

Research shows there can be significant benefits if pregnant women and women with children receive good residential substance abuse treatment, including parenting skills and empowerment skills.

Victims of fetal alcohol syndrome can suffer from mental health problems; legal, alcohol, and drug problems; difficulty caring for themselves and others; as well as homelessness. Early diagnosis may lessen the risk of problems such as learning challenges and substance abuse.

Prevention

Fetal alcohol syndrome and spectrum disorders are totally preventable by abstaining from alcohol consumption, including wine and beer, during pregnancy. There is no safe level of alcohol intake that can be recommended to pregnant mothers, so abstaining from conception to birth is essential.

Targeting at-risk women and providing tailored treatments, plus encouraging pregnancy prevention among those at highest risk for alcohol abuse—especially those who already have a child with fetal alcohol syndrome problems—are also recommended.

Ray Marks

See also: Alcoholism; Epilepsy; Failure to Thrive; Mental Disorders; Social Health; Substance Abuse

Further Reading

Centers for Disease Control and Prevention. (2015, July 27). Fetal alcohol spectrum disorders (FASDs). Retrieved from http://www.cdc.gov/ncbddd/fasd/index.html.

Fetal Alcohol Spectrum Disorders Center for Excellence. (2015, October 30). About FASD. Retrieved from http://fasdcenter.samhsa.gov/aboutUs/aboutFASD.aspx#1.

Mayo Clinic. (2014, June 2). Fetal alcohol syndrome. Retrieved from http://www.mayoclinic.org/diseases-conditions/fetal-alcohol-syndrome/basics/definition/con-20021015.

National Organization on Fetal Alcohol Syndrome. (2015). FAQs. Retrieved from http://www.nofas.org/.

Rodger, E., & Gowsell, R. (2014). *Fetal Alcohol Spectrum Disorder (Understanding Mental Health)*. St. Catharines, Ontario: Crabtree Publishing.

FIBROMYALGIA

Fibromyalgia is a multifaceted, chronic, long-standing pain syndrome that seems to be associated with dysfunction in interpreting pain stimuli within the central nervous system.

Affecting women, for the most part, in their mid-30s to late 50s, the ailment causes a wide range of symptoms and can be extremely debilitating. It is also often associated with chronic fatigue syndrome and can occur in the teenage years or in older adulthood.

People with fibromyalgia often experience great sensitivity not just to pain, but also to loud noises, bright lights, odors, drugs, temperature changes, and chemicals.

Signs and Symptoms

Balance problems
Depression and dizziness
Difficulties in the ability to think clearly, remember, or concentrate
Fatigue that can range from mild to severe to incapacitating
Headaches and intestinal disturbances
Irritable or overactive bladder
Insomnia or waking up feeling tired
Pain in the muscles and ligaments of the neck, shoulders, back, pelvis, and hips
Skin that may burn or feel itchy, and feel numb, and muscles that may cramp or twitch
Sleep problems and fatigue
Stiffness and achiness on waking or after prolonged rest
Tenderness of the muscles and ligaments, which is worse in the morning

These symptoms may fluctuate throughout the day and over time and are worsened by stress.

Causes

There continues to be no known cause for this condition. However, some research suggests that substances that process pain and are involved in transmitting pain messages to the brain may be abnormally high in people with this condition. Others have argued the condition is caused by lack of deep sleep or poor-quality sleep, and this causes a problem with regard to recovery of the muscles overnight from the previous day's activities. Factors that may also play a role in causing the problem include infection, trauma, genetics, and emotional and biochemical factors. People with associated health problems such as rheumatoid arthritis or ankylosing spondylitis may be prone to fibromyalgia.

Psychological disorders are no longer believed to cause fibromyalgia. However, the anxiety and depression brought about by chronic pain and fatigue can make fibromyalgia symptoms worse, creating a cycle of pain, fatigue, anxiety, and maladaptive behaviors leading to more pain, etc.

Diagnosis

There is no definite test for fibromyalgia, and the diagnosis will be made on the basis of a medical and physical examination, followed by blood tests, thyroid tests, urine tests, and x-rays to rule out other diagnoses that produce similar symptoms. A diagnosis is usually confirmed if the pain has been present for longer than three months and is widespread. Pain must also be present at a minimum of 11 of a total of 18 tender spots or trigger points on the body, usually located on the neck and back, which cause additional pain when firm pressure is applied to these spots.

Treatment

Self-care or self-management of the condition is usually required. Included in self-care is the recommendation the individual follow a low-impact exercise program and keep muscles conditioned. Other remedies include heat applications, stretching exercises, yoga, tai-chi, massage, and over-the-counter pain and anti-inflammatory medications. Medications such as muscle relaxants, antidepressant medications, and steroid or lidocaine injections of painful sites may be used. Relaxation therapy and biofeedback to reduce stress levels, acupuncture, and getting adequate sleep may also be recommended. Counseling and cognitive behavioral therapy may also be of help.

Most important, though, is keeping muscles conditioned and healthy by exercising three times a week, which helps to decrease the amount of discomfort. It is also important to try low-stress exercises such as walking, swimming, water aerobics, and biking rather than muscle-straining exercises such as weight training. Besides helping with tenderness, regular exercises can also boost energy levels and help with sleep.

Medical treatment options a physician may offer include Lyrica, Cymbalta, and Savella. These are the only three drugs approved by the FDA for the treatment of fibromyalgia. Lyrica is an antiseizure medication, while Cymbalta and Savella are antidepressants. All three have been shown to reduce the pain of fibromyalgia.

Generally, no single treatment will take away all the symptoms associated with fibromyalgia. But most people do get some relief by trying a combination of therapies.

If an individual has any of the symptoms of fibromyalgia, he or she should contact a physician. If diagnosed with the condition, a skilled provider who is experienced at treating fibromyalgia is recommended.

Prognosis or Outcome

Although no cure exists for fibromyalgia, self-care that focuses on maintaining a healthy lifestyle and pacing oneself may be beneficial. Getting enough high-quality sleep and adopting a positive outlook may be helpful as well. About one-fourth of cases with this condition may be work-impaired. The condition can also interfere with the ability to function normally in daily life due to lack of sleep and/or depression.

Prevention

There is no known way to prevent fibromyalgia because the cause is not fully understood.

Research

According to the Mayo Clinic, researchers believe fibromyalgia is caused by amplification of pain signals due to the way the brain processes pain signals. This may involve abnormal increases of certain chemicals involved in transmitting pain, as well as sensitization of pain receptors to pain signals.

Most researchers agree that the central nervous system in people with fibromyalgia is not functioning properly and that components of the body's stress response are responsible for symptoms.

Ongoing research focuses on identifying the cause of fibromyalgia and testing new drugs to reduce pain.

Ray Marks

See also: Ankylosing Spondylitis; Chronic Fatigue Syndrome; Neurological Disorders; Rheumatoid Arthritis; Self-Management

Further Reading

American College of Rheumatology. (2015). Fibromyalgia. Retrieved from http://www.rheu matology.org/I-Am-A/Patient-Caregiver/Diseases-Conditions/Fibromyalgia.

Arthritis Foundation. (2015). Fibromyalgia. Retrieved from http://www.arthritis.org/about -arthritis/types/fibromyalgia/.

Fibromyalgia Network. (2015). Symptoms. Retrieved from http://www.fmnetnews.com /fibro-basics/symptoms.

Mayo Clinic. (2015, October 1). Fibromyalgia. Retrieved from http://www.mayoclinic.org /diseases-conditions/fibromyalgia/basics/definition/con-20019243.

National Fibromyalgia Association. (2012). About fibromyalgia. Retrieved from http:// fmaware.org/PageServerded3html?pagename=fibromyalgia.

National Institute of Arthritis and Musculoskeletal and Skin Diseases. (July 2014). Questions and answers about fibromyalgia. Retrieved from http://www.niams.nih.gov/Health _Info/Fibromyalgia/default.asp.

Ostalecki, S., ed. (2008). *Fibromyalgia: The Complete Guide from Medical Experts and Patients.* Burlington, MA: Jones & Bartlett Learning.

Starlanyl, D. J., & Copeland, M. E. (2001). *Fibromyalgia and Chronic Myofascial Pain: A Survival Manual*, 2nd ed. Oakland, CA: New Harbinger Publications.

FOOD GUIDES FROM THE U.S. DEPARTMENT OF AGRICULTURE

The U.S. Department of Agriculture (USDA) has created a number of guides for more than a century in order to provide healthful food choices for the American population. Chronic diseases—such as obesity, diabetes, cardiovascular disease, hypertension, and others—have a clear link to foods that people eat.

Although originally established in 1862 to support and monitor agricultural practices, the USDA's mandate was expanded in 1914, with the passage of the Smith-Lever Act, to include oversight of food and nutrient distribution as well as nutrition education. Today, many of the initiatives that promote sound nutrition and provide dietary guidance for Americans are operated by USDA's Center for Nutrition Policy and Promotion.

20th-Century Food Guides

USDA's history of food guidance, in of itself, began in 1916 with the establishment of an instruction sheet that identified food groups and household serving measures. The initial guide focused on the nutrient intake of children, and, thus, the instruction sheet was entitled *Food for Young Children*. This was replaced in 1940 by a new guide, known as the *Basic Seven: A Guide to Good Eating*, which lacked specific serving sizes but included the number of servings needed throughout the day from each of the seven food groups (grain items, meats/legumes, dairy foods, fruits, green vegetables, starchy vegetables, and solid fats). The information in this guide was accompanied by an image designed to convey pictorially the guide's dietary messages.

Critics considered the *Basic Seven* complicated, and, as a result, the guide was modified in 1956 to a simpler version, known as the *Basic Four: Food for Fitness—A Daily Food Guide*. This newer guide consolidated the foods into four groups (grain items, meats/legumes, dairy foods, and vegetables/fruits) and specified the number of servings needed to achieve nutrient adequacy, but it did not address fat, sugar, or calorie intake. This shortcoming was considered in 1979 when the food guide was revised to include a fifth group, known as the combined fats, sweets, and alcohol group, for which consumption was to be moderate. This is illustrated in the 1979 *Hassle-Free Daily Food Guide*.

By the mid-1980s, the USDA adopted a "total diet approach" to food guidance as a result of new research that suggested dietary goals of moderation were as important to health as those that stressed nutrient adequacy; earlier food guides had focused mainly on promoting diets adequate in nutrients. To that end, the *Food Wheel: A Pattern for Daily Food Choices* was developed jointly by the USDA and the American Red Cross, which included similar food groups (grain items, meat/legumes, dairy foods, fruits, vegetables, fats/sweets/alcohol) but also designated, for the first time, three distinct calorie levels. The *Food Wheel* served as the conceptual basis for the *Food Guide Pyramid*, which was introduced to the public in 1992.

The food patterns graphically presented in the 1992 *Food Guide Pyramid* were designed by the USDA to be adequate in meeting nutritional standards but moderate in calories, fat, and sugar. The *Food Guide Pyramid* symbol incorporated the recommendations outlined in the Dietary Guidelines of 1985 and 1990, which were presented at the time by the newly established Office of Disease Prevention and Health Promotion, housed within the Department of Health and Human Services (DHHS). Furthermore, the *Food Guide Pyramid* reflected the updated Recommended Dietary Allowances of 1980 and 1989, which had been established by members of the Dietary Reference Intakes Committee of the National Academy of Sciences. In addition to using scientific information from a variety of sources in the creation of this food guide, the USDA conducted consumer research to identify a symbol that could effectively communicate healthful food patterns. The outcome was a pyramid-shaped design that could easily convey the dietary message of proportion.

In other words, the food groups, identified at the base of the pyramid, were to constitute a larger proportion of the daily diet, and the food groups, identified near the top of the pyramid, were to comprise a smaller proportion of the daily diet. For example, grain products, such as bread, cereal, rice and pasta, were to be the foundation of the diet with individuals consuming 6 to 11 servings. Regarding the other food groups, individuals were encouraged to consume three to five servings of the vegetable group; two to four servings of the fruit group; two to three servings of the dairy group; and two to three servings of the meat, poultry, fish, eggs, nuts, and dried beans group. The range of servings accommodated three calorie levels (1600, 2200, 2800), representing the daily needs of most Americans. The symbol design also included visualization of fats and sugars throughout the five food groups as a cautionary reminder that they were present in varying amounts within these foods. In addition, dots and triangles, representing fats and sugars, were located in the tip of the pyramid alongside text that read "use sparingly."

Subsequent use of the *Food Guide Pyramid* revealed some confusion among individuals in interpreting the USDA's dietary guidance. For instance, during USDA-sponsored market research, focus group participants stated they did not understand the message of the *Food Guide Pyramid*'s dots and triangles. In addition, participants were unclear about how to interpret both number of servings and portion sizes. Furthermore, they mistakenly thought the range of servings allowed for flexibility of choice rather than the varying caloric needs of individuals. Lastly, the Healthy Eating Index, which assesses the population's compliance with national dietary goals, revealed at this time that most Americans were not following the *Food Guide Pyramid* and that their diets needed improvement.

21st-Century Food Guides

In 2005, the USDA modified the pyramid to align its dietary information with recent advances in nutritional science. Thus, the food patterns were adjusted to meet the nutritional goals set forth in the 2005 Dietary Guidelines. The USDA also wanted to provide guidance that was easier for consumers to understand and, in turn, put into practice. The symbol was revised to depict each food group as a unique vertical band housed within a pyramid rather than the horizontal bands used in the earlier design. It was decided that the pyramid shape would be retained because it was widely recognized as an official USDA symbol; the bands, although now in a different direction, were also retained to show proportionality. The terms *sweets* and *fats* were removed from the image so as not to encourage their consumption. The term *oil* was retained because, in an unsaturated liquid form, it represents a more healthful dietary source of lipids than solid fat; a vertical band labeled *oil* was included to represent this food group. In addition, the image of a stair climber was placed alongside the revised pyramid in order to promote physical activity as a way to balance calories. At the recommendation of those involved in USDA's market research, household measures, such as cups, replaced "servings" as the unit of food measurement. Furthermore, focus group participants requested that the guide's nutrition information be individualized, so the USDA arranged for this icon to be linked to a government website that enabled users to interact and retrieve a personalized diet plan. Individual caloric levels and amounts of food needed from each group—based on gender, height, age, and physical activity level—could be determined from the personal information entered. As a result of these revisions, the new symbol was called *MyPyramid* and could be accessed through the website, www.mypyramid.gov.

In 2011, the symbol used to represent the food groups of the American diet, again, underwent a major change. Based on feedback from consumer research, it was clear that in order to simplify the dietary messages it embodies, further modifications of the symbol were needed. It also became apparent that individuals struggled to connect conceptually to the pyramid idea. Consumers, as market-testing showed, were more comfortable with the notion of a plate representing mealtime behaviors, and, thus, a plate-shaped icon was chosen as the 2011 food guide.

The food groups represented on the plate included grains, protein items, dairy foods, fruits, and vegetables; these were not different than the groups identified on MyPyramid. The difference, rather, was in the layout of the design; the plate shape made it easier to describe the new consumption patterns recommended in the 2010 Dietary Guidelines. Dietary messages—such as *make half your plate fruits and vegetables*—could be depicted and conceptualized more clearly. Furthermore, in an effort to collectively promote positive nutrition behaviors, *MyPlate* communications were designed to support the DHHS Dietary Guidelines with action-oriented consumer messages. These included the following: (1) Avoid oversized portions, (2) switch to fat-free or lower fat (1 percent) milk, (3) drink water instead of sugary drinks, and (4) choose foods with lower sodium. As noted earlier, this edition of the Dietary Guidelines placed stronger emphasis on reducing consumption in order to promote health and reduce the risk of chronic diseases, such as overweight, obesity, diabetes, and hypertension. Lastly, in adhering to consumer demand, the interactive and personalized approach from the *MyPyramid* food guidance system was retained in developing the new *MyPlate* symbol. Individuals can access the MyPlate website through the website address www.chooseMyPlate.gov and obtain diet information specifically tailored to their needs as well as many other nutrition resources. It is through this interaction that individuals can learn the precise amounts needed from each food group so they may obtain all their essential nutrients.

Food Guidance Systems

A food guidance system is critical because daily consumption of nutrients is vital to proper body functioning. Nutrients are typically found in food and beverages that individuals consume as part of their diet. Scientists have categorized foods and beverages, based on their nutrient and caloric values, into groups. Dietary guidance, therefore, involves identifying the foods that comprise a group and determining a measurable amount for each item in the food group that, when consumed, can appropriately lead to optimal nutrition. Government scientists gather their information from nutrition research to assist them in establishing nutrient standards and food pattern recommendations like those presented in Dietary Reference Intakes and Dietary Guidelines. Also supplementing this information are studies about food consumption practices and consumer research. Utilizing these resources, a food guide is developed that graphically translates nutrition recommendations into food patterns. Thus, the food guide serves as both a nutrition education tool and a visual cue to assist Americans in selecting healthy food choices. The development of food guidance systems is an ongoing process; revisions, undertaken by the USDA, occur often as there are advances in nutritional science and as more knowledge about health behaviors is gained. In addition, as the need arises, appropriate government agencies should make improvements in the food guide if they enhance consumer understanding and use.

Some critics have charged the USDA with conflicts between promoting and supporting American agriculture and, at the same time, providing recommendations for the best, most nutritious food. There have been concerns, for example, that, especially in the past, the USDA promoted the dairy and meat industries by encouraging milk, cheese, butter, and meat as healthful and nutritious for all people. There have been recommendations that food guidelines be moved to other U.S. agencies, such as the Centers for Disease Control and Prevention or the National Institutes of Health. In 2011, The Harvard T.H. Chan School of Public Health provided an alternative to the *MyPlate* devised by the USDA, called the "Healthy Eating Plate" (2011), which promotes higher standard proportions of fruits and vegetables, for example, than does *MyPlate*, although *MyPlate* is now more interactive online and can be tailored to individuals based on a number of factors.

Gloria Shine McNamara

See also: Cardiovascular Disease; Cholesterol; Diabetes, Type 2; Diet and Nutrition; Environment; Heart Diseases; Obesity; Self-Management; Stroke; Wellness

Further Reading

American Diabetes Association. (2015, October 19). Create your plate. Retrieved from http://www.diabetes.org/food-and-fitness/food/planning-meals/create-your-plate/.

Britten, P., Haven, J., & Davis, C. (2006). Consumer research for development of educational messages for the MyPyramid food guidance system. *Journal of Nutrition Education and Behavior, 38,* S93–S102.

Britten, P., Marcoe, K., Yamini, S., & Davis, C. (2006). Development of food intake patterns for the MyPyramid food guidance system. *Journal of Nutrition Education and Behavior, 38,* S78–S92.

Center for Nutrition Policy and Promotion. (2005, August). Research summary report for MyPyramid food guidance system development. U.S. Department of Agriculture, Center for Nutrition Policy and Promotion, Research Report.

Harvard T.H. Chan School of Public Health. (2011). Food pyramids and plates: What should you really eat? Retrieved from http://www.hsph.harvard.edu/nutritionsource/what-should-you-eat/pyramid/.

Mayo Clinic. (2011, June 18). Nutrition and healthy eating. Retrieved from http://www.mayoclinic.org/healthy-lifestyle/nutrition-and-healthy-eating/in-depth/healthy-diet/art-20044905.

U.S. Department of Agriculture (USDA). (2016). ChooseMyPlate.gov. Retrieved from www.ChooseMyPlate.gov.

Welsh, S., Davis, C., & Shaw, A. (1992, November/December). A brief history of food guides in the United States. *Nutrition Today,* 12–23.

G

GALL BLADDER DISEASE

The gallbladder is a sac-like organ under the liver in the upper right side of the abdomen that plays a part in food digestion. Its function typically goes unnoticed until infection or inflammation causes pain. Some problems require surgical removal of the gallbladder, which results in little impact on daily life.

Sometimes, infection is caused by small, hard deposits that form in the gallbladder called gallstones. Gallstones are formed primarily of bile, which is a mixture of water, bile salts, lecithin (a fat known as a phospholipid), and cholesterol. About 70 percent of gallstones are formed from cholesterol because it is insoluble and depends on a proper mix of bile salts to move efficiently through the gallbladder. An imbalance of bile salts and cholesterol results in sludge and, in worsened cases, the formation of crystals that lead to gallstones.

Gallstones can cause obstruction at any point along the ducts that carry bile, resulting in inflammation and more serious complications. In most cases of obstruction, the stones block the cystic duct, which leads from the gallbladder to the common bile duct (the duct leading to the small intestine). This blockage typically leads to a condition known as acute cholecystitis, which can produce symptoms such as fever and chills, nausea and vomiting, and pain in the upper right abdomen that is severe and constant. The most serious complication of acute cholecystitis is infection. Symptoms include fever, rapid heartbeat, fast breathing, and confusion. Acute cholecystitis almost always requires surgery to remove the gallbladder.

If left untreated, acute cholecystitis can lead to a number of infections that can be life-threatening. If the condition becomes very severe, inflammation can cause abscesses or necrosis (destruction of tissue) in the gallbladder. An estimated 10 percent of acute cholecystitis cases result in a perforated gallbladder, which is a life-threatening condition. The risk for perforation increases with a condition called emphysematous cholecystitis, in which gas forms in the gallbladder, leading to peritonitis (widespread abdominal infection). Infection in the common bile duct from obstruction (cholangitis) is another serious condition. Antibiotics normally clear up the condition, but if cholangitis does not improve, then infection may spread and become life-threatening. Either surgery or a procedure known as endoscopic sphincterotomy is required to open and drain the ducts.

Gallbladder problems are often symptomless, but ultrasound or other imaging techniques can usually detect gallstones. Nonetheless, the symptoms of cholecystitis are similar to those of other conditions that must be ruled out. These conditions include irritable bowel syndrome, pancreatitis (inflammation of the pancreas), acute appendicitis (inflammation of the appendix), kidney stones, and stomach ulcers.

Diet may play a role in preventing gallstones and infection. Although fats have been associated with gallstone attacks, some studies have found a lower risk for gallstones in people who consume foods containing monounsaturated fats or omega-3 fatty acids. High fiber intake has likewise been associated with a lower risk for gallstones. People who consume fruits, vegetables, and nuts may also have a lower risk of developing symptomatic gallstones that require gallbladder removal. On the other hand, diets high in sugar and other carbohydrates (such as pasta and bread) can increase the risk of infection.

Linda Tancs

See also: Abdominal Diseases; Diet and Nutrition; Digestive Diseases; Self-Management

Further Reading

Clavien, P.-A., & Baillie, J., eds. (2006). *Diseases of the Gallbladder and Bile Ducts: Diagnosis and Treatment*, 2nd ed. Boston, MA: Wiley-Blackwell.

Cleveland Clinic. (2015). What is cholecystitis? Retrieved from https://my.clevelandclinic .org/health/diseases_conditions/hic-cholecystitis.

Eachermpati, S. R., & Reed, R. L. (2015). *Acute Cholecystitis*. Philadelphia, PA: Springer.

Mayo Clinic. (2015). Cholecystitis. Retrieved from http://www.mayoclinic.org/diseases -conditions/cholecystitis/basics/definition/con-20034277.

University of Maryland Medical Center. (2015, July 7). Gallstones and gallbladder disease. Retrieved from http://umm.edu/health/medical/reports/articles/gallstones-and-gall bladder-disease.

GANGRENE

Gangrene is the death of bodily tissues. Most commonly affecting the toes, fingers, and limbs, it can also occur in muscles and internal organs. It is a serious condition caused by a lack of blood flow to an affected area or an infection. Anyone can get gangrene, but those most at risk have chronic diseases such as diabetes, atherosclerosis, or other conditions that affect the blood vessels.

Two main types of the disorder are dry gangrene, which develops gradually when the flow of blood is impaired and is notable for discolored skin tissue that dries up and falls off, and wet gangrene, caused by a bacterial infection from a wound, characterized by swelling, blistering, and a wet appearance. Internal gangrene, a type of wet gangrene, affects internal organs. Other rare forms are gas gangrene, caused by the *Clostridia* bacteria that grow in the absence of oxygen; Fournier's gangrene, caused by a genital-area infection; and progressive bacterial synergistic gangrene, which typically follows an operation.

Typical symptoms include discolored skin, pain, numbness, and foul-smelling sores or, if beneath the skin surface, painful swelling and fever. Immediate treatment of gangrene is required, involving surgical removal of the damaged tissues and medications to fight infections.

Symptoms

Symptoms depend on the type of gangrene and the area affected; those present on the skin include coldness and discoloration (such as pale, brown, blue, purple, red, or black); a foul-smelling wound with discharge, numbness, or loss of feeling; and swelling and pain. Symptoms of gangrene inside the body include fever, painful swelling, and a general feeling of illness. If bacteria from gangrene enter the bloodstream, it may result in septic shock, which is life-threatening; symptoms include low blood pressure, change in body temperature, rapid heart rate, pain and rash, lightheadedness, shortness of breath, and confusion.

Causes and Risk Factors

Gangrene is caused by the interruption of blood flow to an affected area that occurs with an underlying illness, injury, or infection. Those most at risk of gangrene have conditions that affect blood vessels and circulation, such as diabetes, atherosclerosis, and Raynaud's phenomenon—a rare condition in which the blood vessels narrow in cold temperatures. Other risk factors include aging; obesity; weakened immune system; tobacco smoking; a severe burn, frostbite, or other injury that damages underlying tissues; and certain blood-thinning medications in rare cases.

Diagnosis

A diagnosis is made on the symptoms present. Tests used to determine the type of gangrene or infection and the progression of the condition include x-rays and CT and MRI scans. Blood tests and cultures of blisters and infected tissues help identify the infection. Dry gangrene may be diagnosed with an arteriogram, which shows arterial blood flow in tissues.

Treatments

Gangrene is a serious condition that requires immediate attention, including surgical removal of dead tissue, antibiotics to fight bacterial infections and prevent further spreading, and treating an underlying illness or condition that caused the disorder to develop. Surgery may be performed to restore or improve blood flow to an area or to repair damaged skin. Occasionally, amputation of an affected limb is necessary. For some cases of wet gangrene, hyperbaric oxygen therapy may be used: Increased levels of pressure and oxygen saturate the blood and promote healing infected wounds.

Prevention

Prevention requires proper wound care and careful monitoring for infection and symptoms of gangrene, as well as identifying underlying illnesses or conditions that can cause interruptions in blood supply. Individuals with diabetes or other blood vessel diseases can routinely examine their feet for any signs of gangrene to prevent further complications. Measures to reduce the risk of getting gangrene include losing weight, avoiding tobacco products, preventing wound infections, and seeking medical care if skin becomes frostbitten.

Prognosis and Outcomes

The prognosis for recovery from gangrene is better if it is identified and treated quickly. Those who have dry gangrene stand the best chance of recovery because this type is not caused by infection and spreads more gradually. But when gangrene caused by an infection is treated quickly, the prognosis for recovery is good. The condition is life-threatening if a gangrenous infection spreads through the bloodstream and goes untreated, if treatment is delayed, or if an infection does not respond to treatment.

Brad Lang

See also: Atherosclerosis; Diabetes, Type 1; Heart Diseases; Raynaud's Phenomenon

Further Reading

Mayo Clinic. (2014, June 7). Gangrene. Retrieved from http://www.mayoclinic.com/health /gangrene/DS00993.

MedicineNet.com. (2014, December 4). Gangrene. Retrieved from http://www.medicinenet .com/gangrene/article.htm.

MedlinePlus. (2015, September 10). Gangrene. Retrieved from http://www.nlm.nih.gov /medlineplus/gangrene.html.

GASTRIC CANCER

Overview

Gastric cancer, also known as stomach cancer, refers to a cancerous tumor that affects the stomach lining. Although this condition is declining in numbers, approximately 21,320 new cases, along with 15,070 deaths, are estimated to occur in 2012 within the United States.

The type of stomach tumor that exists depends on what part of the stomach is affected. If the tumor starts in the glandular part of the stomach, which is the most common site, the type of cancer is referred to as an *adenocarcinoma*.

If it arises in the lymph glands it is called a *lymphoma*. If it arises or involves muscle, fat, or blood vessels, it is called a *sarcoma*.

Stomach cancer or tumors that are malignant can spread to the esophagus above or to the small intestine below and can extend through the stomach wall to nearby lymph nodes in the liver, colon, or pancreas, as well as to the lungs, bones, and ovaries.

Changes in frequency of occurrence have been said to be due to changes in diet and food preparation, which reduce the numbers of cancers in the lower stomach area, known as distal gastric cancer. However, gastric cancer in the upper part of the stomach or proximal gastric cancer is increasing in frequency primarily as a result of obesity.

Stages of gastric cancer are as follows:

Stage 0: Tumor is located at inner layer of stomach.

Stage I: Tumor has invaded the submucosa and may be found in up to six lymph glands; or the tumor has invaded the muscle layer or subserosa and has not spread elsewhere.

Stage II: Tumor has invaded the submucosa and spread to 7 to 15 lymph nodes; or tumor has invaded muscle layer or subserosa and spread to one to six lymph nodes; or the tumor has penetrated the outer wall of the stomach but has not spread elsewhere.

Stage III: Tumor has invaded the muscle layer and cancer has spread to 7 to 15 lymph nodes; or tumor has penetrated outer layer of stomach and spread from 1 to 15 lymph nodes; or tumor has invaded nearby organs, such as the liver, colon, or spleen but has not spread elsewhere.

Stage IV: Cancer has spread to more than 15 lymph nodes; or invaded nearby organs and at least one lymph node; or cancer has spread to distant organs.

Symptoms

If a person has stomach cancer, he or she may not realize this initially because there may be very few symptoms in the early disease stages. If symptoms do occur, they are likely to involve having a bloated feeling after eating, mild nausea, appetite loss, indigestion, heartburn, and stomach discomfort.

As stomach cancer develops, more clear signs emerge as follows:

Abdominal discomfort
Blood in stool
Diarrhea or constipation
Difficulty swallowing
Fatigue
Gastrointestinal bleeding
Pain or bloating after eating
Vomiting
Weakness or fatigue with mild anemia
Weight loss

Causes

The precise cause of stomach cancer remains unknown. There are several possible explanations or risk factors for this condition that have been identified, including age, in that gastric cancer is more likely to be detected and diagnosed when a person is in his or her early 70s. In terms of race, the condition is found to be more common in African Americans and Asians.

Genetics, too, may play a role, and having some forms of inherited cancer may increase the risk for gastric cancer. In terms of geography, stomach cancer is more prevalent in Japan, the former Soviet Union, and parts of Central and South America. While men and women may both suffer from gastric cancer, men are said to have twice the risk for this disease as women. Individuals with certain blood types and a family history of gastric cancer may also be at heightened risk for gastric cancer.

Stomach infections, long-term stomach inflammation, stomach polyps, prior stomach surgery, and certain health conditions such as chronic gastritis and obesity may raise the risk for the condition. Lifestyle factors that may raise the risk of gastric cancer include smoking, drinking alcohol, having a poor diet, and eating smoked foods or nitrate-preserved foods, while work-related factors include exposure to asbestos.

Diagnosis

The presence of stomach cancer in its more advanced stages can be detected by a physical examination, and on the basis of a medical history. In both this stage and earlier stages, x-rays of the stomach area, examination of the stomach via gastroscopy, and biopsy using a thin long tube passed via the mouth to the stomach may be used. Other tests may include CT scans, bone scans, and surgical exploration known as a laparoscopy, fecal occult blood tests, and complete blood cell counts.

Treatments

Treatments depend on size and location of tumor as well as stage of the disease and the patient's general health. Treatments may include chemotherapy, radiation therapy to shrink tumor, laser therapy to destroy cancer cells, targeted drugs to attack abnormalities in cancer cells, and surgery to remove all or part of the stomach, called partial and total gastrectomy, respectively. Medication and supportive care to deal with treatment side effects and disease consequences such as pain are indicated.

Prognosis or Outcome

Malignant tumors may be a threat to life and can grow back even if removed. They can also invade other organs and tissues and spread to other parts of the body.

Prevention

A healthy diet, and treatment of related medical conditions may help, as may avoiding smoking and environments that are hazardous.

Research

Future research may reveal more information on what causes gastric cancer, thus possibly leading to better ways of preventing or treating the condition.

Ray Marks

See also: Abdominal Diseases; Cancer; Digestive Diseases

Further Reading

American Cancer Society. (2015). Stomach cancer. Retrieved from http://www.cancer.org /cancer/stomachcancer/.

Gastric Cancer Foundation. (2015). About gastric cancer. Retrieved from http://www.gastric cancer.org/about-gastric-cancer/.

Mayo Clinic. (2013, April 26). Stomach cancer. Retrieved from http://www.mayoclinic.org /diseases-conditions/stomach-cancer/basics/definition/con-20038197.

MedlinePlus. (2014, November 26). Stomach cancer. Retrieved from http://www.nlm.nih .gov/medlineplus/ency/article/000223.htm.

Memorial Sloan Kettering Cancer Center. (2015). About stomach cancer. Retrieved from https://www.mskcc.org/cancer-care/types/stomach-gastric/about-stomach.

National Cancer Institute. (2015). Stomach (gastric) cancer—for patients. Retrieved from http://www.cancer.gov/types/stomach.

GASTROESOPHAGEAL REFLUX DISEASE (GERD)

Gastroesophageal reflux disease, also known as GERD, is a serious form of gastro-esophageal reflux (GER), which is common. The symptoms of GER occur when the lower part of the esophagus (which is the tube carrying food from the mouth to the stomach) and its sphincter (or the ring of muscle at the bottom of the esophagus that acts like a valve between the esophagus and stomach) open spontaneously for varying periods or do not close properly. As a result, the stomach's contents rise upward into the esophagus. The condition is also called acid reflux or acid regurgitation.

According to information posted at the National Digestive Diseases Information Clearinghouse, when acid reflux occurs, food or fluid can be tasted at the back of the mouth. The condition may cause a burning sensation in the chest or throat, called heartburn or acid indigestion. Occasional GER is common and does not necessarily mean one has GERD, but if the condition persists more than twice a week, the condition is considered to be GERD, which can lead to more serious health problems.

GERD may damage the lining of the esophagus, thereby causing inflammation. Complications of GERD include ulcers and strictures of the esophagus. It may also cause throat and laryngeal inflammation, inflammation and infection of the lungs, a precancerous condition of the esophagus, and a collection of fluid in the sinuses and middle ear.

GERD is a thus a chronic condition of the digestive system that occurs when stomach acid or, occasionally, bile flows back into the food pipe or esophagus. This backwash of acid irritates the lining of the esophagus and causes GERD signs and symptoms.

Once it begins, it commonly continues lifelong. People of all ages can have GERD; more than 60 million American adults experience heartburn at least once a month, and about 25 million adults suffer daily from heartburn. Twenty-five percent of pregnant women experience daily heartburn. Recent studies show that GERD in infants and children is more common than previously recognized and may produce recurrent vomiting, coughing, and other respiratory problems.

Symptoms

The most common symptom of GERD in adults is frequent heartburn, also called acid indigestion. It can also cause nausea, difficulty swallowing, and a burning-type of pain in the lower part of the mid-chest area, behind the breast bone, and in the mid-abdomen. It can cause ulcers, as well.

Most children under age 12, and some adults, have GERD without heartburn. Instead, they may experience a dry cough or asthma symptoms or have trouble swallowing.

Diagnosis

GERD may be diagnosed or evaluated by endoscopy, biopsy, x-ray, examination of the throat and larynx, 24-hour esophageal acid testing, esophageal motility testing, emptying studies of the stomach, and esophageal acid perfusion.

According to Patti (2016), the only way to determine if abnormal reflux is present and if symptoms are actually caused by gastroesophageal reflux is through pH monitoring.

Causes

Why some people develop GERD is still unclear. However, research shows that people with GERD have an esophageal sphincter that relaxes while the rest of the esophagus is working. Abnormal esophageal contractions and slow or prolonged emptying of the stomach may also cause the problem.

It is also thought that anatomical abnormalities, such as hiatal hernias, may contribute to GERD. A hiatal hernia is found when the upper part of the stomach and the esophageal sphincter move above the diaphragm—the muscle wall that separates the stomach from the chest. Normally, the diaphragm helps the sphincter keep acid from rising up into the esophagus. When a hiatal hernia is present, acid reflux can occur more easily. A hiatal hernia can occur in people of any age and is most often a normal finding in otherwise healthy people over age 50. Most of the time, a hiatal hernia produces no symptoms.

A functional or mechanical problem of the esophageal sphincter is the most common cause of GERD. Transient relaxation of the sphincter can be caused by foods, medications, hormones, and nicotine.

Other factors that may contribute to GERD include obesity and pregnancy. Also, people are more prone to develop GERD if they have diseases that weaken the esophageal muscles, such as scleroderma or mixed connective tissue diseases.

Common foods that can worsen reflux symptoms include:

- Citrus fruits
- Chocolate
- Caffeinated or alcoholic drinks
- Fatty and fried foods
- Garlic and onions
- Peppermint or mint flavorings
- Spicy foods
- Tomato-based foods, such as marinara, salsa, chili, and pizza

Treatments

If a person has symptoms of GERD, using antacids or other over-the-counter reflux medications may help. Or a health care provider may refer the person to a gastroenterologist, who specializes in the treatment of stomach and intestinal diseases. Depending on the severity of the condition, treatment may involve one or more of the following lifestyle changes, medications, or surgery.

GERD can be treated by lifestyle changes; histamine antagonists (H2 blockers); proton pump inhibitors (PPIs), which block the secretion of acid into the stomach by the acid-secreting cells; pro-motility drugs that increase the pressure in the lower esophageal sphincter and strengthen the contractions (peristalsis) of the esophagus; and foam barriers, which are tablets that are composed of an antacid and a foaming agent. As the tablet disintegrates and reaches the stomach, it turns into foam that floats on the top of the liquid contents of the stomach. The foam forms a physical barrier to the reflux of liquid. At the same time, the antacid bound to the foam neutralizes acid that comes in contact with the foam.

A second type of endoscopy involves the application of radio-frequency waves to the lower part of the esophagus just above the sphincter. The waves cause damage to the tissue beneath the esophageal lining and a scar (fibrosis) forms. The scar shrinks and pulls on the surrounding tissue, thereby tightening the sphincter and the area above it.

Recommended lifestyle changes include:

- Stopping smoking if you are a smoker
- Avoiding foods and beverages that worsen symptoms
- Losing weight if needed
- Eating small, frequent meals
- Wearing loose-fitting clothes
- Avoiding lying down for at least three hours after a meal
- Raising the head of the bed six to eight inches

Research

According to the National Digestive Diseases Information Clearinghouse, the reasons some people develop GERD while others do not remains unknown. Several factors may be involved, and research is under way to explore risk factors for developing GERD and the role of GERD in other conditions such as asthma and laryngitis.

Participants in clinical trials can play a more active role in their own health care, gain access to new research treatments before they are widely available, and help others by contributing to medical research.

Ray Marks

See also: Abdominal Diseases; Digestive Diseases; Eating Disorders; Esophageal Cancer; Inflammation; Swallowing Disorders

Further Reading

American Gastroenterological Association. (2015). GERD. Retrieved from http://www.gastro .org/patient-care/conditions-diseases/gerd.

International Foundation for Functional Gastrointestinal Disorders. (2015, June 23). About GERD. Retrieved from http://www.aboutgerd.org.

Mayo Clinic. (2014, July 31). GERD. Retrieved from http://www.mayoclinic.org/diseases -conditions/gerd/basics/definition/con-20025201.

National Digestive Diseases Information Clearinghouse. (2015). Gastroesophageal reflux (GER) and gastroesophageal reflux disease (GERD) in adults. Retrieved from http:// digestive.niddk.nih.gov/ddiseases/pubs/gerd/.

Patti, M. G., & Katz, J. (2016). Gastroesophageal reflux disease. *Medscape*. Retrieved from http://emedicine.medscape.com/article/176595-overview

GENETICS AND GENOMICS

Each person is born with a genetic code. Found in each cell's DNA molecules, this unique set of instructions, or genome, tells the body how to function. Passed from parent to child, DNA is inside the body's inherited genes. When a mutation takes place in a gene, it changes the instructions, which can cause a genetic disorder. Genetic mutations can affect anyone. They can be inherited from one or both parents, and they can also occur any time during a person's lifetime due to environmental exposure. But not all gene mutations cause a disorder.

The mapping of the entire set of human genes, called the human genome, has led to the knowledge that most diseases have a genetic component. Scientists have identified three types of genetic disorders: single-gene disorders; chromosomal disorders, where a whole or partial chromosome is missing or mutated (chromosomes are structures that carry genes); and complex disorders with mutations in two or more genes, usually as a result of lifestyle or environment.

Sickle cell disease and cystic fibrosis are genetic disorders caused by inheriting one particular mutated gene passed down through generations. But most genetic disorders are caused by a combination of inherited mutations in numerous genes, often along with environmental factors. Heart disease and diabetes are two such diseases that are common around the world.

Here is a sample of the thousands of disorders with a genetic component, both physical and mental:

- Alzheimer's disease
- Amyotrophic lateral sclerosis (ALS)

- Anxiety
- Attention deficit hyperactivity disorder (ADHD)
- Autism
- Bipolar disorder
- Cancer
- Celiac disease
- Charcot Marie-Tooth disorder
- Crohn's disease
- Cystic fibrosis
- Depression
- Diabetes
- Down syndrome
- Duchenne muscular dystrophy
- Ehlers-Danlos syndrome
- Familial hypercholesterolemia
- Fragile X syndrome
- Heart disease
- Hemophilia
- Huntington's disease
- Macular degeneration
- Marfan syndrome
- Panic disorder
- Parkinson's disease
- Schizophrenia
- Sickle cell anemia
- Tay-Sachs disease
- Thalassemia
- Wilson disease

History

The study of genetics, which focuses on individual genes and how they influence health and disease, began in the mid-19th century when the Austrian monk Gregor Mendel conducted experiments on the genetics of pea plants and described how traits are inherited from one generation to the next. Geneticists continued to study the effects of genes on diseases, launching the Human Genome Project in the 1980s. (A genome is all the genetic information comprising an organism.) The goal was to understand the genetic basis of all diseases. By 2003, geneticists had mapped the location of every gene in the human genome, including decoding the instructions for each one.

The Human Genome Project provided insight into the relatively new field of pharmacogenomics, which examines how inherited genetic differences affect a person's response to drugs. These genetic differences will be studied to predict whether a medication will be effective to create safe effective medications customized to a person's genetic makeup and to prevent adverse drug reactions.

Treatments

Pharmacogenomics is the relatively new area of study that examines how a person's genes affect its response to drugs. By testing how certain drugs are processed by an individual's body, doctors will be able to choose the most effective medicines and doses for a person's genetic makeup that are most likely to prevent negative side effects. The ultimate goal is to develop drugs that can be tailored to treat many diseases. Studies are examining drugs for cardiovascular disease and breast and prostate cancers.

Prevention

Genetic tests can be carried out to discover if adults carry genetic diseases they might pass to their offspring, even if they have no symptoms, or if they are carriers of a gene mutation; some tests find gene mutations that increase the likelihood of developing a disease. Prenatal testing during pregnancy and newborn screening help identify genetic diseases that are known to adversely affect a child's health or development.

Participating in genetic testing for research purposes may not help an individual directly, but it can be useful to those in the future who have genetic disorders.

Prognosis and Outcomes

Because individual genomes differ, the prognosis of any genetic disorder can vary immensely from one person to another, even for those who have the same condition. Some genetic disorders cause problems that are nearly always life-threatening, while others have benefited by the development of drugs that can provide patients with ways to manage their conditions long term.

Future

As genomic research continues, one goal is to create and apply strategies for the early detection, diagnosis, and treatment of genetic disorders. One such strategy is gene therapy, although its effectiveness is unproven, and it's currently only available in clinical trials. Researchers are investigating ways to develop treatments that alter a person's genes inside the cells to cure cancer, heart disease, diabetes, cystic fibrosis, and other diseases or improve the body's ability to fight them.

Jean Kaplan Teichroew

See also: ALS (Amyotrophic Lateral Sclerosis); Alzheimer's Disease; Anxiety Disorders; Attention Deficit Hyperactivity Disorder (ADHD); Autism; Bipolar Disorder; Cancer; Celiac Disease; Charcot Marie-Tooth Disorder; Crohn's Disease; Cystic Fibrosis; Depression; Diabetes, Type 1; Ehlers-Danlos Syndrome; Familial Hypercholesterolemia; Heart Disease; Hemophilia; Huntington's Disease; Macular Degeneration; Panic Disorder; Parkinson's Disease; Schizophrenia; Sickle-Cell Disease; Tay-Sachs Disease; Wilson's Disease

Further Reading

Centers for Disease Control and Prevention. (2013, June 28). Genomic testing. Retrieved from www.cdc.gov/genomics/gtesting/.

Healthline. (2014, March 24). Genomics versus genetics: A close look. Retrieved from http://www.healthline.com/health-slideshow/genomics-vs-genetics.

National Human Genome Research Institute. (2013, November 20). Frequently asked questions about genetic counseling. Retrieved from http://www.genome.gov/19016905.

National Human Genome Research Institute. (2012, February 27). Frequently asked questions about genetic disorders. Retrieved from http://www.genome.gov/19016930.

National Library of Medicine. (2015, July 19). Genetics home reference. Retrieved from http://ghr.nlm.nih.gov/.

GLAUCOMA

Glaucoma is a group of eye conditions that lead to damage of the optic nerve, which carries visual information from the eye to the brain. Damage to the optic nerve leads to progressive, irreversible vision loss, and it is the second leading cause of blindness in the United States, where nearly 3 million adults have some type of glaucoma.

In most cases, the damage to the optic nerve is a result of increased pressure in the eye, also known as intraocular pressure. In people with glaucoma, too much fluid pressure builds up inside the eye. The increased pressure can then damage the optic nerve, which transmits images to the brain, causing a loss of vision. Without treatment, glaucoma can cause total permanent blindness within a few years.

Glaucoma tends to be an inherited disorder that may not show up until later in life. Because most people have no early symptoms or pain from the increased pressure, it is important for those at risk to see an eye doctor regularly so the disorder can be accurately diagnosed and treated before long-term vision loss occurs.

Four major types of glaucoma are diagnosed:

Open-angle, or *chronic*, is the most common type of glaucoma, caused by a slow increase in eye pressure on the optic nerve. Often running in families, those at higher risk are of African descent or have parents or grandparents with the condition.

Angle-closure, or *acute glaucoma*, occurs when the exit for the aqueous humor fluid becomes blocked suddenly, creating a severe and painful increase in the pressure. Dilating eye drops and certain medications can trigger this, and it requires immediate medical attention. An individual who has had acute glaucoma in one eye is at risk for an occurrence in the second eye, which may call for preventive treatment.

Congenital glaucoma, present at birth, often runs in families. The cause is abnormal eye development.

Secondary glaucoma is caused by corticosteroids and other drugs, uveitis and other eye diseases, systemic diseases, and trauma.

Symptoms

Many people with open-angle glaucoma experience no symptoms, including the loss of peripheral vision, which can be unnoticed at first. Symptoms may come and go at first or worsen steadily for those with angle-closure glaucoma. The most common are sudden, severe pain in one eye; decreased, cloudy, or "steamy" vision; nausea and vomiting; the appearance of halos around lights; and eye redness and swelling. Congenital glaucoma symptoms are usually evident at a few months old: hazy or cloudy-looking eyes, red or enlarged eyes, tearing, and light sensitivity.

Causes and Risk Factors

Most often occurring in adults older than 40, glaucoma can also occur in young adults, children, and infants. African Americans experience it more frequently, at an earlier age, and with greater vision loss.

Those at an increased risk are older than 40 and of African American, Irish, Russian, Japanese, Hispanic, Inuit, or Scandinavian descent; have a family history of glaucoma or poor vision; have diabetes, high blood pressure, or heart disease; take prednisone or other steroids or medications that increase pressure inside the eyes; have experienced a physical eye injury; or have thin corneas or chronic eye inflammation.

Diagnosis

A complete eye exam with a detailed medical history is necessary for an accurate diagnosis. A doctor dilates the pupils with drops to look inside the eyes. A tonometry test checks the pressure inside the eyes, but because pressure changes, it may be within normal range for some people who have glaucoma. Additional tests to confirm glaucoma are a gonioscopy, which examines the front part of the eye; imaging of the optic nerve; retinal examination; visual acuity and loss, including of central and peripheral vision; and a slit-lamp examination to examine the parts of the eyes specialized magnifying microscope.

Treatments

Reducing eye pressure is the goal of all glaucoma treatment. Eye drops and laser and microsurgery are the most common treatments for open-angle glaucoma. Eye drops decrease the pressure by helping the fluid in the eye better drain, by decreasing the amount of fluid, or by increasing its ability to flow out. Medications also may be prescribed to reduce eye pressure and prevent damage to the optic nerve.

Laser surgery slightly increases the outflow of the eye fluid for those with open-angle glaucoma, and it eliminates fluid blockage in people who have angle-closure glaucoma. In the several types of surgery available, a laser pulls open the drainage area, creates a tiny hole in the iris to allow the fluid to freely flow, or treats the middle layer of the eye to reduce fluid production.

Microsurgery creates a channel to drain fluid inside the eye, which reduces pressure. Some patients must have the surgery more than once, or have a glaucoma implant to keep the channel open. Complications may include some temporary or permanent loss of vision, bleeding, or infection.

Angle-closure glaucoma is considered a medical emergency because blindness can occur within days if it goes untreated. Eye drops and medications are first-line treatments.

Because congenital glaucoma is caused by an abnormal drainage system, the preferred treatment is surgery. Treatment for secondary glaucoma depends on the underlying illness or other cause.

Prevention

No form of glaucoma cannot be prevented, but regular eye exams are the key to detecting it early enough for successful preventive treatment. If diagnosed and treated early, glaucoma can be controlled. Because most people have no early symptoms from increased eye pressure, it is important to make visits to an ophthalmologist, or eye doctor, for complete eye exams. The American Academy of Ophthalmology recommends a comprehensive eye exam for adults starting at age 40; every three to five years after that if an individual has diabetes, a family history of glaucoma, or other risk factors; and annually after age 60. Those at high risk for angle-closure glaucoma may consider eye surgery to prevent an attack.

Prognosis and Outcome

Open-angle glaucoma cannot be cured, but symptoms can be managed along with regular visits to a doctor to prevent loss of vision. Angle-closure glaucoma is a medical emergency requires immediate treatment to save vision. Babies with congenital glaucoma usually do well when surgery is done early. How well a person with secondary glaucoma does depends on the disease causing the condition.

Loss of vision caused by glaucoma is irreversible and cannot be restored. However, successfully lowering eye pressure can prevent further visual loss. Most people with glaucoma do not go blind as long as they follow their treatment plan and have regular eye exams

Future

According to the Glaucoma Research Foundation, the identification of a metabolic marker indicating tissue injury has the potential to help predict glaucoma in patients who don't show symptoms of vision loss.

Ray Marks

See also: Colorblindness; Diabetes, Type 1; Eye Diseases; Hyperopia; Macular Degeneration; Myopia; Sjögren's Syndrome

Further Reading

American Optometric Association. (2014). Glaucoma. Retrieved from http://www.aoa.org /Glaucoma.xml.

Glaucoma Research Foundation. (2012). Learn about glaucoma. Retrieved from http://www
.glaucoma.org/.

Mayo Clinic. (2012, October 2). Glaucoma. Retrieved from http://www.mayoclinic.com
/health/glaucoma/DS00283/.

National Eye Institute. (2012). Glaucoma. Retrieved from http://www.nei.nih.gov/glau
coma/.

GLOBAL HEALTH

Definitions of global health have been developed by many agencies and institutions. *Global health*, as defined by the Institute of Medicine (IOM, 1997) for example, involves the "health problems, issues, and concerns that transcend national boundaries, may be influenced by circumstances or experiences in other countries, and are best addressed by cooperative actions and solutions." In addition to being a term referencing a distinct field of study, global health is also used to refer to the state of health worldwide, as well as a goal to be achieved. Global health (also sometimes referred to as *international health*) is a growing field within the larger domain of public health and is presently viewed as a key area of public health practice, with academicians, researchers, and clinicians now focusing their study and research on global health issues and topics.

Recognition of the importance of global health issues increased significantly in the last decade of the 20th century, in large part due to the need for greater understanding of the global context of the AIDS crisis. In more recent history, and prompted in part by the emergence and reemergence of several virulent communicable diseases (including SARS, H1N1, and bovine spongiform encephalopathy, more commonly known as mad cow disease, among others), international focus on global health issues has grown steadily in the new millennium.

Scientists, clinicians and the media have given much attention to the communicable diseases that have the potential to cross borders easily and relatively undetected. Advances in public health infrastructure and delivery in the past 100 years—including the recognition of the importance of sterile procedures; the development of antibiotics, vaccines, and pharmaceutical prophylaxis; and the increased emphasis on sanitation and hygiene—have collectively succeeded in decreasing the burden posed by infectious diseases globally. This has resulted in a significant improvement in both the quality and quantity of life for people worldwide measured by several critical health indicators, including maternal mortality, infant life expectancy, childhood growth, and overall life expectancy. In general, people today live longer than people did at any other point in human history.

Nonetheless, health indicators remain poor in many countries in sub-Saharan Africa, Central America, and Southeast Asia where communicable diseases—most importantly HIV/AIDS, malaria, and tuberculosis—remain major public health threats, particularly for the most vulnerable (infants, children, and the elderly). Fortunately, the international public health community has never been better positioned to respond to these threats at the local, regional, and global levels. As evidence of this, in 2003 the Gates Foundation announced its plan to fund the "Grand Challenges in Global Health" medical research initiative to encourage investigation into solutions that would address and remove the barriers to progress against the diseases that were disproportionately affecting developing nations. This initiative identified seven specific "grand challenges," five of which directly included goals related to infectious disease control, treatment, and eradication.

In 2000, the United Nations developed the Millennium Development Goals (MDGs) as a framework for understanding and addressing critical global health challenges. This framework identified eight goals to be met by the year 2015. Several of these MDGs documented the role that poverty plays in health status at the individual, community, and national levels specific to childhood mortality, maternal health, and infectious diseases. While some improvement has been made in these areas, particularly in relation to childhood mortality, these goals were not fully met by the target deadline. In May 2011, the World Health Organization released the following progress statement relative to the MDGs: "While some countries have made impressive gains in achieving health-related targets, others are falling behind. Often the countries making the least progress are those affected by high levels of HIV/AIDS, economic hardship or conflict."

Communicable diseases have received a great deal of attention from professionals working in the field of global health. In this past decade, there has been increased attention focused on chronic disease and injury in the global context, particularly in the developed nations where chronic illnesses (also commonly referred to as noncommunicable diseases, or NCDs) including obesity, cardiovascular disease, cancer, stroke and diabetes have replaced communicable diseases as the greatest factors in morbidity and mortality. The growth of NCDs in developed countries is due to myriad reasons, most notably a growing and aging population that has adopted a number of disease-promoting unhealthy lifestyle behaviors.

Strikingly, while the burden caused by infectious disease remains high in many developing nations, NCDs have begun to rival infectious diseases as a major contributor to overall morbidity and mortality in many areas of the developing world. In fact, in 2008 it was estimated that 60 percent of the 57 million deaths worldwide were caused by NCDs. In 2009, the World Health Organization verified these earlier estimates by reporting that 6 out of every 10 deaths worldwide was caused by an NCD. Of the remaining four deaths, three were due to infectious agents with the final death due to injury.

In an attempt to better understand those health conditions that are most critical to address to ensure future success in combating global health challenges, researchers use various methodologies to measure and create projected estimates of the burden of disease worldwide. For example, initiated in 1992 with the first results published in 1996, the "Global Burden of Disease Study" used the DALY metric (disability-adjusted life years) to estimate the disease burden posed by the major causes of illness worldwide. This study provided rank-order estimates for the year 1990, where the top eight leading causes of disease worldwide were lower respiratory infections, diarrheal diseases, conditions arising during the perinatal period, major depression, ischemic heart disease, cerebrovascular disease, tuberculosis, and measles. The study then projected a baseline scenario for the year 2020 in which ischemic heart disease rose from fifth position to first, major depression rose from the fourth to second position, and cerebrovascular disease rose from the sixth to the fourth position. This trend of increased burden was true for all NCDs measured. Conversely, projections indicated decreased burden related to nearly all infectious diseases. Lower respiratory infections, for example, fell six rankings, diarrheal diseases fell seven rankings, and measles fell from the eighth position to 25th.

These estimates should not be surprising, however. Decreased rates of infant and child mortality and better treatment of infectious disease across the lifespan have contributed to the increase in life expectancy seen in the modern world. Therefore, if it is true that a longer life increases the likelihood of developing a chronic illness, it is natural that NCDs will be responsible for a greater share of the global disease burden.

In addition to the aforementioned role of poverty as a determinant of health status globally, pollution and population growth are also often cited as significant challenges to making improvements in global health indicators. The uncertainties presented by global climate change present yet another critical issue that must remain a priority in the study of global health. As globalization—with the resultant trends toward rapid urbanization and increased international trade—continues to influence the ways in which in the modern world responds to critical global health issues, the need for sustained and cooperative efforts in research, prevention, and treatment of chronic disease remains a high priority.

William D. Kernan

See also: Centers for Disease Control and Prevention (CDC); Health; Healthy People 2020; World Health Organization

Further Reading

Holtz, C. (2013). *Global Health Care: Issues and Policies.* Burlington, MA: Jones and Bartlett Learning.

Institute of Medicine (IOM), Board on International Health. (1997). America's vital interest in global health: Protecting our people, enhancing our economy, and advancing our international interests. National Academy of Sciences.

Lopez, A. D., & Murray, C. C. J. L. (1998). The global burden of disease, 1990–2020. *Nature Medicine, 4*(11), 1241–1243.

Merson, M. H., Black, R. E., & Mills, A. J. (2012). *Global Health: Diseases, Programs, Systems, and Policies.* Burlington, MA: Jones and Bartlett Learning.

Skolnik, R. (2008). *Essentials of Global Health.* Burlington, MA: Jones and Bartlett Learning.

Skolnik, R. (2012). *Global Health 101.* Burlington, MA: Jones and Bartlett Learning.

U.S. Department of Health and Human Services, Global Health Initiative (Office of Global Affairs) Retrieved from http://www.globalhealth.gov.

Varmus, H., Klausner, R., Zerhouni, E., Acharya, T., Daar, A. S., & Singer, P. A. (2003). Grand challenges in global health. *Science, 302,* 398–399.

World Health Organization. Retrieved from http://www.who.int/en.

GONORRHEA

Gonorrhea is a sexually transmitted disease, or STD, that is caused by the bacterium called *Neisseria gonorrhoeae.* The bacteria grow in warm moist areas of the body and infect the mucous membranes of the cervix, uterus, and fallopian tubes in women and the urethra in women and men. They can also infect the mucous membranes of the mouth, throat, eyes, and anus, as well as grow in the eyes.

Gonorrhea is among the most commonly sexually transmitted diseases. Estimates from the Centers for Disease Control and Prevention indicate that in the United States, more than 700,000 people get new gonorrheal infections every year; 334,826 cases were reported in 2012.

Easily spread, this contagious disease may exhibit no symptoms. Any sexually active person can become infected, although infection is more common among some specific populations: adolescents and young adults; those who use drugs; people living in poverty in urban areas and Southern states; and African Americans, particularly young women. The infection rate for women is higher for women than men.

Symptoms

Most often symptoms appear within 14 days of infection, although men and women may exhibit no symptoms at all. Or mild symptoms may appear only in the morning, a reason many people do not know they are infected.

In men, the most common sign of infection is a white, yellow, or green pus-like discharge from the penis. Other common symptoms are painful, burning, or more frequent urination; red or swollen opening of the penis; tender or swollen testicles.

Symptoms in women may be mild and be mistaken for a bladder or vaginal infection. Common symptoms include severe lower abdomen pain, indicating the infection has spread to fallopian tubes and stomach area; vaginal bleeding between menstrual periods; menstrual irregularities; painful urination and a greater urge to urinate; painful intercourse; swollen and tender genitals; vomiting; sore throat; and fever. Infected women are at risk of developing serious complications regardless of the symptoms or their severity.

Both men and women may experience rectal infection, including anal discharge, itching, soreness, bleeding, and painful bowel movements. They may also have symptoms of an oral infection called gonococcal pharyngitis, which is a sore throat often accompanied by itching and trouble swallowing. Many times, though, rectal and oral infections exhibit no symptoms. If the infection spreads to the bloodstream, fever, rash, and arthritis-like symptoms may be evident.

Untreated gonorrhea can cause serious and chronic problems in women and men. In women, gonorrhea can spread into the uterus or fallopian tubes and cause pelvic inflammatory disease (PID), which may lead to internal abscesses and chronic pelvic pain. Damage to the fallopian tubes can cause infertility or increase the risk of ectopic pregnancy. During pregnancy, untreated gonorrhea can cause premature labor and stillbirth.

In men, gonorrhea can cause epididymitis, a bacterial infection of the epididymis (the coiled duct behind the testicle), rarely but possibly leading to infertility. If epididymitis and other infections are also present, men are likely to feel pain in the testes or scrotum.

When gonorrhea spreads to the blood it can cause disseminated gonococcal infection (DGI). Women, especially adolescents, are more likely than men to get this condition and experience its symptoms of fever, arthritis, skin sores, joint pain, and inflammation of tendons. DGI is easily treated, although if untreated, it can cause permanent joint damage and become life-threatening.

Causes and Risk Factors

Gonorrhea is transmitted through sexual contact with the penis, vagina, anus, or mouth of an infected partner; oral sex can transmit gonorrhea from the genitals to the throat and vice versa. An infected mother can pass the disease to her baby during childbirth, which may cause infections in the blood, joints, and eyes. Antibiotic drops are routinely put into the eyes of newborns immediately after delivery to prevent infection.

People who have had gonorrhea and received treatment are at greater risk of reinfection, particularly if they have sexual contact with an infected person. In addition, those who are more likely to develop the infection have numerous sexual partners, do not use a condom during sex, abuse alcohol or illegal substances, are under age 25, or engage in sex work.

Diagnosis

A doctor tests for gonorrhea by taking a sample from an infected area, usually fluid from the urethra in men and the cervix in women. Samples for testing can also be taken from the blood, a skin lesion, throat, anus, and fluid from the joints. At a laboratory, the culture—or the sample's cells growing in a petri dish—gets analyzed for the presence of bacteria. Results are often available within 24 to 72 hours. Women may receive a complete pelvic examination. Other tests may be used to check urine samples for the presence of the gonorrhea bacteria.

Treatment

Gonorrhea can be cured with two antibiotics taken orally or injected. In cases of pelvic inflammatory disease, a hospital stay and intravenous antibiotics are recommended. Because gonorrhea may not exhibit symptoms, it is important to notify sexual partners, who should then get treatment. Antibiotics will stop infection, but the medication does not repair any permanent damage.

Prevention

The only way to completely avoid getting or passing on gonorrhea is by abstaining from sexual intercourse. Other preventive measures are using a latex condom consistently and correctly during sexual intercourse; remaining in a long-term, monogamous relationship with an uninfected partner; avoiding sexual contact with high-risk partners; and making sure infected sexual partners are treated and tested before re sexual relations.

Prognosis

When treated with the appropriate antibiotics, gonorrhea can be quickly cured up to 99 percent of the time. Some types of gonorrhea bacteria have grown resistant to certain antibiotics that were successful in the past, making treatment of gonorrhea more difficult. Follow-up tests will ensure that the infection has cleared. It is important to return to a doctor or other health care provider if symptoms continue for more than a few days after receiving treatment.

Ray Marks

See also: Men's Health; Pelvic Inflammatory Disease; Sexually Transmitted Diseases; Women's Health

Further Reading

Avert. (2014). Gonorrhea: Including signs and symptoms. Retrieved from http://www.avert.org/gonorrhea.htm.

Centers for Disease Control and Prevention. (2014, December 16). Gonorrhea—CDC fact sheet (detailed version). Retrieved from http://www.cdc.gov/std/gonorrhea/stdfact-gonorrhea-detailed.htm.

Mayo Clinic. (2014, January 2). Gonorrhea. Retrieved from http://www.mayoclinic.com/health/gonorrhea/DS00180.

New York Times Health Guide. (2013, April 25). Gonorrhea. Retrieved from http://health.nytimes.com/health/guides/disease/gonorrhea/overview.html.

GOUT

Gout is a painful and potentially disabling form of arthritis. It was first described by ancient Greek writers. Traditionally, gout was believed to be connected with excessive consumption of rich foods and drinks, receiving the nickname "king of diseases and disease of kings." Gout is actually the result of excessive uric acid in the blood, which collects in joints. Although very painful, gout is not life-threatening, but it might cripple a person through the destruction of joint surfaces.

The term *gout* is derived from the Latin word "gutta," meaning a drop. It was believed that drops of harmful material gathered around the joints. The first record of gout comes from Egyptian hieroglyphics from 2600 BCE, discussing arthritis in the big toe. In 400 BCE, the Greek physician Hippocrates identified the disease and recognized that it rarely occurred in children or premenopausal women. Hippocrates also noted that gout did not usually attack those who refrained from consuming wine and other forms of alcohol.

Although gout does not just attack the wealthy and overindulgent, some causes are related to what an individual consumes. Some foods, including red meat and seafood, are rich in a substance known as purine. The purine can help form uric acid crystals in the blood. Those likely to develop gout should also avoid overindulgence in alcohol, especially beer. Sugary drinks and foods that are high in fructose may increase the chances of gout. Some medications, such as aspirin, should be avoided, along with medications that reduce the amount of salt and water in the body. Illnesses and medical conditions like rapid weight loss may cause attacks of gout. Surgery and some genetic conditions can also cause high uric acid levels in one's body, making gout likely.

Uric acid is a normal waste product of the body. Excessive amounts are usually removed by the kidneys and excreted in urine. However, if excessive uric acid builds up in the blood, it may form needle-like crystals. The crystals can accumulate in joints. The most common is the joint at the base of the big toe. Other commonly affected joints include the fingers. The crystal deposits in the joints are called tophi. If left untreated, they can continue to grow and damage the joints, causing arthritis and permanent distortion. The tophi may burst and drain through the skin.

Gout's symptoms often take the form of a painful attack and swelling in the night. One reason for this is that the body's system for removing uric acid slows down when you are asleep. The least amount of pressure on swollen areas can be unbearable. The skin around the affected joint may turn reddish or purple, giving it an infected appearance. Movement of the joint is limited. Mild attacks may last for several hours up to one to two days. Severe attacks can last up to several weeks, with soreness in the joint for a month. Attacks of gout will occur more often as time passes.

The diagnosis of gout can be done by checking the level of uric acid in the blood. Elevated amounts of uric acid, however, may occur in people without gout. Fluid can be drawn from inflamed joints and examined under a microscope. Trained observers should be able to see the needle-like crystals.

Gout's treatment consists mostly of relieving the symptoms. To relieve the pain and reduce the inflammation, nonsteroidal anti-inflamatory drugs (NSAIDs) are often used. Similar to aspirin, indomethacin and naproxen are the common choices. High doses of NSAIDs can give quick relief but may cause upset stomach or irritate ulcers. Colchicine can reduce the pain if given early in a flare-up of gout. However, it can also cause nausea, vomiting, diarrhea, and other side effects. Patients suffering from kidney problems or taking blood thinners can be treated with corticosteroids by their doctors. Home remedies that provide some relief include cold compresses or ice applied to the affected joint for 20 to 30 minutes at a time.

For long-term relief from gout, doctors try to reduce the amount of uric acid in the blood. Some drugs, such as febuxostat, block the production of uric acid, while others help the kidneys to remove more uric acid. Success usually requires months of treatment. Failure to prevent attacks of gout can increase blood pressure, cause heart disease, or result in kidney failures. High uric acid levels can also result in painful kidney stones.

Tim J. Watts

See also: Arthritis; Kidney Diseases

Further Reading

American College of Rheumatology. (2016). Gout. Retrieved from http://www.rheumatology .org/Practice-Quality/Clinical-Support/Clinical-Practice-Guidelines/Gout.
American College of Rheumatology. (2016). Gout: Fast facts. Retrieved from http://www .rheumatology.org/I-Am-A/Patient-Caregiver/Diseases-Conditions/Gout.

Arthritis Foundation. (2015). What is gout? Retrieved from http://www.arthritis.org/about
-arthritis/types/gout/what-is-gout.php.

Centers for Disease Control and Prevention. (2015). Arthritis types: Gout. http://www.cdc
.gov/arthritis/basics/gout.html.

Emmerson, B. (2003). *Getting Rid of Gout*. New York: Oxford University Press.

English, J. (2013). *The Gout Book*. Greybull, WY: Pronghorn Press.

Mayo Clinic. (2015). Gout. Retrieved from http://www.mayoclinic.org/diseases-conditions
/gout/basics/definition/con-20019400.

GRAVES' DISEASE

The thyroid gland is a small, butterfly-shaped gland located in the front of the neck that makes thyroid hormones, which are sent throughout the body. Thyroid hormone helps the body use energy; stay warm; and keep the brain, heart, muscles, and other organs working as they should via the hormones thyroxine (T4) and triiodothyronine (T3), which control metabolism. Graves' disease is an autoimmune thyroid condition produced by abnormal stimulation of the thyroid gland. It is a common cause of hyperthyroidism, or overactive thyroid condition, where the thyroid makes more thyroid hormone than the body needs. This causes the function of the body to speed up, including the heart rate. It affects the rate at which food is converted into energy as well. In Graves' disease, the patient's own immune system attacks the thyroid gland, which results in excessive thyroxine production, a hormone involved in helping to regulate growth and control body metabolism.

Women are generally affected more often than men, and the disease can occur in people of all ages, but it commonly starts in the 20s or 30s. Graves' disease may go into remission or disappear completely after several months or years. Because untreated symptoms may have long-term detrimental consequences, it is recommended that symptoms be treated early in with good medical care.

History

Graves' disease is named after an Irish physician, Robert J. Graves, who lived between 1796–1853.

Symptoms

People with Graves' disease may present with an enlarged thyroid known as a goiter. They may have sleeping problems, act in an irritable manner, and be highly sensitive to heat. They may suffer from hand tremors, a rapid heartbeat, and weight loss without dieting.

They may feel weak or fatigued, show thinning of the skin, or redness and thickening of the skin on the shins and top of the feet, as well as exhibiting fine brittle hair or thinning of the hair.

Other changes include inflammation, redness, and swelling of the eyes, causing them to bulge; double vision or reduced or blurred vision; extreme sensitivity to light; and eye irritation and swelling of the eyelids and tissues around the eyes.

Causes

Causes of Graves' disease include genetic factors, gender, stress, pregnancy, smoking, and possibly infections.

Having other autoimmune diseases such as rheumatoid arthritis, diabetes, or pernicious anemia may serve as a risk factor.

The disease may also be triggered by both genetics and environmental factors.

Diagnosis

Blood thyroid tests to measure thyroid hormones, serum thyroid tests, antibody tests, hair tissue mineral analysis, a medical history, and physical examination are used to diagnose Graves' disease.

The general practitioner, primary care physician, or specialist may examine the thyroid area to determine whether it is enlarged, as well as the patient's eyes to see whether they are bulging or irritated. Physicians may also check the patient's heart rate and blood pressure, as well as presence of any trembling of the hands or fingers. During the interview, they may inquire about their symptoms and medical and family histories.

Other tests include radioactive iodine uptake tests, tests to detect the presence and volume of thyroid-stimulating immunoglobulins, and an orbit CT scan.

The radioactive iodine thyroid nuclear test shows the rate at which the thyroid gland takes up iodine over a set period. If the uptake of radioactive iodine is high, it means that the patient's thyroid gland is producing excessive amounts of thyroxine as occurs in Graves' disease.

A CT scan of the orbit is an imaging technique that uses x-rays to create detailed pictures of the eye sockets (orbits) and eyes.

Treatments

There are no current medications or treatments that can stop the patient's immune system from attacking the thyroid gland and causing Graves' disease. However, much can be done to ease the disease symptoms and lower the production of thyroxine or block its action.

The condition is primarily treated with anti-thyroid medications to reduce excess thyroid hormone production. Most commonly used is a drug called Methimazole, which interferes with the conversion of T4 to T3. Because T3 is more potent than T4, this also reduces the activity of thyroid hormones. The FDA approved Methimazole in March 1999.

It can also be treated through the introduction of radioactive iodine that damages the thyroid by giving it radiation, followed by thyroid hormone replacement medication for life or along with anti-thyroid medication.

Surgery may be used to remove all or part of the thyroid gland, followed by replacement of oral thyroid hormone for life.

The secondary conditions that may accompany Graves' disease may need to be treated medically as well.

Treating the eye-related problems may also be necessary and may involve the use of steroid therapy to reduce any swelling or irritation, eye muscle surgery, orbital radiotherapy, and eye lubricating medications.

Chinese researchers have reportedly successfully applied a technique known as thyroid arterial embolization, in which the blood supply to the thyroid is blocked as a treatment to disable the thyroid's hormone-producing capabilities.

Prognosis

Untreated Graves' disease can lead to a condition known as thyrotoxicosis and its severe form called thyroid storm, which can lead to death. It can also lead to heart problems, such as atrial fibrillation and weak and brittle bones.

Poorly treated Graves' disease during pregnancy can result in miscarriage, as well as health problems for the baby and mother, including low birth weight and heart failure, respectively.

Other complications may arise if either too little or too much thyroid hormone is given or if patient is intolerant to anti-thyroid medication.

Radioactive iodine treatment may increase the eye problems associated with Graves' disease.

Complications from surgery can include damage to the nerves supplying the voice box, damage to the surrounding parathyroid glands, and scarring of the neck.

Prevention

There is no known approach for preventing Graves' disease. Women with Graves' disease can become pregnant but should be under medical supervision.

Research

Researchers are examining the natural history, clinical presentation, and genetics of thyroid function disorders. According to the Mayo Clinic website, Mayo Clinic alone has been researching and treating Graves' disease and its associated eye-related changes, called Graves' ophthalmopathy, for more than 100 years. It is continuing to actively investigate the causes of Graves' disease and Graves' ophthalmopathy as well as new potential treatments.

Ray Marks

See also: Autoimmune Disease; Thyroid Disease

Further Reading
American Thyroid Association. (2015). Graves disease FAQs. Retrieved from http://www.thyroid.org/graves-disease/.
Graves Disease & Thyroid Foundation. (2015). About Graves' disease. Retrieved from http://www.gdatf.org/about/about-graves-disease/.

Mayo Clinic. (2014, July 1). Graves' disease. Retrieved from http://www.mayoclinic.org/diseases-conditions/graves-disease/basics/definition/con-20025811.

National Institute of Diabetes and Digestive and Kidney Diseases. (2012, August 10). Graves' disease. Retrieved http://www.niddk.nih.gov/health-information/health-topics/endocrine/graves-disease/Pages/fact-sheet.aspx.

WomensHealth.gov. (2012, July 16). Graves' disease fact sheet. Retrieved from http://www.womenshealth.gov/publications/our-publications/fact-sheet/graves-disease.html?from=AtoZ#a.

HANSEN'S DISEASE (LEPROSY)

Hansen's disease, and commonly called *leprosy*, is a disease dating back to antiquity. Egyptian historical records from approximately 4000 BC made reference to leprosy. Pejoratively called *lepers*, people with this health condition suffered from disfiguring skin nodules and loss of their limbs as a result of nerve-related sensory loss. To be a leper was to be ostracized from society because the disease was linked to notions of uncleanliness, being cursed, or being evil. In public, lepers wore bells around their necks to signal their approach and to warn others to stay clear.

Even in modern times, Hansen's disease treatment has often occurred in separate hospitals and live-in colonies called "leprosariums" because of the stigma of the disease. In the United States, there was such a facility located in Carville, Louisiana, but it stopped caring for those with Hansen's disease in 1998. Today, due to effective drug treatment and living conditions, there are fewer than 100 to 200 new cases a year in the United States (National Institute of Allergy and Infectious Disease 2015).

Leprosy is now described as a slowly developing, progressive chronic disease that damages the skin and nervous system, upper respiratory tract, eyes, and nasal mucosa (lining of the nose). It is caused by bacterial infection from the bacillus bacterium known as *Mycobacterium leprae*. It is more commonly called Hansen's disease, named for Armauer Hansen, a 19th-century Norwegian doctor, who observed, identified, and published information the bacteria in 1874 when working at a leper hospital in Bergen, Norway. Before Hansen's evidence and description of leprosy as a disease spread by bacteria, it was commonly thought to be inherited.

Leprosy-related disability, however, is a challenge to public health and social and rehabilitation services in countries where it is common. This disability is more than a mere physical dysfunction; it includes activity limitations, stigma, discrimination, and social participation restrictions (van Brakel et al. 2012).

Leprosy mainly affects the skin and nerves. It also affects muscles. If untreated, there can be progressive and permanent damage to the skin, nerves, limbs, and eyes. Children are more likely than adults to get the disease. Susceptibility to getting leprosy may be due to certain human genes.

Currently, there are several areas (India, East Timor) of the world where the World Health Organization (WHO) and other agencies (e.g., the Leprosy Mission) are working to decrease the number of clinical cases of leprosy. Official figures show that more than 213,000 people—mainly in Asia and Africa—are infected, with approximately 249,000 new cases reported in 2008.

Reducing the Problem

In 1991, the WHO's governing body, the World Health Assembly (WHA), passed a resolution to eliminate leprosy as a public health problem by the year 2000. The target was achieved on time, and the widespread use of multidrug therapy reduced the disease burden dramatically.

- Over the past 20 years, data show more than 14 million leprosy patients have been cured.
- The prevalence rate of the disease dropped by 90 percent, from 21.1 per 10,000 inhabitants to less than 1 per 10,000 inhabitants in 2000.
- There was a dramatic decrease in the global disease burden at the end of 2008.
- Leprosy has been eliminated from 119 countries out of 122 countries where the disease was considered as a public health problem in 1985.
- So far, there has been no resistance to antileprosy treatments.
- Efforts currently focus on eliminating leprosy at a national level in the remaining endemic countries.

Signs and Symptoms

Signs of leprosy include the presence of painless ulcers, skin lesions of hypopigmented macules (flat, pale areas of skin), and eye damage (dryness, reduced blinking). Later, large ulcerations, loss of digits, skin nodules, and facial disfigurement may develop.

Tuberculoid leprosy symptoms include a few well-defined skin lesions that are numb. Lepromatous leprosy symptoms include a chronically stuffy nose and many skin lesions and nodules on both sides of the body.

Treatment and Diagnosis

The majority of sufferers report problems in all components of disability. The reported physical impairment after release from treatment justifies ongoing monitoring to facilitate early prevention. Stigma is a major determinant of social participation, and therefore disability. Stigma reduction activities and socioeconomic rehabilitation are thus urgently needed in addition to strategies to reduce the development of further physical impairment after release from leprosy treatment (van Brakel et al. 2012).

Leprosy must be diagnosed through skin biopsy performed by health care providers.

Effective medications are a combination of antibiotics. The dosage and length of time of administration depends upon which form of leprosy the patient has. Isolating people with this disease in "leper colonies" is not needed once medication is started.

Prognosis

Early diagnosis and treatment reduce damage and prevent a person from spreading the disease. They allow the affected individual to have a normal lifestyle. Complications include disfigurement, weakness of the muscles, and permanent damage to arm and leg nerves. People with long-term leprosy may lose the use of their hands or feet due to repeated injury because they may lack feeling in those areas.

Ray Marks

See also: Neurological Diseases; Skin Conditions; World Health Organization

Further Reading

American Leprosy Missions. (2015). Learn about leprosy. Retrieved from http://www.leprosy .org/learn-about-leprosy/.

Centers for Disease Control and Prevention. (2013, April 29). Hansen's disease (leprosy). Retrieved from http://www.cdc.gov/leprosy/.

National Institute of Allergy and Infectious Diseases. (2015, September 15). Leprosy (Hansen's disease). Retrieved from https://www.niaid.nih.gov/topics/leprosy/Pages/Default .aspx.

van Brakel, W. H., Sihombing, B., Djarir, H., Beise, K., Kusumawardhani, L., Yulihane, R., Kurniasari, I., Kasim, M., Kesumaningsih, K. I., & Wilder-Smith, A. (2012). Disability in people affected by leprosy: The role of impairment, activity, social participation, stigma and discrimination. *Global Health Action*, 5, published online. Retrieved from http://www.ncbi.nlm.nih.gov/pmc/articles/PMC3402069/.

World Health Organization. (2015, May). Leprosy. Retrieved from http://www.who.int /mediacentre/factsheets/fs101/en/.

HASHIMOTO'S DISEASE

Hashimoto's disease, also known as Hashimoto's thryroiditis, is an autoimmune disorder in which the body's immune system attacks the thyroid gland. As a result, the thyroid does not produce enough hormones for the body to function properly. Symptoms of Hashimoto's disease include depression, chronic fatigue, muscle pain, and dry skin. It can be easily treated with synthetic hormones after being diagnosed. Women are more likely to develop Hashimoto's disease than men, particularly when they become middle-aged.

Hashimoto's disease was discovered by Dr. Hakaru Hashimoto, a faculty member of the medical school at Kyushu University. He described the symptoms of patients he found with intense concentrations of lymphocytes within the thyroid in 1912. Lymphocytes are white blood cells that ordinarily attack bacteria and other foreign bodies, but in the case of Hashimoto's disease, they instead attack the thyroid. As a result, the thyroid becomes inflamed and fails to produce enough hormones to adequately control the body's metabolism, as well as heart and nervous system functions, muscle strength, weight, and cholesterol levels. This condition is known as *hypothyroidism*.

Symptoms of Hashimoto's disease include fatigue; limited weight gain; and joint and muscle pain in the shoulders, hips, knees, and small joints in the hands. In addition, patients usually have constipation with three or fewer bowel movements per week, dry and thinning hair, pale and dry skin, a hoarse voice, and sensitivity to the cold. Women suffer from heavy or irregular menstrual periods and have difficulty getting pregnant. Most people also experience depression and memory problems.

The causes of Hashimoto's disease remain uncertain. One theory is that a virus or bacteria might trigger the autoimmune system to overreact, while another is that genetic factors lead to Hashimoto's disease. Certain factors are known to contribute to the likelihood of developing the disorder. Women are up to eight times more likely than men to develop Hashimoto's disease. Although it may strike young people, Hashimoto's disease usually attacks middle-aged people. Another factor is whether a relative has suffered from thyroid or other autoimmune disorders. Finally, if a patient has had another autoimmune disease—such as lupus, rheumatoid arthritis, or Type 1 diabetes—he or she is more likely to develop Hashimoto's disease. Likewise, someone with Hashimoto's disease is also more likely to develop other autoimmune disorders. Environmental factors such as exposure to pesticides or consuming too much iodine increase the likelihood of getting the condition.

Doctors can diagnose Hashimoto's disease by a number of tests. The thyroid-stimulating hormone (TSH) test measures the level of TSH produced by the pituitary gland in the brain. Higher levels of TSH indicate Hashimoto's disease. Tests for the T4 hormone, as well as for anti-thyroid antibodies, are also used.

Hashimoto's disease can usually be treated with synthetic thyroxine, a hormone. In the past, replacement hormones made from pig thyroids were used. They are rarely prescribed today, however, because their levels of hormones vary. Hormone treatments will remain necessary for the rest of a patient's life.

Hashimoto's disease progresses slowly. Failure to treat it, however, can have health implications. These include the enlargement of the thyroid, known as a goiter. A goiter can affect a person's appearance and may make swallowing and breathing difficult. Heart problems have been associated with Hashimoto's disease, as well as birth defects in babies born to mothers with the condition. Mental health can also suffer, as well as a patient's sex drive.

Tim J. Watts

See also: Autoimmune Disease; Hypothyroidism; Thyroid Disease

Further Reading

Mayo Clinic. (2016). Hashimoto's disease. Retrieved from http://www.mayoclinic.org/diseases-conditions/hashimotos-disease/basics/definition/con-20030293.

National Institute of Diabetes and Digestive and Kidney Diseases. (2015). Hashimoto's disease. Retrieved from http://www.niddk.nih.gov/health-information/health-topics/endocrine/hashimotos-disease/Pages/fact-sheet.aspx.

O'Rourke, M. (August 26, 2013). What's wrong with me? *The New Yorker*. Retrieved from http://www.newyorker.com/magazine/2013/08/26/whats-wrong-with-me.

Shomon, M. J. (2005). *Living Well with Hypothyroidism: What Your Doctor Doesn't Tell You That You Need to Know.* New York: William Morrow.

HEAD AND NECK CANCER

Head and neck cancer is the abnormal, uncontrolled multiplication of cells in the head or neck. These types of cancers can develop in the nasal cavity or paranasal sinuses, the oral cavity (including the lips, gums, inner cheeks, and floor or hard palate of the mouth), the salivary glands, the pharynx (throat), the larynx (voice box), or other sites in the head or neck. Most such cancers arise in the squamous cells that line the moist, mucosal surfaces inside the head and neck, especially in the mouth, nose, and throat.

Cancer that affects the brain, eyes, esophagus, and thyroid gland are usually classified as forms of cancer separate from head and neck cancers.

Prevalence and Mortality

Cancers of the head and neck account for about 3 percent of cancer cases in the United States. Approximately 60,000 new cases of head and neck cancer are diagnosed each year in the United States, with about 12,000 annual deaths attributed to these cancers. Head and neck cancers are more than twice as common in men than in women. These cancers are most common in people who are older than age 50.

The five-year survival rates for head and neck cancer vary substantially, depending on the specific nature, stage, and location of the individual's cancer. For example, if lip cancer is diagnosed when it is still localized, 93 percent of patients will be alive five years after diagnosis. However, only 52 percent of lip-cancer patients will survive five years if their cancer had spread to distant regions of the body at the time of diagnosis. For patients with cancer of the mouth floor, the five-year survival rate is 75 percent for localized cancer and 20 percent for metastasized cancer.

Risk Factors

The risk of head and neck cancer increases with excessive use of tobacco or alcohol. The main tobacco product contributing to this risk is chewing tobacco. Roughly 75 percent of all head and neck cancers are caused by tobacco or alcohol.

Previous infection with human papillomavirus (HPV), a family of viruses that make up the most common sexually transmitted infections, raises the risk of head and neck cancer. The main type of HPV responsible for head and neck cancer is HPV-16. HPV-associated oropharyngeal cancers are increasing in prevalence in the United States. Also raising the risk level for head and neck cancer is previous infection with the Epstein-Barr virus.

Poor oral hygiene and missing teeth have been associated with oral cancers. Eating certain preserved or salted foods has been linked to nasopharyngeal cancer, and drinking a tea-like South American beverage called maté is linked with cancers of the mouth, pharynx, and larynx.

Individuals who are exposed to large amounts of wood dust, metal dust, asbestos, formaldehyde, or certain other substances often encountered in the construction, textile, food, or chemical industries may be at elevated risk for head or neck cancer. Exposure of the head or neck to large amounts of radiation also increases this risk.

Genetic factors may play some role in head and neck cancer. For example, individuals of Chinese ancestry seem to face an elevated risk for nasopharyngeal cancer.

Symptoms and Diagnosis

People with head or neck cancer usually notice a lump or sore somewhere on the head or neck (such as in the mouth, nose, or throat) that does not heal or go away, a persistent sore throat and difficulty swallowing, or a hoarseness or other change to the voice. Among the more common oral cancer symptoms are a white or red patch on the gums, the tongue, or mouth lining; swelling of the jaw; and unusual bleeding or pain in the mouth. Common pharynx cancer symptoms include difficulties in breathing or speaking, frequent headaches, and trouble with hearing.

Symptoms specific to nasal cavity cancer include blocked sinuses, chronic sinus infections, nasal bleeding, frequent headaches, eye swelling, and pain around the upper teeth. Salivary gland cancer is characterized by swelling under the chin and along the jaws, as well as facial numbness and neck pain.

A diagnosis of head or neck cancer is based on the evaluation of a patient's medical history, a physical examination of the patient, and a microscopic examination of biopsy tissue samples. Additional laboratory and x-ray procedures are used to determine the stage of cancer development and, thus, the type of treatment that would be most effective.

Treatment

Because of the wide variety of head and neck cancer types, the treatments for individual patients vary widely. Besides the patient's cancer type, stage, and location, treatment also depends on the patient's age and overall health. In general, however, treatment for head and neck cancer includes some combination of surgery, radiation therapy, and chemotherapy.

The surgical removal of cancerous tissue from the head or neck may result in long-term facial or neck swelling or other changes in the patient's appearance. The surgery is also likely to affect the patient's chewing, swallowing, and speaking. Radiation and drug therapy may have adverse affects ranging from skin irritation to jaw stiffness to changes in taste and appetite.

After treatment, many patients are advised to pursue certain forms of rehabilitation, including physical therapy, speech therapy, feeding and dietary guidance, and caring for a stoma (an opening in the trachea through which a patient must breathe after removal of the larynx). Some patients may choose to undergo reconstructive cosmetic surgery to rebuild facial tissue and bones that were removed. The use of facial prostheses may be necessary if the face cannot be properly reconstructed.

A. J. Smuskiewicz

See also: Alcoholism; Cancer; Squamous Cell Carcinoma; Substance Abuse

Further Reading

American Cancer Society. (2015). Oral cavity and oropharyngeal cancer. Retrieved from http://www.cancer.org/cancer/oralcavityandoropharyngealcancer/detailedguide/oral-cavity-and-oropharyngeal-cancer-survival-rates.

Cleveland Clinic. (2015). Head & neck cancer facts. Retrieved from http://my.clevelandclinic.org/services/head-neck/diseases-conditions/head-neck-cancer-faqs.

Johns Hopkins Medicine. (2015). HPV and head and neck cancer. Retrieved from http://www.hopkinsmedicine.org/kimmel_cancer_center/centers/head_neck/HPV/.

National Cancer Institute. (2015). Head and neck cancer. Retrieved from http://www.cancer.gov/cancertopics/types/head-and-neck.

Ward, E. C., & van As-Brooks, C. J. (2014). *Head and Neck Cancer: Treatment, Rehabilitation, and Outcomes*. San Diego, CA: Plural Publishing.

HEALTH

Health is a difficult concept to put into words. The most cited definition of health comes from the World Health Organization (WHO): "Health is a state of complete physical, mental, and social well-being and not merely the absence of disease or infirmity" (World Health Organization 1946). Thus, the WHO recognized three elements of health in its definition, illustrating that health is a multidimensional concept (Simons-Morton et al. 1995). Despite being difficult to define and having multiple dimensions, many people agree that health is crucial. In fact, the common saying "health is wealth" serves as a testament to the high value placed on health. Health is greatly valued because being healthy allows us to function, gives us control, and grants us a sense of independence in life (Siegel & Lotenberg 2007).

The earliest notions of the idea of "health" most likely date back to the earliest societies and every culture has its own conception of what it means to be healthy. In the western context, specifically in the English language, the word "health" first appeared around approximately 1000 AD and it was a broad-encompassing definition referring to the quality of "wholeness," which included aspects of intelligence, physical ability, and spirituality (Dolfman 1973). Then, with the rise of modern science in the Western world and the increased medicalization of health, by the early 1900s, the concept of health was reduced to only the absence of disease or physical illness. Nevertheless, the conception of health began to widen again as the fields of sociology and psychology gained respectability, and consequently, social and psychological aspects of health resurfaced in the definition. To date, the 1946 WHO definition still stands as one of the most widely accepted modern definitions of health. Although the WHO definition is often used, many other definitions of health exist. A couple of other common definitions of health include: (1) successfully adapting to environmental challenges (Dubos 1965) and (2) the degree of functioning and maximizing of one's potential (Dunn 1977). In fact, the act of defining health has been compared to trying to define an aesthetic concept like music: Such concepts are extremely difficult to put into words because they are understood through experience. Nonetheless, researchers have not given up on trying to accurately describe health or measure health.

Traditional measurements of health reflect the traditional notion of health as the absence of disease or illness. Certain measurements indicate the presence of disease or illness. Measurements of health occur on at least two different scales: individual and group. Individual-level measurements (also known as clinical measures) include collecting data on basic anthropometric measurements, such as weight and height; blood levels of certain substances or elements, like sugar, cholesterol, and iron; body temperature; and symptoms, which are physical and mental manifestations of illness. Group-level measurements (also known as epidemiological measures) can very immensely in scale from the community level to the global level. Nonetheless, typical group-level measurements include death rates, called mortality rates (e.g., infant and cause-specific mortality rates); average life expectancy; and measures of disease in a population, called morbidity rates, which include such measures like (1) the number of new cases of a specific disease in a population over time (incidence rate) and (2) the number of existing cases of a specific disease over time (prevalence rate). Much of the traditional indices of health are tied to physical symptoms and physical manifestations of disease, but they do not capture a broader, more holistic view of health.

Hence, researchers have recently created new indices—like years of healthy life, quality-adjusted years of life, and self-assessment of health—to reflect a more inclusive definition of health. Years of healthy life is an indicator of health that assesses the number of functional years of life: Although the average lifespan in the United States since the 1900s has increased from 47 years to 75 years, an extension of age does not necessarily mean better health (Simons-Morton et al. 1995). Many people suffer from decreased functionality because of some form of age-related disability, chronic disease(s), or both. Quality-adjusted life years (QALY) is a financial measure of health that uses both quantity and quality of added years of life to assess the monetary value of a health intervention. Self-assessment refers to simply asking individuals, "How healthy do you feel?" (Simons-Morton et al. 1995). Researchers find that report via self-assessment may be the single, greatest measure of individual overall health status.

Using various measures of health, scientists have tracked the United States' health status for more than a century. The United States experienced a dramatic shift in health status during the 20th century. In fact, in the realm of public health and health promotion, the 1900s have been referred to as "a century of progress"; with the rapid advancement of science and technology, many of the hazards to health that were of primary concern were extinguished or effectively managed (Simons-Morton et al. 1995). Many of the threats to health were eliminated with significant achievements such as vaccination, family planning, safer foods, and safer workplaces. The 20th century was also a time in which the United States witnessed greater control of infectious diseases, motor vehicle safety, and maternal–child health. Although significant progress has been made on these fronts and their impact on society has produced greater life expectancies, an epidemiological shift has occurred. Now, the greatest threats to health are chronic diseases stemming from unhealthy behaviors and lifestyles, declining economic and social conditions, and differential access to health care (Siegel & Lotenberg 2007).

With the emergence of preventable chronic diseases such as coronary heart disease (CHD), Type 2 diabetes, high blood pressure, and obesity, new fields were created to study how to stem the spread of such diseases and how to promote health. Therefore, health promotion and health education—entirely new realms of study— were recently established: Both are dedicated to furthering the health and wellness of individuals, communities, and populations. In these fields, the term *health determinants* is often used to describe the complex relationship among various factors that influence health to explain the health disparities. Health disparities are differential health statuses that exist between two or more groups of people (groups may be organized in any number of ways, including socioeconomic status, race/ethnicity, and age). Determinants of health are typically classified into four broad categories: (1) biological, (2) environmental (physical and social), (3) behavioral, and (4) health care (Simons-Morton et al. 1995). *Biological* determinants include one's genetics because much of a person's body size, susceptibility to disease, and disposition may be attributable to a person's genetic makeup. *Physical environment* refers to the physical surroundings of an individual, including temperature, the presence of pollutants and allergens in the air, and the structural layout of one's surroundings. *Social environment* refers to the matrix of cultural customs and policies that create economic and political circumstances at all levels of society (community, national, and international). *Behavioral* determinants include the personal choices with respect to exercise, diet, sexual behavior, substance use, and myriad other lifestyle factors. *Health care* refers to the quality and availability of health services, including medical and dental, to individuals. These determinants of health are so coined because they independently and interactively work together to promote or hamper health. Importantly, these determinants are not mutually exclusive. For example, a largely known determinant of health is socioeconomic status (SES), which may be classified as a social environmental determinant of health. However, SES also affects a person's educational attainment, which, in turn may influence a person's behavior and personal choices. Furthermore, it has been well established that people with lower SES have reduced access to quality health care. Thus, all these determinants of health are highly interrelated and are typically not mutually exclusive.

Many people investigate health determinants, and many more individuals and institutions fall under the vast umbrella of "health." People who study health include sociologists, epidemiologists, biostatisticians, economists, and researchers, who are among many others that engage in academic studies. Many more people contribute to our health by practically applying knowledge about health. Practitioners include doctors, pharmacists, nurses, occupational therapists, physical therapists, physician assistants, dentists, ophthalmologists, psychologists, therapists, and chiropractors, among many others. Myriad institutions also exist that are devoted to health. Some of the major institutions include the Centers for Disease Control and Prevention (CDC), the National Institutes of Health (NIH), the U.S. Department of Health and Human Services (HHS), the Food and Drug Administration (FDA), and the World Health Organization (WHO). Thus, the fields, people, and institutions involved in the study and practice of health are quite diverse—indeed, health itself is recognized as incredibly multidisciplinary.

Looking ahead, much of the future of health research will focus on preventing chronic diseases and promoting a holistic sense of wellness. Avenues through which prevention and promotion may occur are via educational efforts designed to produce behavioral and lifestyle changes and policy efforts to create the framework within which health may be promoted. As the Western paradigm increasingly accepts a more holistic concept of health, research on health will continue to cut across disciplines, and researchers with diverse backgrounds will coalesce to study how to best protect and promote this integral quality of human life.

Sukhminder Kaur

See also: Access to Health Services; Centers for Disease Control and Prevention (CDC); Diet and Nutrition; Family Health; Food Guides from the USDA; World Health Organization

Further Reading

Dolfman, M. L. (1973). The concept of health: An historic and analytical examination. *Journal of School Health, 43*(8), 491–497.

Dubos, R. (1965). *Man Adapting.* New Haven, CT: Yale University Press.

Dunn, H. L. (1977). What high-level wellness means. *Health Values, 1,* 9–16.

Siegel, M., & Lotenberg, L. D. (2007). *Marketing Public Health: Strategies to Promote Social Change,* 2nd ed. Boston, MA: Jones and Bartlett Publishers.

Simons-Morton, B. G., Greene, W. H., & Gottlieb, N. H. (1995). *Introduction to Health Education and Health Promotion,* 2nd ed. Long Grove, IL: Waveland Press.

World Health Organization. (1946). *Constitution of the World Health Organization.* Geneva, Switzerland.

HEALTH DISPARITIES

Health disparities or inequities refer to differences among health of and treatment for groups of people. These differences can affect how frequently a disease affects a group, how many people get sick, or how often the disease causes death. Health disparities are preventable differences in the burden of disease, injury, violence, or opportunities to achieve optimal health that are experienced by socially disadvantaged populations.

According to the American Medical Association (AMA), recent studies have shown that despite the steady improvements in the overall health of the United States, racial and ethnic minorities experience a lower quality of health services, are less likely to receive routine medical procedures, and have higher rates of morbidity and mortality than nonminorities. Disparities in health care exist even when controlling for gender, condition, age, and socioeconomic status. Thus, despite dramatic achievements in health and health care over the past century, evident racial/ethnic and rural/urban health disparities continue to exist.

These inequities are often due to the historical and current unequal distribution of social, political, economic, and environmental resources.

They can thus result from multiple factors, including:

- Poverty
- Environmental threats
- Inadequate access to health care
- Individual and behavioral factors
- Educational inequalities—for example, lack of education or dropping out of school is associated with multiple social and health problems, and individuals with limited education are more likely to experience a number of health risks, such as obesity, substance abuse, and intentional and unintentional injury, compared with individuals with more education

Many different populations are affected by disparities, including:

- Racial and ethnic minorities
- Residents of rural areas
- Women, children, the elderly
- Persons with disabilities

As outlined by the Centers for Disease Control and Prevention (CDC), health inequities are reflected in differences in length of life; quality of life; rates of disease, disability, and death; severity of disease; and access to treatment.

Health Disparities and Chronic Disease

Chronic diseases account for three-quarters of the health care expenditures in the United States, including a majority of early deaths and lost years of productive life. Health disparities exist among the common chronic diseases, such as hypertension, diabetes mellitus, HIV/AIDS, cancer, cardiovascular disease, and obesity, with ethnic minorities and the poor having higher incidence or worse outcomes.

It has been noted that behavioral risk factors—such as tobacco smoking, physical inactivity, and poor diet—are likely to play a big role in explaining these health disparities. However, health disparities are also reflected in differing levels of access to health care and the quality of medical care and reflect disparities in income and educational attainment.

Disparities in health outcomes, health determinants, access, and quality of health care are ongoing policy priorities in the United States because the excess burden of disease arising from this unequal situation is generally preventable. There are many organizations actively involved in achieving this goal.

For example, at the New York Academy of Medicine—where it is accepted that urban environments give rise to health disparities that cannot be explained by an individual's behavior alone, but are directly related to differences in the physical and social characteristics of neighborhoods—vulnerable populations, including the working poor, homebound older adults, injection drug users, and currently and formerly incarcerated individuals, are targeted. In this regard, one program has been designed to specifically address the persistent problem of low vaccination rates among minorities and people living in poverty. Another provides free seasonal influenza vaccination clinics at community-based organizations in East and Central Harlem and spreads awareness about influenza in those communities.

The National Institutes of Health (NIH) in the United States specifically has put in place efforts to eliminate health disparities that include the following key programs:

- *Centers of Excellence*—conducts research on health disparities in areas such as cancer, cardiovascular diseases, stroke, diabetes, nutrition, obesity, and maternal and infant health.
- *Community-Based Participatory Research*—enables partnerships among scientists and communities to conduct research and improve the health of communities.
- *Loan Repayment Program*—assists scientists to advance their careers in basic, clinical, and behavioral research focused on minority health or health disparities.
- *Minority Health and Health Disparities International Research Training*—supports young scientists conducting scientific research abroad.
- *The Bridges to the Future Program*—helps students in an associate's or master's degree program make the sometimes-difficult transition to the next level of training.
- *Minority Biomedical Research Support, Building Research Infrastructure and Capacity, Research Centers in Minority Institutions, and Research Endowment*—support research and strengthen the biomedical research capability of the eligible institutions.
- *Competitive Research (SCORE) Programs*—support the biomedical and behavioral research of faculty at institutions that serve minority populations.
- *Clinical Trial Networks*—enroll a diverse population to ensure access and representation of the populations most affected by and vulnerable to the spread of HIV/AIDS (NIAID's HIV/AIDS Research Program).

Future

The Census Bureau predicts that racial and ethnic minority populations in the United States will grow to become half of the U.S. population in three decades. NIH's research agenda described earlier to address the increasing health needs of racial and ethnic minorities, rural and urban poor, and other medically underserved populations in the midst of efforts to strengthen the health care system and improve access to care for millions of Americans is expected to be successful. Eliminating health disparities is a priority for the NIH, and involving diverse communities and partners is critical in its effort to achieve health equity in America. However, as outlined by the CDC, *health equity* will only be achieved when every person in the United States has the same opportunity to "attain his or her full health potential" and no one is "disadvantaged from achieving this potential because of social position or other socially determined circumstances."

To assist in meeting this goal, the CDC's National Center for Chronic Disease Prevention and Health Promotion (NCCDPHP) is addressing its goal of health equity through its programs, research, tools and resources, and leadership.

Throughout the next decade, Healthy People 2020, the National Health Promotion Initiative of the United States, will assess health disparities in the U.S. population by tracking rates of illness, death, chronic conditions, behaviors, and other types of outcomes in relation to demographic factors, including:

- Race and ethnicity
- Gender
- Sexual identity and orientation
- Disability status or special health care needs
- Geographic location (rural and urban)

Importantly, the AMA has encouraged physicians to examine their own practices to ensure equality in medical care.

As well, the AMA's Ethics Standards Group is committed to helping eliminate racial and ethnic health disparities. It focuses on academic research and training programs to help increase awareness and improve understanding of issues related to ethics and health disparities, as well as providing resources for others working on these issues.

Many disparities arise because of communication problems and personal biases; thus, it is noteworthy that the AMA is encouraging physicians to examine their own practices to ensure equality in medical care. Thus, as patient advocates and agents of change, primary care physicians are playing a critical role in efforts to eliminate disparities in health care. This will undoubtedly help reduce the excess suffering of minorities and the disadvantaged they presently experience from chronic health conditions.

The Affordable Care Act, a new health law in the United States, specifically contains several provisions that address health disparities as a priority in awarding various grants, developing research priorities, gathering accurate data, and evaluating community preventive services.

Summary

Health disparities adversely affect groups of people who experience greater obstacles to health on the basis of their racial or ethnic group; religion, socioeconomic status; gender; age; mental health; cognitive, sensory, or physical disability; sexual orientation or gender identity; geographic location; or other characteristics historically linked to discrimination or exclusion, as well as greater health-related problems, as a whole.

To reduce health disparities, improving education for all, and reducing socioeconomic barriers—along with strengthening health systems and reducing barriers to health services (e.g., lack of patient-centered care, use of evidence-based clinical guidelines)—can improve access to timely, quality care.

Ray Marks

See also: Access to Health Services; Centers for Disease Control and Prevention (CDC); Healthy People 2020; Poverty; Substance Abuse; World Health Organization

Further Reading

American Medical Association. (2012). Eliminating health disparities. Retrieved from http://www.ama-assn.org/ama/pub/physician-resources/public-health/eliminating-health-disparities.page.

American Public Health Association. (2012). Eliminating health disparities. Retrieved from http://www.apha.org/advocacy/priorities/issues/disparities/.

Centers for Disease Control and Prevention. (2012). Health equity. Retrieved from http://www.cdc.gov/chronicdisease/healthequity/index.htm.

Crook, E. D., & Peters, M. (2008). Health disparities in chronic diseases: Where the money is. *American Journal of Medical Science, 335*, 266–270.

Healthy People 2020. (2012). Retrieved from http://www.healthypeople.gov/2020/about/disparitiesAbout.aspx.

Institute for Health and Metrics Evaluation. (2012). Monitoring disparities in chronic conditions study: The MDCC study. Retrieved from http://www.healthmetricsandevaluation.org/research/project/monitoring-disparities-chronic-conditions-study-mdcc-study.

LaVeist, T. A., & Isaac, L. A. (eds.). (2013). *Race, Ethnicity, and Health: A Public Health Reader.* Hoboken, NJ: John Wiley and Sons.

National Institutes of Health. (2012). Health disparities. Retrieved from http://report.nih.gov/NIHfactsheets/ViewFactSheet.aspx?csid=124.

New York Academy of Medicine. (2012). Eliminating health disparities. Retrieved from http://www.nyam.org/urban-health/eliminating-health-disparities/.

Strategic directions. Elimination of health disparities. (2012). Retrieved from http://www.healthcare.gov/prevention/nphpphc/strategy/health-disparities.pdf.

Williams, D. R., & Williams-Morris, R. (2000). "Racism and mental health: The African American experience. *Ethnicity and Health, 5*(314), 243–268.

HEALTH LITERACY

Health literacy is a complex concept that directly influences a patient's access to necessary information about his or her health care, whether it involves following instructions, taking medicine, comprehending disease-related information, or learning about health promotion activities or accessing health care (Baker et al. 1996). It is defined as "the degree to which individuals have the capacity to obtain, process, and understand basic health information and services needed to make appropriate health decisions" (U.S. Department of Health and Human Services 2001, 16).

History

Historically, the literature regarding health literacy focused exclusively on readability of health and medical information (Bettman 1975). As early as 1980, Eaton and Halloway suggested that package inserts be written at reading levels between grades 5 and 7. However, in 1994, when 63 package inserts from pharmaceutical companies were analyzed, the average readability was scored at grade 10 (Basara & Jeurgens 1994). Many studies have shown that typical handouts used to educate patients, including those from many professional organizations, are written at a 9th-grade or higher level (Glazer et al. 1996; Guidry & Fagan 1997; Meade et al. 1992). Readability of other disease categories yielded similar results. Cholesterol education materials (Glanz & Rudd 1990), prenatal education materials (Primas et al. 1992), and diabetes education materials (Leichter et al. 1981) were all scored at well above 9th grade reading levels.

Health literacy and literacy are related but not identical. Literacy is often defined as having skills related to reading, writing, math (including numeracy), and comprehension. Studies have shown that nearly 9 out of 10 Americans have difficulties understanding and utilizing health information on a daily basis (Kutner et al. 2006). In 2004, researchers took a look at national literacy assessments (NALs and IALs), and in a report entitled "Literacy and Health in America," researchers provided the first of its kind description of health literacy skills among at-risk or vulnerable population groups. It also demonstrated how health-related skills are connected to health status, among other things, and that individuals with inadequate literacy skills come from a variety of backgrounds, including all races, socioeconomic classes, education levels, and cultural background (Rudd et al. 2004).

Consequences of Inadequate Health Literacy

Issues such as trouble navigating the health care system, providing health care professionals with inaccurate or incomplete personal medical histories, or missing appointments are a few of the problems that individuals with low health literacy face. All of these issues have been corroborated in a variety of health care research settings. A landmark study of 2,500 patients at two public hospitals by Williams et al. (1995) found that 42 percent of patients could not understand directions for taking medications on an empty stomach and 26 percent could not understand an appointment slip. These patients were also at a greater risk of misunderstanding the diagnosis and self-care instructions.

Studies have found that patients with low health literacy have more outpatient visits, a greater likelihood of hospitalization, higher expenses for health care, and poorer health (Baker et al. 2002; Weiss et al. 1994). Baker and colleagues (1996) examined the relationship of functional health literacy to self-reported health and use of health services. This cross-sectional, retrospective study included a sample of 979 English-speaking patients presenting for nonurgent care at the emergency care centers and walk-in clinics at two public hospitals. Patients with inadequate functional health literacy were more likely than patients with adequate literacy to report their health as poor.

Health Knowledge. Low health literacy can also pose an obstacle to effective health communication, or a patient's ability to manage his or her health and screening decisions. Patients with poor health literacy are disadvantaged in their capacity to obtain, process, and understand both written and verbal information. Davis and colleagues (1993) assessed the relationship between health literacy levels and knowledge and attitudes toward screening mammography with a convenience sample of 445 low-income women, 40 years of age and older, from two outpatient clinics in Louisiana. The researchers concluded that limited literacy skills and lack of knowledge about screening mammography may contribute considerably to the underutilization of mammography by low-income women. A similar study by Bennett et al. (1998) examined the relationship among literacy, race, and stage of presentation among 212 low-income men diagnosed with prostate cancer and found that men with lower literacy levels were more likely to present with advanced-stage prostate cancer.

Disease Prevention and Health Promotion. Appropriate health literacy is also important to health promotion in both primary and secondary prevention. Studies have shown that patients with low health literacy and chronic diseases may also be less well informed about the basics of their care. Williams and colleagues (1998a) assessed the relationship between functional health literacy and knowledge of chronic disease in a cross-sectional survey of patients with hypertension and diabetes. Almost half of the patients were at inadequate functional health literacy levels and were less likely to know basic information about their diseases and essential self-management skills than those with high functional health literacy scores. Only 50 percent of the low literacy patients with diabetes knew the symptoms of hypoglycemia compared with 94 percent of those patients with adequate literacy levels. Another study published by Williams and colleagues (1998b) examined the relationship between literacy and asthma knowledge and self-management skills. In this convenience sample of 483 patients, lower literacy levels, as measured by the Rapid Estimate of Adult Literacy in Medicine (REALM), were associated with lower asthma knowledge scores and improper asthma self-management.

Health Care Costs. Based on the research, it is feasible to assume that low literacy levels might be associated with higher health care costs. One study estimated that between 106 and 236 billion are spent per year in the health care system because of low health literacy (Vernon et al. 2007); however, little research has been done in this area.

Current Trends in Health Literacy

Professional medical organizations and government agencies are beginning to realize the importance of health literacy on the public's health. In 1998, the American Medical Association (AMA) became the first national medical organization to adopt a policy recognizing that limited health literacy affects diagnosis and treatments.

In two separate reports, released by the Institute of Medicine (IOM) in 2003 and 2004, health literacy was expressly identified as a key issue in improving the health and quality of the population of the United States. In the 2003 report, "*Priority Areas for Nation Action: Transforming Health Care Quality,*" health literacy is identified as one of the country's top priorities for improving the quality of care. Of the 20 health-related issues listed in the report, health literacy is one of only two health-related issues classified as "cross-cutting" because it affects patients suffering from all types of medical conditions. The report continues on by describing efforts to improve health literacy as "essential for effective self-management and collaborative care" (Institute of Medicine 2003).

In 2004, the Institute of Medicine convened a committee to examine the issues associated with health literacy and released their findings and recommendations in a report, *Health Literacy: A Prescription to End Confusion.* The committee developed a framework for health literacy and outlined potential influences on health literacy as individuals interact with educational systems, health systems, and cultural and social factors. Healthy People 2020 also includes a health literacy objective, representing a significant step in raising public awareness of this critical issue (U.S. Department of Health and Human Services 2001).

Several health care accreditation agencies, including the Joint Commission on Accreditation of Healthcare Organizations (JCAHO) and the National Committee for Quality Assurance, now require providers to take steps to ensure that patients understand the medical information they receive (JCAHO 1996). Since 1993, health organizations are also scored on how well their patients understand the (1) safe and effective use of medication and/or medical equipment, (2) potential food-drug interactions, and (3) when and how to obtain further treatment.

Tools for Measuring Health Literacy

There have been specific health literacy assessment tools that have been designed to assess the health literacy of individuals, and not just their reading ability. The most commonly referenced health literacy assessment tools are the Rapid Estimate of Adult Literacy in Medicine (REALM) (Davis et al. 1991, 1993) and the Test of Functional Health Literacy in Adults (TOFHLA) (Parker et al. 1995). For the REALM test, participants read from a list of 125 common medical terms, arranged in four columns according to the number of syllables they contain (Davis et al. 1991). The test of functional health literacy in adults (TOFHLA) was developed in English and Spanish and uses actual hospital materials, such as the patients' rights and responsibilities section of a Medicaid application form, instructions for preparing for a gastrointestinal series, a standardized hospital consent form, and labeled prescription vials (Parker et al. 1995).

Rachel Torres

See also: Access to Health Services; Centers for Disease Control and Prevention (CDC); Healthy People 2020; World Health Organization

Further Reading
Baker, D. W., Parker, R. M., Williams, M. V., Pitkin, K., Parikh, N. S., Coates, W., & Mwalimu, I. (1996). The health experience of patients with low literacy. *Archives of Family Medicine, 5,* 329–334.
Baker, D. W., Gazmararian, J. A., Williams, M. V., Scott, T., Parker, R. M., Green, D., Ren, J., & Peel, J. (2002). Functional health literacy and the risk of hospital admission among Medicare managed care enrollees. *American Journal of Public Health, 92*(8), 1278–1283.
Basara, L. R., & Juergens, J. P. (1994). Patient package insert readability and design. *American Pharmacy, 34*(Suppl. 8), 48–53.
Bennett, C. L., Ferreira, M. R., Davis, T. C., Kaplan, J., Weinberger, M., Kuzel, T., Seday, M. A., & Sartor, O. (1998). Relation between literacy, race, and stage of presentation among low-income patients with prostate cancer. *Journal of Clinical Oncology, 16*(9), 3101–3104.
Bettman, J. R. (1975). Issues in designing consumer health information environments. *Journal of Consumer Research, 2,* 169–177.

Davis, T. C., Crouch, M. A., Long, S. W., Jackson, R. H., Bates, P., George, R. B., & Bairns-father, L. E. (1991). Rapid assessment of literacy levels of adult primary care patients. *Family Medicine, 23*(6), 433–435.

Davis, T. C., Long, S. W., Jackson, R. H., Mayeaux, E. J., George, R. B., Murphy, P. W., & Crouch, M. A. (1993). Rapid estimate of adult literacy in medicine: A shortened screening instrument. *Family Medicine, 25*(6), 391–395.

Eaton, M. L., & Holloway, R. L. (1980). Patient comprehension of written drug information. *American Journal of Hospital Pharmacy, 37*(2), 240–243.

Glanz, K., & Rudd, J. (1990). Readability and content analysis of print cholesterol education materials. *Patient Education and Counseling, 16*(2), 109–118.

Glazer, H. R., Kirk, L. M., & Bosle, F. E. (1996). Patient education pamphlets about prevention, detection, and treatment of breast cancer for low literacy women. *Patient Education and Counseling, 27*(2), 185–189.

Guidry, J. J., & Fagan, P. (1997). The readability levels of cancer-prevention materials targeting African Americans. *Journal of Cancer Education, 12*(2), 108–113.

Institute of Medicine. (2003). *Priority areas for national action: Transforming health care quality.* Washington, DC: The National Press.

Institute of Medicine. (2004). *Health Literacy: A Prescription to End Confusion.* Washington, DC: The National Press.

Joint Commission on Accreditation of Healthcare Organizations (JCAHO). (2004). 2004 standards for home care and hospitals. Retrieved October 2004 from https://www.jointcommission.org/

Kutner, M., Jin, Y., Greenberg, E., & Paulsen, C. (2006). The health literacy of America's adults: Results from the 2003 National Assessment of Adult Literacy (NCES 2006–483). Washington, DC: U.S. Department of Education, National Center for Educational Statistics.

Leichter, S. B., Nieman, J. A., Moore, R. W., Collins, P., & Rhodes, A. (1981). Readability of self-care instructional pamphlets for diabetic patients. *Diabetes Care, 4*(6), 627–630.

Meade, C. D., Diekmann, J., & Thornhill, D. G (1992). Readability of American Cancer Society patient education literature. *Oncology Nursing Forum, 19*(1), 51–55.

National Academy on an Aging Society. (1998). Understanding health literacy: New estimates of the costs of inadequate health literacy. Presented at the Pfizer Conference on Health Literacy, "Promoting Health Literacy: A Call to Action." Washington, DC.

Parker, R. M., Baker, D. W., Williams, M. V., & Nurss, J. R. (1995). The test of functional health literacy in adults: A new instrument for measuring patients' literacy skills. *Journal of General Internal Medicine, 10*(10), 537–541.

Primas, P., Lefor, N., Johnson, J., Helms, S. M., Coats, L., & Coe, M. K. (1992). Prenatal literature testing: A pilot project. *Journal of Community Health, 17*(1), 61–67.

Rudd, R., Kirsch, I., & Yamamoto, K. (2004). *Literacy and Health in America.* Princeton, NJ: Educational Testing Services.

U.S. Department of Health and Human Services. (2001). Health communication. *Healthy People 2010.* Retrieved from http://www.health.gov/healthypeople.

Vernon, J. A., Trujillo, A., Rosenbaum, S., & DeBuono, B. (2007). Low Health Literacy: Implications for National Health Policy. University of Connecticut.

Weiss, B. D., Blanchard, J. S., McGee, D. L., Hart, G., Warren, B., Burgoon, M., & Smith, K. J. (1994). Illiteracy among Medicaid recipients and its relationship to health care costs. *Journal of Health Care for the Poor and Underserved, 5*(2), 99–111.

Williams, M. V., Parker, R. M., Baker, D. W., Parikh, K., Coates, W. C., & Nurss, J. R. (1995). Inadequate functional health literacy among patients at two public hospitals. *Journal of the American Medical Association, 2714*(21), 1677–1682.

Williams, M. V., Baker, D. W., Parker, R. M., & Nurss, J. R. (1998a). Relationship of functional health literacy to patients' knowledge of their chronic disease. A study of patients with hypertension and diabetes. *Archives of Internal Medicine, 158*(2), 166–172.

Williams, M. V., Baker, D. W., Honig, E. G., Lee, T. M., & Nowlan, A. (1998b). Inadequate literacy is a barrier to asthma knowledge and self-care. *Chest, 114*(4), 1008–1015.

HEALTHY LIFESTYLES AND RISKY BEHAVIORS

How many answers appear if you search online for the term "healthy lifestyle"? More than 77 million hits (in early 2016). At least numerically, healthy lifestyle is a hot topic. Now, search the term "risky behavior." The number of hits is dramatically fewer, only 2.95 million. A *healthy lifestyle* is one whose health behaviors promote health and fitness; *risky behavior* includes those nonsupportive behaviors that compromise our health status. In simple terms, healthy lifestyles are the DOs and risky behaviors are the DON'Ts of health and well-being.

For three decades, the U.S. government's Healthy People program has led efforts to educate the nation that health is about more than the absence of disease and is created through the conditions of our daily lives—not at the doctor's office. The Healthy People initiative reiterates that individuals can exercise greater control over their health and well-being. Underscoring this notion, McKenzie, Pinger, and Kotecki (2014) reported the common causes of death in the United States for 2006 in rank order. The number-one cause of death is *diseases of the heart*. For this same period, the actual cause of death is listed as tobacco. Is there a relationship between diseases of the heart and tobacco? Absolutely! National Heart, Lung, and Blood Institute, NIH (2015) reported the medical consequences of tobacco use as conclusively linked to pneumonia, cancers, and cardio-respiratory illnesses. The NIH estimates suggest that tobacco use kills more people than illegal drug use, homicide, suicide car accidents, and AIDS combined.

Central to discussions of a healthy lifestyle or risky behaviors is "locus of control." This psychological theory maintains there is a positive relationship between internal locus of control and decision making, self-empowerment, and positive outcomes. Essentially, locus of control orientation is a belief about whether the outcomes of our actions are contingent on what we do (internal control orientation) or on events outside our personal control (external control orientation) (Rotter 1966; Zimbardo 1992). More recently, research in health psychology demonstrates the relationship between locus of control and performance of a variety of health-related behaviors. Recent studies report internal locus of control has been associated with information seeking, autonomous decision making, and having a sense of well-being. According to Nir and Neuman (1995), individuals exhibiting an internal locus of control tend to respond better than externals to programs involving self-change.

The Healthy People Initiative (1979) brought together in one place what we know of the relationship between personal behavior and health status: without doubt, 50 percent of all deaths were (and remain) related to personal lifestyle or health behavior. Healthy People continues to advocate informed health decisions and behaviors about diet, physical activity, alcohol and drug use, smoking, sexual and reproductive practices, and safety precautions.

The Youth Risk Behavior Surveillance System (YRBSS), a social epidemiologic surveillance system established by the Centers for Disease Control and Prevention (CDC), monitors health-risk behaviors among high school students. Between 1990 and 1999, multiple separate studies were conducted. YRBSS monitors six types of health-risk behaviors that contribute to the leading causes of death and disability among youth and adults. These include inadequate physical activity, unhealthy dietary behaviors, tobacco use, alcohol and other drug use, sexual behaviors that contribute to unintended pregnancy and sexually transmitted diseases (including HIV infection), and behaviors that contribute to unintentional injuries and violence. Clearly, these risk behaviors are the DON'T list of health and well-being.

Adopting a positive perspective—the DOs as opposed to the DON'Ts—is generally believed to be psychologically sound, empowering, and supportive to our *health locus of control*. Individual health behavior plays a role in health outcomes. For example, if an individual quits smoking, his or her risk of developing heart disease is greatly reduced. These five healthy lifestyle behaviors are simple and straightforward.

> *Get physical.* The health and fitness benefits of regular physical activity are numerous and include decreased risk of obesity, heart disease, hypertension, and diabetes mellitus; improved body mass index (BMI); blood glucose and cholesterol control; improved stress management; and reduced depression and anxiety.
>
> As general rule of thumb, aerobic physical activities are recommended three times per week. Vary the length and intensity of your activity, but for better results (fitness and weight control), spread your physical activities out over the week. For more detailed information and suggestions, visit http://www.health.gov/paguidelines/toolkit.aspx.
>
> *Don't smoke.* Tobacco and smoking behaviors affect everyone: the smoker and the bystander. According to the National Cancer Institute (2011), secondhand smoke are as dangerous as firsthand smoke. Cigarette smoke gases and particles cling to smokers' hair and clothing, as well as to cushions, carpeting, drapes, and wallpaper. The residues include heavy metals, carcinogens, and radioactive materials that are dangerous to anyone who breathes or ingests them. The negative health effects of smoking range from breathing problems and heart disease to increased rates of colds and flu and a greater risk for sudden infant death syndrome (SIDS). Smoking cessation programs are numerous and available in almost every community. For more detailed information, visit https://a816-nycquits.nyc.gov/pages/programs.aspx.
>
> *Eat healthily.* The film *Super Size Me* by independent filmmaker Morgan Spurlock documented his odyssey with fast food. In 30 days, his fast-food diet resulted in weight gain (obesity), increased cholesterol levels (hypercholesterolemia), depressed libido, and mood swings. The U.S. Surgeon General has sounded the alarm that obesity is an epidemic; it is related to prediabetes and diabetes—both of which are preventable. To view the updated and newest government food guidelines on the MyFood Plate program, see www.ChooseMyPlate.gov.
>
> *Make healthy sexual choices.* Making smart, informed choices about sex is important. Because choices about sex are never straightforward, having clear, concise, and accurate information and knowing your values are essential. People have sex for all sorts of different reasons. Their reasons include being horny or "in love," wanting to

lose their virginity, feeling lonely, just wanting to be close to someone, wanting to feel emotionally connected, or because they were drunk or "out of it." Healthy sexual choices range widely. Some questions may include: Do I really want to be sexually active? What is *safe* sex? How do I politely refuse without alienating anyone? How do I protect myself? Who am I as a sexual being? To make healthy sexual choices people need to know themselves, have access to information and services, and be comfortable with their decisions.

Wash your hands. Keeping hands clean is one of the best ways to prevent the spread of infection and illness. The Centers for Disease Control and Prevention provides tips for hand-washing.

Linda R. Barley

See also: Alcoholism; Diet and Nutrition; Environment; Healthy People 2020; Physical Activity; Risk Factors; Substance Abuse

Further Reading

Center for Young Women's Health. (2015, April 30). Making healthy sexual decisions. Retrieved from http://youngwomenshealth.org/2013/05/23/making-healthy-sexual-decisions/.

Centers for Disease Control and Prevention. (2015, September 3). Physical activity. Retrieved from http://www.cdc.gov/physicalactivity/index.html.

Centers for Disease Control and Prevention. (2015, September 3). Wash your hands. Retrieved from http://www.cdc.gov/features/handwashing/.

Hamann, B. (2006). *Disease: Identification, Prevention and Control*, 3rd ed. New York: McGraw-Hill Humanities/Social Sciences/Languages.

HealthyPeople.gov. (2015, November 5). About healthy people. Retrieved from http://www.healthypeople.gov/2020/About-Healthy-People.

McKenzie, J. F., Pinger, R. R., & Kotecki, J. E. (2014). *An Introduction to Community & Public Health*, 8th ed. Sudbury, MA: Jones & Bartlett Learning.

National Cancer Institute. (2011). Secondhand Smoke and Cancer. Retrieved from http://www.cancer.gov/about-cancer/causes-prevention/risk/tobacco/second-hand-smoke-fact-sheet.

National Heart, Lung, and Blood Institute. (2015). How does smoking affect the heart and blood vessels? Retrieved from http://www.nhlbi.nih.gov/health/health-topics/topics/smo.

Nir, Z., & Neumann, L. (1995). Relationship among self-esteem, internal-external locus of control, and weight change after participation in a weight reduction program. *Journal of Clinical Psychology*, 51(4), 482–490.

NSW Government. (2014, July 10). Sexual health plus. Retrieved from http://www.health.nsw.gov.au/publichealth/sexualhealth/sex_choices.asp.

Rotter, J. B. (1966). Generalized expectancies for internal versus external control of reinforcement. *Psychological Monographs*, 80(609).

Zimbardo, P. G. (1992). *Psychology and Life*. New York, NY: Harper Collins.

HEALTHY PEOPLE 2020

Healthy People 2020 establishes national goals and objectives for policy, programs, and activities to address the major health challenges facing our country today and seeks to assure conditions in which people can be healthy, both now and for generations to come. This essential planning document is based on four previous, science-based, 10-year national objectives to improve the health of all Americans.

Initiated with the 1979 Surgeon General's Report, *Healthy People: The Surgeon General's Report on Health Promotion and Disease Prevention*, the Healthy People initiative evolved into a decanal report on the health status of Americans and a proposal for future health goals and objectives. Since its inception, the initiative produced *Healthy People 1990: Promoting Health/Preventing Disease: Objectives for the Nation*, *Healthy People 2000: National Health Promotion and Disease Prevention Objectives,* and *Healthy People 2010: Objectives for Improving Health*.

Promoting the health of a nation is a collaborative effort that goes beyond providing health services once a person reaches the doctor's office. *Healthy People* has established health status benchmarks and worked to monitor progress. To achieve these benchmarks, key tasks have been planned and implemented, including encouraging collaborations across communities and health delivery sectors, empowering individuals toward making informed health decisions, and measuring the impact of prevention activities.

Because the values of a nation are reflected in its willingness to secure better health, well-being, and vitality for all, the *vision* of Healthy People 2020—"a society in which all people live long, healthy lives"—is a live document. Its five-part mission seeks to strengthen policy and practice. Specifically to:

- Identify nationwide health improvement priorities.
- Increase public awareness and understanding of the determinants of health, disease and disability, and the opportunities for progress.
- Provide measureable objectives and goals that can be used at the national, state, and local levels.
- Engage multiple sectors to take actions that are driven by the best available evidence and knowledge.
- Identify critical research and data collection needs.

Ultimately, *Healthy People 2020* seeks to eliminate preventable disease and death, achieve health equity, create social and physical environments that promote good health for all, and promote healthy development and healthy behaviors across every stage of life. To achieve these doable goals, Healthy People brings communities and individuals into partnerships that acknowledge need, foster cooperation, and implement solutions.

Encourage Collaborations across Communities. Community organizing and building has becoming a signature of the *Healthy People* initiative. The U.S. Department of Health and Human Services (DHHS) produced *Healthy People in Health Communities*—a five-step framework that mobilizes a community, collects and organizes data, chooses a heath priority, develops and implements the intervention, and monitors the community's progress.

Empowering Individuals toward Making Informed Health Decisions. The 1979 Surgeon General's Report, *Healthy People: The Surgeon General's Report on Health Promotion and Disease Prevention*, brought together in one place what was known of the relationship between personal behavior and health status. Without doubt, the report revealed that 50 percent of all deaths were (and remain) related to personal life-style or heath behavior. *Healthy People* advocates informed health decisions and behaviors about diet, physical activity, alcohol and drug use, smoking, sexual and reproductive practices, and safety precautions.

Measure the Impact of Prevention Activities. The past three decades have produced a wealth of evidence-based health promotion programs—informed and supported by community collaboration and the outcomes of fostering informed decision mak-ing. These evidenced-based studies encompass individual health choices, commu-nity interventions, and policy implementation by city, state, and national health providers.

Societal Determinants of Health. The Secretary's Advisory Committee stated, "Healthy People envisions a day when preventable death, illness, injury, and disabil-ity, as well as health disparities, will be eliminated and each person will enjoy the best health possible" (2010). Societal determinants of health are broadly defined as those social, physical, and economic environments in which people are born, live, work, and age. These environments also include policies, institutions, government, and community factors that touch on all aspects of life—home, school, worship, recreation, work, and public and national safety—and the values that guide how we treat ourselves and others.

Physical Determinants of Health. The physical environment includes our natural environment and our built environment—plants, water, atmosphere, rivers, oceans, forests and homes, buildings, bridges, schools, energy plants, and our modes of transportation. The impact and relationship among and between nature and the built environment cannot be underestimated. Environmental health is a key deter-minate of health.

Implementing Healthy People 2020. Based on a simple but powerful mode—*establish national health objectives and provide data and tools to enable states, cities, com-munities, and individuals across the country*—the *MAP-IT* framework is the "how" of *Healthy People 2020.*

MAP-IT stands for mobilize, assess, plan, implement, and track. For a more de-tailed discussion of MAP-IT, visit http://www.healthypeople.gov/2020/implementing /planning.aspx.

Leading health indicators address access to health care, preventive health services, environmental quality, and a comprehensive topical area. Topics and objectives are organized alphabetically, opening with "Access to Health." The *new* topics did not appear in Healthy People 2010. These new topics are robust additions and include Adolescent Health; Blood Disorders and Blood Safety; Dementias and Alzheimer's Disease; Early and Middle Childhood Health; Genomics; Global Health; Health Care-Associated Infections; Health-Related Quality of Life and Well-Being; Lesbian, Gay, Bisexual, and Transgender Health; Older Adult Health; Preparedness; Sleep Health; and Social Determents of Health. For a complete listing of topics and objec-tives, visit http://www.healthypeople.gov/2020/topicsobjectives2020/default.aspx.

Good nutrition, physical activity, and a healthy body weight are essential to a person's overall health and well-being regardless of age, gender, or ethnicity. Together, these can help decrease a person's risk of developing serious health conditions, such as high blood pressure, high cholesterol, diabetes, heart disease, stroke, and cancer. A healthful diet, regular physical activity, and achieving and maintaining a healthy weight also are paramount to managing health conditions so they do not worsen over time.

A Simple, Direct and Effective Intervention: Physical Activity. Since the inception of the Healthy People initiative, one common thread is repeated: Improve health, fitness, and quality of life through daily physical activity. Released in 2008, the *Physical Activity Guidelines for Americans* (PAG) was the first-ever publication of *national* guidelines for physical activity. The Physical Activity objectives for Healthy People 2020 reflect the strong state of the science supporting the health benefits of regular physical activity among youth and adults, as identified in the PAG. Regular physical activity includes participation in moderate and vigorous physical activities and muscle-strengthening activities.

Healthy People 2020 targets a multidisciplinary approach to increasing the levels of physical activity and improving health in the United States. The Physical Activity Guideline objectives for 2020 include positive structural environments (sidewalks, bike lanes, trails, and parks), policies targeting younger children in child care settings, and legislative policy that support physical activity for kindergarten through grade 12 learners. Healthy children become healthy adults!

Linda R. Barley

See also: Access to Health Services; Centers for Disease Control and Prevention (CDC); Health; Health Disparities; Poverty; Substance Abuse; World Health Organization

Further Reading

www.HealthyPeople.gov.
http://www.health.gov/PAGuidelines/.
http://www.healthypeople.gov/2020/topicsobjectives2020/default.aspx.
http://www.physicalactivityplan.org/theplan.htm.
http://healthypeople.gov/2020/about/advisory/PhaseI.pdf.
http://healthypeople.gov/2020/about/default.aspx.
http://www.healthypeople.gov/2020/about/advisory/SocietalDeterminantsHealth.pdf.

HEART DISEASES

About the size of a fist, the heart is the strongest muscle in the body. It pumps six quarts of blood rich in oxygen and nutrients throughout the body's circulatory system every minute by expanding and contracting 100,000 times each day. The term *heart disease* includes many different conditions that affect its structure and function. Also known as *cardiac diseases*, they are the leading cause of death for men and women in the United States, killing more than 600,000 people each year, as well as a significant cause of disability. Related to or included in the term heart disease are cardiovascular diseases, which are conditions that involve the narrowing or blockage of blood vessels as well as the heart.

The most common type of heart disease is coronary artery disease, and it occurs over time when the arteries supplying the heart with blood become stiff and narrow when plaque—or cholesterol and other fatty material—builds up inside them. This blocks or limits blood flow in the process known as atherosclerosis, contributes to the heart receiving less oxygen, and can lead to heart attack or angina (pain in the chest). Eventually, after weakening the heart muscle, coronary artery disease can lead to heart failure, in which the heart cannot pump enough blood, and arrhythmias (irregular heartbeats). Other cardiac diseases include congenital heart defects, genetic heart disorders, diseases of the heart valves and blood vessels, weak heart muscle, and those caused by infections.

Although they are often different for men and women, symptoms common to many forms of heart disease include chest pain or discomfort; shortness of breath; dizziness, lightheadedness, and fainting; fluttering in the chest due to an irregular heartbeat; weakness or fatigue; and swelling in the legs, feet, ankles, or abdomen.

People of all ages can develop heart diseases, and some children are born with heart defects. But risk factors for developing for the most common types of heart disease include smoking, high blood pressure, high LDL ("bad" cholesterol), being overweight, diabetes, aging, and lack of exercise.

Because heart diseases have a great variety of causes, treatments depend on the specific form. But most people can make lifestyle changes to reduce their risk of developing heart disease.

Symptoms

Heart disease symptoms depend on the type of heart disease, but the most common of coronary artery disease is angina, often described as heaviness in the center of the chest that radiates to the left arm or jaw. Other symptoms include shortness of breath; sweating; numbness, weakness, or coldness in the areas of the body where blood vessels have narrowed; pain in the upper abdomen, back, or shoulder; and nausea or indigestion. Symptoms of heart disease may differ for men, who typically have chest pain, and women, who often experience shortness of breath, nausea, and extreme fatigue.

Causes and Risk Factors

The most common cause of heart disease is the narrowing or blockage of the coronary arteries, which usually takes place very slowly over time. The risk of heart disease and heart attacks increases with the number and severity of risk factors any individual has. Many risk factors start during childhood, including in the first 10 years of life.

Key risk factors that lead to this condition include smoking, high blood pressure, and high LDL ("bad" cholesterol); about half the adults in the United States have at least one of these. Other significant risk factors include being overweight, physical inactivity, diabetes, poor diet high in high in saturated fats, excessive alcohol use, family history of heart disease, stress, and age (over 55). In general, men have a slightly higher risk, but the risk for women increases following menopause.

Other risk factors may include poverty and social isolation, and major depression and bipolar disorder can increase the risk for teenagers.

Diagnosis

No single test can confirm a diagnosis of coronary artery disease. After taking medical and family histories and conducting a physical examination, a cardiologist may employ diagnostic tests, including an EKG (or electrocardiogram), which tests the heart's electrical activity; a stress test to examine how the heart responds to exertion; echocardiography, a moving picture of the heart that can show areas of poor blood flow and muscle abnormalities; chest x-rays that may reveal symptoms of heart failure; blood tests for abnormal levels of fats, cholesterol, sugar, and proteins in the blood; coronary angiography, showing the insides of the coronary arteries; a cardiac computerized tomography (CT) scan or cardiac magnetic resonance imaging (MRI); and nuclear imaging, or the placement of a radioactive tracer to assess blow flow to the heart.

Treatments

Treatment of coronary artery disease focuses first on managing symptoms to reduce the risk of developing a heart attack, including eating a healthful diet, increasing physical activity, quitting smoking, maintaining a healthy weight, and learning to cope with stress.

Medication may also be prescribed to enable the heart muscle to function more efficiently, including aspirin and other medicines to reduce or prevent clots, blood thinners (anticoagulants), ACE inhibitors and beta blockers to lower high blood pressure, calcium channel blockers to help the heart muscle work more efficiently, nitroglycerin for angina, statins to lower cholesterol, and fish oil and other supplements high in heart-healthy omega-3 fatty acids.

Procedures for coronary artery disease include nonsurgical angioplasty, which opens narrowed or blocked arteries, and coronary artery bypass graft surgery, which improves blood flow to the heart by using arteries from elsewhere in the body to bypass the damaged arteries. Medically supervised cardiac rehabilitation provides individualized exercise programs to help strengthen muscles and improve stamina for those with heart disease. It also provides education about heart conditions and teaches people how to reduce their risk for future disease, cope with stress, and adjust to lifestyle changes.

Prevention

The risks of developing heart disease can be reduced or prevented by quitting smoking, lowering LDL or "bad" cholesterol, controlling high blood pressure, maintaining a healthy weight, increasing physical activity, limiting alcohol intake, reducing stressful triggers, and managing diabetes, if necessary.

Prognosis and Outcomes

The prognosis of heart disease improves the sooner a diagnosis is made and treatment begins. Increased knowledge of symptoms experienced by women, older adults, and others who do not exhibit the classic male symptoms has improved diagnosis and saved lives, as have educational efforts to raise awareness of risk factors and when to seek emergency medical care with the development of chest pain.

Future

Among its many clinical trials, the National Heart, Lung, and Blood Institute has conducted research studies exploring the comparison of coronary artery bypass grafting with angioplasty and stenting in those who have diabetes and blockages in numerous coronary arteries, how well patients do after surgery or angioplasty, whether exercise helps treat depression in people who have heart disease, and how the risk factors for heart disease affect aging in healthy people.

Ray Marks

See also: Angina; Arrhythmias/Dysrhythmias; Atherosclerosis; Cardiomyopathy; Cardiovascular Disease; Cerebral Vascular Disease; Cholesterol; Circulation Disorders; Congenital Heart Disease; Congestive Heart Failure; Coronary Artery Disease; Diabetes, Type 2; Endocarditis; High Blood Pressure; Hypertension; Prediabetes; Stroke; Tachycardia

Further Reading

American Heart Association. (2015, May 18). What is cardiovascular disease? Retrieved from http://www.heart.org/HEARTORG/Caregiver/Resources/WhatisCardiovascularDisease/What-is-Cardiovascular-Disease_UCM_301852_Article.jsp#.

Centers for Disease Control and Prevention. (2015, September 1). Heart disease. Retrieved from http://www.cdc.gov/HeartDisease/.

Esselstyn, C. B., Jr. (2007). *Prevent and Reverse Heart Disease: The Revolutionary, Scientifically Proven, Nutrition-Based Cure.* New York: Avery.

Granato, J. E. (2008). *Living with Coronary Heart Disease: A Guide for Patients and Families.* Baltimore, MD: Johns Hopkins University Press.

Mayo Clinic. (2014, July 29). Heart disease. Retrieved from http://www.mayoclinic.org/diseases-conditions/heart-disease/basics/definition/CON-20034056?p=1.

National Heart Lung and Blood Institute. (2014, August 26). What is heart disease? Retrieved from http://www.nhlbi.nih.gov/health/educational/hearttruth/lower-risk/what-is-heart-disease.htm.

HEART MURMUR

A heart murmur is the sound of turbulent blood in or near the heart made during the heartbeat cycle, meaning the blood flow is not smooth. The sounds—whistling, whooshing, or swishing—are heard when listening to the heart with a stethoscope. An innocent, or functional, murmur is harmless, and some adults and children have a healthy heart and this type of murmur. Murmurs are common, and most are normal. They can develop later in life or occur at birth; some 25,000 babies a year are born with heart defects. Functional murmurs are often present in adults older than 50, as well as when exercise, pregnancy, or fever causes the blood to temporarily flow harder and faster than usual.

An abnormal heart murmur isn't a disease, but it may suggest an underlying heart problem, such as an impaired heart valve or heart chamber or an abnormal connection of two parts within the heart. Treatment may not be necessary for an abnormal murmur, but medications or surgery may be used to treat the underlying problem. Murmurs present at birth or occurring during the first six months may require medical care by a pediatric cardiologist.

Symptoms

Harmless murmurs do not create any noticeable symptoms. But abnormal murmurs exhibit a variety of symptoms, including chest pain; chronic coughing; dizziness; shortness of breath; excessive sweating, even with little or no exertion; an enlarged liver or neck veins; sudden weight gain or swelling; and a bluish skin color, most visible on the lips and at the fingertips. Infants with congenital heart have trouble breathing and are cyanotic (have a blue skin color) because the heart can't circulate blood and oxygen from the lungs to the rest of the body; they may also have trouble feeding, developing, and growing normally.

Causes and Risk Factors

The reasons some people have innocent heart murmurs is not known, but these commonly occur temporarily during a fever, physical activity, pregnancy, or a period of rapid adolescent growth. The conditions that can cause such murmurs are anemia, or inadequate number of red blood cells to move oxygen throughout the body, and hyperthyroidism, or an excessive amount of thyroid hormone.

Abnormal heart murmurs signal a heart problem, and a very common cause is a congenital heart defect, or one present at birth, such as an impaired heart valve or a hole between two heart chambers. Risk factors that increase a baby's risk of developing a heart murmur are uncontrolled diabetes or rubella infection or using alcohol, drugs, and some prescription medications during the mother's pregnancy.

Damage to the heart valves (caused by mitral valve prolapse, mitral valve or aortic stenosis, aortic sclerosis and stenosis, and mitral or aortic regurgitation) are the usual cause in adults as a result of injury to the heart or disease, including heart attack, uncontrolled high blood pressure, and heart failure; rheumatic fever, endocarditis, and other infections; as well as the normal process of aging.

Risk factors may include an abnormally thick heart muscle that impedes the flow of blood, atherosclerotic heart disease, aortic aneurysm, and the connective tissue disorder systemic lupus erythematosus. Others are a family history of a heart defect, hyperthyroidism, pulmonary hypertension, rheumatoid arthritis, and cardiomyopathy.

Diagnosis

If a doctor hears a heart murmur during a physical exam, its loudness, location in the heart, and type of sound indicate if it is innocent. If it is not, diagnostic tools will determine its cause and severity. Echocardiography shows the heart structure, and Doppler echocardiography shows its blood flow. An electrocardiogram, commonly called an EKG, checks the heart's electrical activity. Blood tests may be taken to check for heart infections. An x-ray shows the heart's shape, size, and location of its large arteries and checks for congenital abnormalities, and a cardiac catheterization checks for defects.

Treatments

Innocent heart murmurs may disappear over time, or they may endure a lifetime without causing any health problems. Treatment depends on the underlying cause of an abnormal murmur. Heart valve problems may require medication to control blood pressure or an irregular heartbeat or to treat an infection, or surgery may be required to repair a valve or correct another type of defect.

Prevention

In general, heart murmurs, especially congenital, are not preventable. But managing high blood pressure or avoiding a heart valve infection may help prevent a murmur from developing. Because they are at high risk, people who have had rheumatic fever may be prescribed antibiotics when they get other infections; those at risk of the infection endocarditis are prescribed these medications before dental work or surgery takes place. Heart valve diseases cannot be cured with medications, but along with lifestyle changes, symptoms can be treated.

Prognosis and Outcomes

Mostly harmless and not a disease, an innocent heart murmur exhibits no symptoms that limits any physical or other activities. The prognosis for abnormal heart murmurs depends on the type and severity of the underlying heart problem.

Ray Marks

See also: Congestive Heart Failure; Heart Diseases; Heart Valve Disorders; Rheumatic Fever; Systemic Lupus Erythematosus

Further Reading

CardioSmart. American College of Cardiology. (2015). Heart murmur. Retrieved from https://www.cardiosmart.org/Heart-Conditions/Heart-Murmur.

Cleveland Clinic. (2015). Heart murmur. Retrieved from http://my.clevelandclinic.org/heart/disorders/valve/murmur2.aspx.

Mayo Clinic. (2015). Heart murmurs. Retrieved from http://www.mayoclinic.com/health/heart-murmurs/DS00727.

National Heart, Lung, and Blood Institute. (2012, September 12). What is a heart murmur? Retrieved from http://www.nhlbi.nih.gov/health/health-topics/topics/heartmurmur/.

HEART VALVE DISORDERS

Heart valves open and close at regular intervals to foster blood flow and to prevent blood flow from flowing backward. There are four heart valves—the aortic, the mitral, the tricuspid, and pulmonary valves. For the heart to function successfully, all four of its chambers must beat in an organized way, and the valves, which are thin flexible flaps of connective tissue, must let the blood flow in only one direction.

The two main types of problems that affect heart valves are stenosis and regurgitation or valvular insufficiency. In people with stenosis, their valve openings are usually too narrow and interfere with the forward flow of blood, so the heart may have to work harder to pump blood across the valve. In people with problems of regurgitation, the valves do not close properly and can produce leaks that cause a significant backflow of blood, which can also cause the heart to work too hard and eventually weaken over time.

Valve problems may be isolated to a single valve or can affect multiple valves. Roughly 90 percent of all valve disorders are chronic in nature, having developed slowly over time. The remaining 10 percent are usually caused by complications of recent heart attacks or infections and are considered acute.

Heart valve disease is diagnosed in about 5 million Americans each year.

Causes and Risk Factors

Heart valve problems may occur at birth, or after birth.

Genetic predisposition and family background of heart valve disorders may increase the risk of a congenital heart defect.

Other factors include the health of the mother during pregnancy and exposure to certain environmental factors, including health conditions such as diabetes, and use of certain drugs, such as lithium.

Heart valve disorders can also be acquired in response to aging, untreated rheumatic fever, a complication of untreated throat infection, inflammation and infection of the heart valves known as endocarditis due to a bacterium or fungus, autoimmune disorders, metabolic disorders, tumors of the digestive tract, injury, radiation therapy, syphilis, high blood pressure or coronary heart disease, arteriosclerosis, connective tissue disorders, overweight or obesity, or a condition seen in the elderly called idiopathic calcific aortic stenosis.

Signs and Symptoms

Many individuals with heart valve disorders may not experience symptoms if the condition is mild. In more severe cases, symptoms may vary depending on the nature of the valve or valves involved.

Some common symptoms

Chest pain
Cyanosis, where the skin becomes bluish
Dizziness
Fainting spells
Fatigue
Heart murmur
Palpitations
Rapid weight gain
Shortness of breath
Sweating
Swelling of the ankles, feet, or abdomen
Weakness

Diagnosis

Diagnosis includes a medical history; a physical examination; the use of diagnostic tests, such as an electrocardiogram; a chest x-ray; blood tests; an echocardiogram, or ultrasound of the heart; and cardiac catheterization or angiogram, radionuclide scan, or cardiac MRI to provide detailed images of the heart.

Treatment

Mild heart valve problems may require monitoring but no active treatment.

Those suffering from symptoms for which there is effective treatment may benefit from surgery to widen a narrowed valve, known as percutaneous balloon valvoplasty, or valvotomy, where the surgeon tries to separate valve components that are fused together (known as fused valve leaflets), remove, or reshape valve tissue, or add tissue. Replacing defective valves through total valve replacement, followed by anticoagulant medications that prolong the clotting time of blood, may be indicated depending on the severity of the disease, the person's age and general health, and need for other forms of heart surgery.

Blood thinning agents; diuretics, which remove fluid from the tissues and bloodstream; a low-salt diet; ACE inhibitors, which are a type of vasodilator used to treat high blood pressure and heart failure; and avoiding vigorous exercise and severe stress may be recommended in persons with mild symptoms.

Overall goals of treatment are to prevent, treat, or relieve symptoms of related heart conditions; protect the valves from further damage; or repair or replace faulty valves in life-threatening situations.

Prognosis

Problems with heart valves are generally irreversible and persist across the lifespan. They may worsen over time and be especially severe if the valves become infected. Surgery for improving the health status of those with heart valve disorders is generally successful, but many patients still have problems of breathlessness on exertion and reduced exercise tolerance.

Lifestyle changes and medications can relieve many of the symptoms and complications of heart valve disease.

Prevention

There is very little that can be done to prevent heart valve disorders. Pregnant women, however, can reduce the risk for their child by minimizing their use of alcohol.

Preventing the onset of rheumatic fever may also prove beneficial as may the prevention of infection in those with valve disease.

Ray Marks

See also: Coronary Artery Disease; Heart Disease; Heart Murmur; Liver Diseases; Rheumatic Fever

Further Reading

American Heart Association. (2015, August 26). Understanding heart valve problems and causes. Retrieved from http://www.heart.org/HEARTORG/Conditions/More/Heart ValveProblemsandDisease/Understanding-Heart-Valve-Problems-and-Causes_UCM _450360_Article.jsp#.Vj4d5GtKjwo.

Cleveland Clinic. (2014). Heart valve disease. Retrieved from http://my.clevelandclinic.org /services/heart/disorders/heart-valve-disease.

Johns Hopkins Medicine. (2015). Heart valve diseases. Retrieved from http://www .hopkinsmedicine.org/healthlibrary/conditions/cardiovascular_diseases/heart_valve _diseases_85,P00210/.

National Heart, Lung, and Blood Institute. (2015). What is heart valve disease? Retrieved from http://www.nhlbi.nih.gov/health/health-topics/topics/hvd.

HEMOCHROMATOSIS

Hemochromatosis is the most common disease stemming from a condition called iron overload. It causes the body to absorb and store too much iron. Instead of absorbing 10 percent of iron in foods eaten, those with hemochromatosis tend to absorb about 30 percent of the available iron. Over time, this may cause them to absorb and retain 20 times as much iron as the body needs. The extra iron that builds in the tissues of the body can damage the tissues and body organs. The condition most commonly affects Caucasians of northern European descent and is less common in other ethnic groups. In general, men develop symptoms between 30 and 50 years of age, while women develop the condition around 50 years of age.

If the disease is not treated, the individual can experience liver, heart, and pancreatic failure.

History

The condition gets its name from the term "hemo," meaning blood, and "chroma," meaning color.

Types

If hemochromatosis occurs as a primary condition, the disease is called hereditary hemochromatosis, and this occurs as an inherited disorder. If the disease arises due to another health condition such as anemia or alcoholism, then the condition is known as a secondary disorder.

The other two forms of the disease are neonatal hemochromatosis and juvenile hemochromatosis. In the neonatal form, the buildup of excess iron in the baby's liver can lead to death. In juvenile hemochromatosis, the presence of a severe iron overload can lead to liver and heart disease in young adults ages 15 to 30.

Symptoms

The most common problem of people with this condition is joint pain in the fingers, knees, hips, and ankles. Other symptoms include the following:

Abdominal pain, often on the right upper portion of the abdomen
Depression, disorientation, or memory problems
Enlarged liver
Fatigue
Heart problems
Impotence
Increased susceptibility to infections
Loss of body hair
Lack of energy
Loss of sex drive
Premature menopause
Skin darkening, known as bronzing
Stomach swelling
Weakness
Weight loss

Causes

Most forms of hemochromatosis are due to defective genetic regulation of iron absorption mechanisms of the body. Different types of hemochromatosis are due to different types of genetic defects or mutations and are commonly passed from parents to children.

Diagnosis

Diagnostic tools may include blood tests to measure the amount of iron in the blood attached to a protein called transferrin, another test that measures the amount of iron stored in the liver, a thorough medical history, a physical exam, a liver biopsy, and abdominal ultrasound. Genetic tests may be done to confirm the diagnosis.

Treatment

Hemochromatosis can be treated by removing the blood from the body of the affected individual to lower the iron level of the body—a process called *phlebotomy*. If this is not possible, certain medications can help the body expel some iron from the blood, and dietary changes may be recommended. Individual problems such as heart failure, liver failure, and arthritis will be treated separately as indicated.

Prevention

Early detection of the condition before organ damage has occurred may be helpful. Regular checkups and avoiding iron supplements, food with added iron, and vitamin C, which increases iron absorption, as well as avoiding using iron cookware, may help to reduce complications. For those with liver damage, avoiding alcohol and periodic screening for liver cancer may help. Shellfish, which can carry bacteria, should be avoided because people with hemochromatosis are susceptible to infections.

Prognosis and Outcome

If the disease is not detected early on, and treated, the accumulation of iron in the tissues can produce several health problems, including:

Abnormal skin pigmentation
Adrenal gland damage
Arthritis
Early menopause
Gall bladder disease
Heart abnormalities, such as congestive heart failure
Impotence
Liver cancer, cirrhosis, or failure
Pancreatic damage, which can cause diabetes
Skin color changes because too much iron can cause skin to appear gray or bronze in color
Thyroid deficiency

If the iron overload caused by hemochromatosis is detected early and treated before organ damage has occurred, the affected individual can lead a normal, healthy life.

Future

Because the genetic defect causing hemochromatosis is common, and early detection and treatment are effective, some researchers and advocacy groups have suggested widespread screening for hemochromatosis should be forthcoming. However, the genetic test for providing a definite diagnosis is very expensive for purposes of screening. The blood test, which is inexpensive, often requires repeated testing because it is not a perfect measure. Scientists are hoping they will better understand why the factors involved in iron metabolism, and how iron in excess, cause organ damage. Various research projects include examining how the gene that regulates iron levels produces the disease, how many people have this defective gene and go on to develop symptoms, and why some do not.

Ray Marks

See also: Iron Overload; Liver Diseases; Substance Abuse

Further Reading

American Liver Foundation. (2015, January 14). Hemochromatosis. Retrieved from http://www.liverfoundation.org/abouttheliver/info/hemochromatosis/.

Hemochromatosis.org. (2015). What is hemochromatosis? Retrieved from http://www.hemochromatosis.org/#overview.

Johns Hopkins Medicine. (2015). Hemochromatosis. Retrieved from http://www.hopkinsmedicine.org/healthlibrary/conditions/adult/digestive_disorders/hemochromatosis_22,Hemochromatosis/.

Mayo Clinic. (2015, February 18). Hemochromatosis. Retrieved from http://www.mayoclinic.org/diseases-conditions/hemochromatosis/basics/definition/con-20023606.

National Institute of Diabetes and Digestive and Kidney Diseases. (2014, March 19). Hemochromatosis. Retrieved from http://www.niddk.nih.gov/health-information/health-topics/liver-disease/hemochromatosis/Pages/facts.aspx.

HEMOPHILIA

Hemophilia is an inherited bleeding disorder in which the blood does not clot properly because it lacks enough clotting factor, or a protein that controls bleeding. Those with the disorder may bleed longer after an injury or surgery or bleed spontaneously or internally, which may damage bodily organs and tissues and be life-threatening. Hemophilia can range from mild to severe, depending on the amount of clotting factor present. The disorder is rare: Only about 1 in 5,000 boys are born with it, but it can occur among all racial and ethnic groups. About 20,000 males in the United States have hemophilia. Worldwide, an estimated 400,000 people have hemophilia.

Of the two types of hemophilia, most people have hemophilia A, caused by a lack or too little clotting factor VIII, and most people experience moderate or severe symptoms; it is also known as classic hemophilia or factor VIII deficiency. Less common hemophilia B, also known as Christmas disease or factor IX deficiency, is caused by lack or too little clotting factor IX. Treatment involves replacing insufficient clotting factor into the blood, usually by infusion, or administration through a vein. It is lifelong disorder that has no cure.

Symptoms

Symptoms of hemophilia A and B are the same, including big bruises; bleeding into muscles and joints; spontaneous bleeding; prolonged bleeding after being cut, tooth removal, or surgery; and prolonged bleeding, especially after an injury to the head. The extent of bleeding externally and internally depends on the severity of the disorder, which is based on the deficiency of the clotting factors. Moderately low levels may lead to bleeding only after surgery or trauma, while very low levels may lead to spontaneous bleeding, which is sudden bleeding inside the body for no obvious reason.

External symptoms may include bleeding in the mouth from a cut, from a bite, or from cutting or losing a tooth; nosebleeds; heavy bleeding from a small cut; and bleeding that resumes after stopping. Internal bleeding may include blood in the urine or stool; large bruises, indicating bleeding into the large muscles; and bleeding in the knees, elbows, or other joints without obvious injury. Bleeding in a joint can cause scarring, and repeated bleeds may lead to a loss of mobility, joint deformity, and susceptibility to further bleeding. Bleeding into the muscles of the legs can also be severely disabling. Internal bleeding in the brain is a severe complication that can occur after a small bump on the head or a more serious injury. Symptoms include long-lasting headaches or neck pain or stiffness, repeated vomiting, sleepiness, changes in behavior, sudden weakness or clumsiness in the arms or legs, problems walking, double vision, convulsions or seizures, and extreme fatigue.

Causes

The cause of hemophilia is a mutation in one of the genes that provides the instructions for making the clotting factor necessary to form blood clots; these genes are located on the X chromosome. Females have two X chromosomes, and males have one X and one Y. A male who has a hemophilia gene on his X chromosome will have hemophilia. A female with a hemophilia gene on only X chromosome is a carrier who can pass the mutated gene to her offspring.

Diagnosis

Hemophilia is diagnosed by testing with a blood sample to measure the level of clotting factor activity (factor VIII for hemophilia A; factor IX for hemophilia B) and the length of time for a clot to form, as well as a complete blood count. On average, hemophilia is diagnosed when a child is about nine months old because most babies do not experience injuries that would cause bleeding. Almost all children are diagnosed by age two, as they become more active, which may result in easily bruising and excessive bleeding from injuries. If a mother is a known carrier of hemophilia, prenatal testing can be done at 9 to 11 weeks by chorionic villus sampling (CVS) or by fetal blood sampling at 18 or more weeks. Family history can also help determine if relatives have had a bleeding disorder or have experienced symptoms.

Treatments

No treatments are known to cure hemophilia. Clotting factor replacement therapy is the most effective treatment. It involves the slow infusion of concentrates of the appropriate clotting factor either dripped or injected into a vein; with instruction and training, it can be done at home. Depending upon severity, replacement therapy may be given on demand or as a regular prophylactic to prevent bleeding. Other types of treatment include those to help stimulate or increase a person's own clotting factor and those to prevent clots from breaking down. Once it takes place, bleeding should be treated as quickly as possible to reduce pain and damage to the joints, muscles, and internal organs; also, less blood replacement product is needed. Prompt treatment also reduces the risk of life-threatening bleeding episodes and the severity of long-term joint damage. Acetaminophen is the preferred pain reliever because those containing aspirin or nonsteroidal anti-inflammatory drugs can lead to increased bleeding.

Prevention

Hemophilia is an inherited genetic disease that cannot be prevented. Genetic counseling can identify carriers who do not have symptoms, and prenatal counselors can explain the risk of having a child with the disorder.

Prognosis and Outcomes

Hemophilia is known as a lifelong disease. But with treatment and good self-care, most people with hemophilia can maintain active lives. Before concentrates of clotting factor were developed, those with hemophilia had a significantly decreased life expectancy; before the 1960s, it was age 11 for those with a severe case of the disorder. The current mortality rate for males with hemophilia is twice that of healthy males. Without treatment, most children with severe hemophilia die young.

Future

Medical researchers are working on ways to insert improved clotting factor genes into the cells of people with hemophilia so their blood will clot more effectively; others are examining the possibility of gene therapy to replace the defective genes in hemophilia. Some new treatment technologies are being tested, including genetically manufactured alternatives to clotting factors produced from little to no human blood products with high purity standards that would eliminate the possibility of infection. In the future, people with hemophilia may be able to continually infuse clotting factors under the skin or in pill form.

Ray Marks

See also: Bleeding Disorders; Genetics and Genomics; Men's Health

Further Reading

Mayo Clinic. (2014, September 26). Hemophilia. Retrieved from http://www.mayoclinic.org
    /diseases-conditions/hemophilia/basics/definition/con-20029824.

Jones, P. (2002). *Living with Haemophilia*, 5th ed. New York: Oxford University Press.

National Heart, Lung, and Blood Institute. (2013, July 13). What is hemophilia? Retrieved
    from http://www.nhlbi.nih.gov/health/health-topics/topics/hemophilia.

National Hemophilia Foundation. (2015). Bleeding disorders. Retrieved from http://www
    .hemophilia.org.

HEPATITIS

Hepatitis is a term used to describe the inflammation of the liver. It is frequently caused by viral infections, and there are five types of hepatitis: A, B, C, D, and E. The B and C types lead to chronic disease for millions of people and form the most common cause of liver cancer and liver cirrhosis. Hepatitis A and E are usually caused by eating contaminated foods or drinking contaminated water. Hepatitis B, C, and D are commonly transmitted through contact with infected individuals through direct contact or contact with tainted blood, blood products, or equipment. Hepatitis B can be passed from a mother to a baby at birth if the mother is infected and from an affected family member to a child. Drug or alcohol use can cause hepatitis, and on occasion it may occur due to autoimmune factors, where the body attacks its own tissues. The most common form is Hepatitis A. Hepatitis C kills more people, however, than AIDS/HIV.

About 250 million persons are said to be affected worldwide by hepatitis C, and another 300 million are carriers of hepatitis B. In the United States, hepatitis A still occurs, but not as frequently as in the past. The estimated 373,000 new infections in 1990 dropped to 143,000 by 2000, possibly as a result of the vaccination of children and people at risk for this health condition. The number of acute hepatitis B virus infections has also been declining each year, possibly also due widespread vaccination of children. However, up to 1.4 million people may have chronic hepatitis B, many of whom are unaware of their infection. There are fewer than 19,000 cases of hepatitis C in the United States currently.

The term *chronic hepatitis* is used to describe hepatitis that has existed for more than six months. It is not a single disease, but as outlined earlier, has several causes and is characterized by varying degrees of liver destruction and inflammation depending on the cause and the duration of this disease.

Symptoms

A person who is infected may show few or no symptoms. Symptoms that do occur may be mild and overlooked and may include jaundice of the skin and eyes, dark urine, itchy skin, nausea, appetite loss, vomiting, diarrhea, mild fever, weight loss, and abdominal pain. As the condition worsens, the individual may experience dizziness, drowsiness, an enlarged spleen, headaches, and hives, depending on the cause of the condition. People with chronic hepatitis may feel very fatigued.

Diagnosis

The diagnosis of hepatitis may include the use of physical examinations, laboratory tests including abdominal ultrasound, liver function tests, liver biopsy, and blood tests.

Treatments

Treatments for hepatitis depend on the type of problem. In some cases, such as for hepatitis A, there is no specific treatment. The physician may advise the patient to avoid alcohol and fatty foods, get plenty of rest, and eat a nutritious diet while they recuperate. Those with severe symptoms may have to be hospitalized for a short period. In cases of weight loss, high calorie diets may be recommended. Support groups for the different types of hepatitis, where people who are affected can interact with others, may be helpful.

In hepatitis B, rest, high-protein and -carbohydrate diets, and an antiviral agent called interferon may be used.

Hepatitis C may be treated with interferon and ribavirin medications.

There is no effective treatment for hepatitis D or E.

Prevention

You can prevent some forms of hepatitis through vaccination. Avoiding drug use and needle sharing, unprotected sex, and eating raw shellfish, plus hand-washing and avoiding tattoos or body piercing with unsterilized needles are recommended.

Prognosis and Outcomes

On occasion, hepatitis may disappear spontaneously. It can be effectively treated in some cases with drugs. In others, it may last a lifetime.

Complications include liver cancer, liver failure, scarring of the liver tissues, and permanent liver damage in long-term cases.

Future

A gene-based vaccine engineered to stimulate the body's immune system to prevent hepatitis C is being developed.

An experimental drug called *telaprevir* is showing good results in trials where the goal is to eliminate hepatitis C in the bloodstream.

Ray Marks

See also: Abdominal Diseases; Liver Cancer; Liver Diseases; Vaccines

Further Reading

Centers for Disease Control and Prevention. (2015, May 31). Viral hepatitis. Retrieved from http://www.cdc.gov/hepatitis/.

National Institute of Diabetes and Digestive and Kidney Diseases. (2012, April 23). Viral hepatitis: A through E and beyond. Retrieved from http://www.niddk.nih.gov/health-information/health-topics/liver-disease/viral-hepatitis-a-through-e/pages/facts.aspx.

World Health Organization. (2015, July). What is hepatitis? Retrieved from http://www.who.int/features/qa/76/en/.

HERPES

The term *herpes* refers to a large number of diseases in humans and other animals caused by one of more than a dozen different viruses. Eight of those diseases affecting humans are caused by viruses classified as human herpesvirus 1 through 8, which are responsible for diseases such as chickenpox and shingles (human herpesvirus 4), infectious mononucleosis (human herpesvirus 5), and Kaposi's sarcoma (human herpesvirus 8).

The two sexually transmitted forms of the disease are caused by human herpesvirus 1 and 2, better known as herpes simplex virus type 1 and type 2 (HSV-1 and HSV-2). HSV-1 and HSV-2 are very similar to each other, sharing about 50 percent of their DNA. The most important difference between the two types is their preferred sites in the body. HSV-1 most commonly resides in nerve cells near the ear, while HSV-2 tends to become established in nerve tissue at the base of the spine. When HSV-1 becomes active, it most commonly causes the painful but relatively harmless condition known as cold sores or fever blisters. When HSV-2 becomes active, it is responsible for the development of the condition known as genital herpes, a painful infection of the genital area. Either form of the virus can cause an infection in either part of the body, although the distribution described here tends to be most common.

As with all sexually transmitted infections (STIs), herpes infections are spread by intimate contact between an infected person and an uninfected person. The first signs of the disease include blister-like sores that may be very painful and may be accompanied by fever and flu-like symptoms. In many cases, symptoms do not appear, and a person may not be aware that she or he has been infected with the virus. According to some estimates, more than one in five American adults have been infected with HSV-2 at some time in their lives, most of whom are not aware of that fact.

The incubation period for the disease is about two weeks, and any sores that appear tend to disappear another two to four weeks later. As with other STIs, the disappearance of symptoms is not an indication that the disease has been cured, however. Instead, the viruses responsible for the disease remain embedded in nerve tissue and may become activated again at a future date. The number and severity of additional outbreaks vary significantly from person to person and appear to be dependent on three major factors: (1) the severity of the first outbreak (i.e., the ability of a person's immune system to combat the first appearance of the virus), (2) the length of time a person has been infected (the number and severity of infections tend to decrease over time), and (3) the variety of virus causing the infection (HSV-1–caused genital herpes tends to be less severe than HSV-2–caused genital herpes).

Genital herpes tends to receive bad press from the general public, largely because people are embarrassed to have sexual partners or others find out about their condition. From a medical standpoint, however, the disease is usually no more serious (although just as uncomfortable and inconvenient) as a cold sore. Somewhat uncommonly, genital herpes may progress to more serious conditions and, perhaps, may be associated with increased risk for other viral infections, especially HIV/AIDS. The most serious consequence of genital herpes is potential infection of a newborn child during birth to a woman with the infection, a condition that is potentially fatal for the child.

There is currently no cure for genital herpes, although medications are available to relieve its symptoms. Three commonly recommended drugs are the antivirals famciclovir, acyclovir, and valacyclovir.

David E. Newton

See also: Kaposi's Sarcoma; Sexually Transmitted Diseases; Shingles

Further Reading

Centers for Disease Control and Prevention. (2014). Genital herpes. CDC fact sheet. Retrieved from http://www.cdc.gov/std/herpes/stdfact-herpes.htm.

Fortenbury, J. (2014, July 14). The overblown stigma of genital herpes. *The Atlantic.* Retrieved from http://www.theatlantic.com/health/archive/2014/07/the-overblown-stigma -of-genital-herpes/374757/.

Mayo Clinic. (2015, May 15). Cold sore. http://www.mayoclinic.org/diseases-conditions /cold-sore/basics/causes/con-20021310.

MedlinePlus. U.S. National Library of Medicine. (2014). Herpes simplex. Retrieved from https://www.nlm.nih.gov/medlineplus/herpessimplex.html.

HODGKIN DISEASE

The condition known as Hodgkin disease is a type of cancer that affects lymph tissue found in several regions of the body, including the liver, spleen, bone marrow, and lymph nodes; it starts in white blood cells known as lymphocytes. Once the disease starts, it can affect any of these areas as it spreads, as well as the lungs. There is no noncancerous form of Hodgkin disease—all forms of the disease are cancerous or malignant and can reduce the body's ability to fight infection. It is also known as Hodgkin lymphoma.

Both children as well as adults can develop Hodgkin disease. It is more common in Caucasians than African Americans and in males compared to females. Estimated cases in the United States in 2012 were 9,060, with 1,190 deaths.

Types

There are two types of lymphoma, Hodgkin disease and non-Hodgkin disease, and the two different forms of Hodgkin disease are called *classic Hodgkin disease*, which includes several subtypes, and *nodular predominant Hodgkin disease*.

Classic or classical Hodgkin disease represents about 95 percent of all cases in developed countries. Its four subtypes are based on the types of cells involved in the disease and include:

- Nodular sclerosis Hodgkin disease, which is the most common and mainly occurs in younger people
- Mixed cellularity Hodgkin disease, the second most common type, mostly found in adults
- Lymphocyte-rich Hodgkin disease, which is rare, and accounts for 5 percent of diseases cases
- Lymphocyte-depleted Hodgkin disease, making up 1 percent cases

Nodular lymphocyte predominant Hodgkin disease accounts for about 5 percent of Hodgkin disease and is more common in men than women. It usually involves the neck and armpit lymph nodes, and contains large cells known as popcorn cells.

History

Hodgkin disease is named after Dr. Thomas Hodgkin, who recognized this disease in 1832. In the 20th century, the disease was renamed Hodgkin lymphoma after it was realized the disease was a cancer of the lymph system.

Symptoms

The first sign of Hodgkin disease may be an enlargement or swelling of a lymph node, very often in the upper part of the body, such as the chest, neck, or arm pits. There may also be a fever coupled with chills, appetite and weight loss, sweating at night, coughing, trouble breathing or chest pain, increased sensitivity to the effects of alcohol or lymph node pain after drinking, and itchiness of the skin.

Causes

There is no known cause of this condition. Risk factors include age either 15 to 35 or over 55; a family history of lymphoma; being male; previous Epstein-Barr infections; and having a weakened immune system, especially those who have HIV.

Diagnosis

The diagnosis of Hodgkin disease is commonly verified using a biopsy that involves removing a small quantity of tissue and examining the cells of the tissue under the microscope. Other tests may involve a physical examination; blood tests; imaging tests such as x-rays, CT scans, or MRIs to stage the disease; bone marrow testing; or biopsy to check for cancer in the bone marrow.

Stages of the disease include:

Stage 1, where the disease is limited to one lymph node area or organ; survival rates are 90 percent.

Stage II, which involves two different lymph nodes or a portion of tissue or organ plus lymph nodes; it also has a 90 percent survival rate five years after diagnosis.

Stage III, occurs when the cancer affects lymph nodes above and below the diaphragm; it has an 84 percent five-year survival rate.

Stage IV, the most advanced stage, where several portions of more than one region and lymph nodes are affected; there is a 65 percent survival rate.

Refractory or *recurrent Hodgkin disease* are terms used when the disease either does not respond to initial therapy or has responded but has come back after being treated, respectively.

Treatments

The treatment will depend on the stage of the disease and how far it has spread, as well as age and tumor size. The key treatments involved in treating Hodgkin's disease are vaccine therapy, chemotherapy, and radiation therapy.

Prevention

No form of prevention is yet identified.

Prognosis and Outcomes

If Hodgkin disease is diagnosed early on, and treated, it can be cured. Patients are recommended to have regular checkups after treatment. They may, however, have an increased risk of developing other cancers later in life, especially leukemia.

Future

Stem cell transplant is a method for replacing diseased bone marrow with healthy stem cells. The affected person's own blood stem cells are removed, frozen, and stored. High-dose chemotherapy and radiation are used to destroy the cancerous tissue; then the stem cells are thawed and returned to the patient's body to build healthy bone marrow.

A new drug called Adcetris is being used to treat patients whose disease has progressed after stem cell therapy or those who have had two chemotherapy treatments but are not eligible for stem cell transplantation.

Other areas of research include a search for the causes of Hodgkin lymphoma, treatment using biological therapy, and combinations of drugs.

Ray Marks

See also: Brain Cancer; Cancer Survivorship; Childhood Cancer; Leukemia; Lymphoma; Non-Hodgkin Lymphoma

Further Reading

American Cancer Society. (2015, March 4). What is Hodgkin disease? Retrieved from http://www.cancer.org/cancer/hodgkindisease/detailedguide/hodgkin-disease-what-is-hodgkin-disease.

Mayo Clinic. (2014, August 15). Hodgkin's lymphoma. Retrieved from http://www.mayoclinic.org/diseases-conditions/hodgkins-lymphoma/basics/definition/con-20030667.

National Cancer Institute. (2015). Lymphoma—for patients. Retrieved from http://www.cancer.gov/types/lymphoma.

HPV (HUMAN PAPILLOMAVIRUS)

Papillomaviruses are viruses that are widely distributed throughout animal species. Human papillomavirus, or HPV, is the virus that infects humans. HPV commonly causes proliferations at cutaneous and mucosal surfaces. HPV is transmitted sexually and is the most common STD in the United States. The Centers for Disease Control and Prevention states that almost all sexually active people will have HPV at some point in their lives. Infections with HPV are generally not serious and may go away with time, but because HPV can also cause cancer, prevention, such as vaccines for young people and screening for cervical cancer through performing the Pap test, are extremely important and life-saving.

Types of HPV

There are more than 100 types of different HPV. There are more than 40 HPV types that infect the central areas of males and females. Some infect cutaneous sites, while others infect mucosal surfaces. This includes the cervix, vagina, vulva, rectum, urethra, penis, and anus. HPV can also infect the mouth and throat. People who are infected may not know it. A person can be infected with more than one type of HPV.

How Do You Get HPV?

HPV is passed through genital and skin-to-skin contact, which includes vaginal, anal, and oral contact. Sexual behavior is the most common way of acquiring this infection.

HPV is more common in:

- Sexually active men and women
- Men who have sex with men
- Women and men with multiple sex partners
- Women

The growth of the infection is approximately eight months. The virus may remain in a dormant state and won't be detected. It can reactivate many years later. If and when acquired, it can be fought off by the body immune system within two years.

Symptoms of HPV include genital warts and warts in throat (RRP). Other types of HPV cause normal cells to turn abnormal, which may lead to cervical cancer and other HPV-related cancers of the throat, vulva, vagina, penis, anus, head, and neck. HPV that causes warts is not the same as the HPV that causes cancer.

Prevention

Methods of prevention from contracting HPV include refraining from sexual activity, being familiar with the health of sexual partners, and using condoms. More significant, there are now vaccines that can prevent cancer caused by HPV. The Centers for Disease Control and Prevention (CDC) recommends that all boys and girls ages 11 or 12 years be vaccinated. And catch-up vaccines are recommended for males through age 21 and for females through age 26 if they did not get vaccinated when they were younger (National Institute of Allergy and Infectious Diseases 2014). This vaccine has been controversial among some parents who believe that receiving it encourages sexual behavior at much too young an age; doctors and researchers say that it simply protects children from contracting HPV, which, because the virus can lead to cancer, is a very good step to take. A study in 2016 in the journal *Pediatrics* found that the rate of HPV infection was reduced by 64 percent among 14- to 19-year-old girls when they had received the vaccine (Markowitz et al. 2016).

HPV can lead to cancer—primarily cervical cancer, but also other cancers in the genital area as well as the anus, the back of the throat, the tonsils, and the tongue. Regular cervical cancer screenings are still necessary for both vaccinated and unvaccinated women because

1. The vaccine provides protection against all types of HPV that causes cervical cancer.
2. Women may not receive the full benefits of the vaccine if they do not complete the vaccine series.
3. Women may not receive the full benefits of the vaccine if they receive the vaccine after they already acquired a vaccine HPV type.

HPV and Genital Warts

Genital warts are caused by genital HPV, which is very common in sexually active men and women. There are 40 types of genital HPV. The presence of genital warts is not associated with the development of cervical cancer.

Screening

The American Cancer Society states that screening should begin approximately three years after vaginal intercourse but no later than age 21. A Pap test should be done annually or every two to three years for women 30 and younger. For genital warts, a visual inspection can be done and be confirmed by having a biopsy done.

Treatment

There are no treatments for HPV, only treatments for the conditions it causes. The immune system may fight off the infection naturally, but sometimes HPV does not go away on its own.

If left untreated, signs of HPV such as genital warts may go away on their own, increase in size or number, or remain unchanged. For the removal of warts, consult a physician.

Prescribed treatments include Podofilox solution or gel, Imiguimod cream, Trichloracetic acid, and Podophylin resin, which can be prescribed by a health care provider. Treating genital warts will not stop transmission of the virus to other people sexually.

Ray Marks

See also: Cervical Cancer; Sexually Transmitted Diseases; Squamous Cell Carcinoma; Vaccines; Women's Health

Further Reading

American Academy of Pediatrics. (2015, August 20). Human papillomavirus (HPV). Retrieved from https://www.healthychildren.org/English/health-issues/vaccine-preventable-diseases/Pages/Human-Papillomavirus-%28HPV%29.aspx.

American Cancer Society. (2014, December 12). What is HPV? Retrieved from http://www.cancer.org/cancer/cancercauses/othercarcinogens/infectiousagents/hpv/humanpapillomavirusandhpvvaccinesfaq/hpv-faq-what-is-hpv.

Centers for Disease Control and Prevention. (2015, September 30). Human papillomavirus (HPV). Retrieved from http://www.cdc.gov/hpv/parents/whatishpv.html.

Holpuch, A. (2016, February 22). HPV rates drop 64% in decade since recommended CDC vaccination. *The Guardian.* Retrieved from http://www.theguardian.com/us-news/2016/feb/22/hpv-rates-drop-vaccination-cdc-human-papillomavirus.

Markowitz, L. E., Liu, G., Hariri, S., Steinau, M., Dunne, E. F., & Unger, E. R. (2016, March). Prevalence of HPV after introduction of the vaccination program in the United States. *Pediatrics.* Retrieved from http://pediatrics.aappublications.org/content/early/2016/02/19/peds.2015-1968.

National Institute of Allergy and Infectious Diseases. (2014, January 23). Genital HPV infection—fact sheet. Retrieved from http://www.niaid.nih.gov/topics/genitalwarts/Pages/default.aspx.

U.S. Food and Drug Administration. (2015, September 28). HPV (human papillomavirus). Retrieved from http://www.fda.gov/ForConsumers/ByAudience/ForWomen/ucm118530.htm.

HYPERLIPIDEMIA

Overview and Facts

Hyperlipidemia is a term used to describe an excessive amount of fat or fats known as *lipids* in the blood. The condition can be caused either as a result of genetic factors or as a result of dietary factors or the presence of underlying diseases such as obesity.

At appropriate levels, lipids perform important body functions, but in excess, they can cause health problems. The two key fats involved in this condition are cholesterol and triglycerides. An excess amount of a certain type of cholesterol known as "bad cholesterol" or low-density lipoprotein can lead to blockages of the blood vessels if this occurs in excessive amounts, and this subcategory of hyperlipidemia is called hypercholesterolemia. The other subcategory of hyperlipidemia is called hypertriglyceridemia, which is due to high levels of triglycerides in the blood. High levels of low-density lipoprotein increase the risk for heart attacks, regardless of gender, age, or race. High triglyceride levels can increase the risk for hardening of the arteries and coronary heart disease.

Risk factors other than genetics and diet associated with hypercholesterolemia are hypothyroidism, pregnancy, and kidney failure.

Risk factors for hypertriglyceridemia include obesity, excess intake of alcohol, diabetes, smoking, and certain medications such as estrogen.

You have an increased chance for developing hyperlipidemia if you are a male over age 45 or a female older than 55. If a close relative had early onset of heart disease, you may have an increased risk as well. Inactivity, higher age, environment, sugary drinks, being ethnic and adopting a Western diet, and smoking are additional risk factors.

Evidence suggests children with high cholesterol may develop high cholesterol levels as adults, especially if there is a family history of this condition.

Symptoms

The condition of hyperlipidemia may go unnoticed and may only be discovered in a routine medical examination. Individuals who suffer from this condition as a result of genetic factors may, however, exhibit fatty deposits under the skin in the ankle region or under the eyes known as xanthomas. People with very high levels of triglyceride in their blood may develop pancreatitis, or inflammation of the pancreas, and exhibit pimple-like lesions over large areas of their body.

Diagnosis

The standard methods for detecting hypercholesterolemia are physical examinations, blood tests to develop a lipid profile, and a medical history.

Treatments

Treatment is based on what type of lipid appears to be too high and or/if there are secondary health conditions contributing to the problem. Making healthy food choices, weight reduction, avoiding or limiting alcohol intake, controlling your blood pressure, getting periodic health checks, and increasing exercise levels are commonly recommended strategies for lowering high cholesterol. Medication to reduce cholesterol is said to be effective in conjunction with health eating and exercise. Other medications may be used to treat hypertriglyceridemia.

Prevention

Consulting a physician to analyze blood lipid level can help prevent selected problems associated with hyperlipidemia and help direct the physician provide the right type of treatment to prevent or slow the progression of any disease. For example, those with high triglyceride levels may benefit from not using alcohol, whereas those with high cholesterol may benefit from small daily alcohol doses.

The National Cholesterol Education Program in the United States suggests people get tested for cholesterol every five years.

Teaching children healthy dietary and exercise behaviors may prevent problems later on.

Prognosis and Outcomes

Hyperlipidemia is reversible in many cases if a healthy diet and exercise are pursued.

Ray Marks

See also: Cholesterol; Coronary Artery Disease; Heart Disease; Hypothyroidism; Kidney Failure

Further Reading

American Heart Association. (2012). Hyperlipidemia. Retrieved from http://www.heart.org/HEARTORG/Conditions/Cholesterol/AboutCholesterol/Hyperlipidemia_UCM_434965_Article.jsp.

Cincinnati Children's. (2012). Hyperlipidemia/cholesterol problems in children. Retrieved from http://www.cincinnatichildrens.org/health/h/hyperlipidemia/.

Mayo Clinic. (2011). High cholesterol. Retrieved from http://www.mayoclinic.com/health/high-blood-cholesterol/DS00178.

North Shore Pediatric Therapy. (2012). What is hyperlipidemia. Retrieved from http://nspt4kids.com/health-topics-conditions/hyperlipidemia-2/.

HYPEROPIA

Hyperopia (farsightedness) is a common vision problem in which a person is able to see distant objects with clarity but has blurred sight when focusing on objects that are nearby. Many people have some degree of farsightedness; in the United States alone, more than 12 million people ages 40 and up are afflicted with the issue, and statistics show it to be among the most common vision problems in children. Altogether, some 5 to 10 percent of the U.S. population has hyperopia. The condition is usually present from birth and tends to be genetic, although some people do not experience any vision problems until later in life.

Hyperopia is a type of refractive error, which means that the eye shape prevents the light entering the eye from focusing correctly and forming clear images. Typically, hyperopia occurs because the eyeball is shorter than normal; however, the problem can also occur if the cornea (the clear surface on the front of the eyeball) does not curve as much as it should or if the lens is abnormally shaped. In a person with hyperopia, images focus behind the retina rather than on the retina as they would in a person with normal vision. In addition to having blurred vision when focusing on close-up objects, a person with hyperopia may also experience headaches or eyestrain after spending a prolonged period of time focusing on such close tasks as reading or drawing. Another potential sign of hyperopia is squinting to try to focus more clearly.

An eye care professional can usually detect hyperopia through a basic eye exam. To confirm a diagnosis, a more complete exam is often conducted, at which time the eye is dilated with special eye drops and a bright light and specialized magnifying glass are used to examine the retina. Once farsightedness has been determined, a specific course of treatment will be decided. In many cases, younger people do not require any medical intervention because their eyes are still flexible and their eyesight is still strong enough to compensate for the hyperopia. In adults and those who cannot compensate, corrective lenses are typically recommended. Such lenses include eyeglasses and a variety of contact lenses. In recent years, several refractive surgical procedures have also become popular in the treatment of farsightedness. LASIK or LASEK surgeries both use specialized lasers to reshape all or part of the cornea and correct vision. Another surgery called photorefractive keratectomy can also be used to correct hyperopia. This procedure involves removing the cornea's protective cover, called the epithelium, and allowing it to grow back naturally to conform to a reshaped cornea. If the surgical procedures are successful, patients will no longer need corrective lenses. But they do come with risk of such issues as infection, overcorrection or undercorrection of the vision problem, and in rare cases, total vision loss.

Tamar Burris

See also: Colorblindness; Diabetes, Type 1; Eye Diseases; Glaucoma; Macular Degeneration; Myopia; Sjögren's Syndrome

Further Reading

Adams, N. (2014). *Healthy Vision: Prevent and Reverse Eye Disease through Better Nutrition.* Guilford, CT: Lyons Press.

American Optometric Association. (2015). Hyperopia (farsightedness). Retrieved from http://www.aoa.org/patients-and-public/eye-and-vision-problems/glossary-of-eye-and-vision-conditions/hyperopia?sso=y.

Kellogg Eye Center. (2015). Hyperopia (farsightedness). Retrieved from http://www.kellogg.umich.edu/patientcare/conditions/hyperopia.html.

Kitchen, C. K. (2007). *Fact and Fiction of Healthy Vision: Eye Care for Adults and Children.* Westport, CT: Praeger.

Mayo Clinic. (2015). Farsightedness. Retrieved from http://www.mayoclinic.org/diseases-conditions/farsightedness/basics/definition/con-20027486.

HYPERTENSION (HIGH BLOOD PRESSURE)

Overview

High blood pressure (BP), or *hypertension*, is a common condition afflicting approximately 75 million teens and adults in the United States. A common name for this condition is hypertension. No known symptoms are associated with hypertension, hence the nickname "silent killer." Two classes of hypertension exist: essential and secondary. About 95 percent of high blood pressures cases with unknown causes are classified as *essential hypertension*. Direct causes of hypertension are termed *secondary hypertension*. Promotion of a healthy lifestyle and pharmacologic medications provide treatment options for those diagnosed with hypertension.

History

Greek and Egyptian physicians more than 2,000 years ago inferred blood circulated through the body. The theory of circulation posited by the physicians challenged future scientists to identify the source that propelled blood. The source that drives blood was proven to be pressure and quantified in the late 19th century. Carl Ludwig recorded the first human blood pressure in 1847 using a catheter hooked to a kymograph. This recording inspired noninvasive techniques captured by the sphygmomanometer, by Samuel Karl Ritter von Basch in 1881, and Scipione Riva-Rocci improved the invention in 1896 by adding an inflatable cuff. Normal blood pressure went mainstream in American after neurosurgeon Harvey Cushing returned from Italy with a plan to standardize blood pressure. In 1905, Nikolai Korotkoff developed the method to capture sounds in the arteries to determine blood pressure that medical personnel apply today.

Types

Essential hypertension develops over time with no identifiable symptoms of high blood pressure. A combination of factors and conditions may contribute to essential hypertension occurrence. Secondary hypertension develops from known medical conditions or medications that cause high blood pressure. Some diseases are kidney disease, changes in hormone levels, narrowing of arteries, various pills (birth control, diet, and cold medications), pregnancy, and congenital defects in blood vessels.

A normal blood pressure recognized by the medical community is below 120/80 mmHg. *Systolic blood pressure* (SBP) represents the top number and contraction and bottom number denotes relaxation of the heart termed *diastolic blood pressure* (DBP). Cardiovascular or kidney disease may develop if changes in pressure increase in either.

Table 5   Blood Pressure Classification

Blood Pressure Classification	Systolic Blood Pressure (mmHg)	Diastolic Blood Pressure (mmHg)
Normal	Below 120	Below 80
Prehypertension	120–139	80–89
Stage 1 hypertension	140–159	90–99
Stage 2 hypertension	160 or higher	100 or higher

Table 5 displays the classification and management of blood pressure for adults adapted from National Heart, Lung, and Blood Institute. (2015, September 10). Description of high blood pressure. http://www.nhlbi.nih.gov/health/health-topics/topics/hbp.

Symptoms

Generally, high blood pressure patients display no signs or symptoms. Signs of dull headaches or dizzy spells may be associated with early-stage high blood pressure. Malignant hypertension represents a severe or even life-threating form of high blood pressure that exhibits more than normal symptoms such as

Severe headache
Nausea or vomiting
Confusion
Changes in vision
Nosebleeds

Causes

High blood pressure displays no identifiable symptoms for most adults with primary (essential) hypertension. The cause is multifactorial and accounts for about 95 percent of primary hypertension cases. For example, high intake of salt (5.8 g/ daily) in groups or societies has been recognized as a potential cause. Furthermore, prominence of genetic factors may contribute, but more evidence is needed to substantiate. Secondary hypertension accounts for about 5 percent and causes kidney problems, adrenal gland tumors, and certain birth defects, and certain medications and illegal drugs pose problems. Specific disorders are associated with a particular organ or blood vessels stimulate secondary hypertension to take place. Risk factors associated with hypertension include:

- Age
- Race
- Family history
- Being overweight
- Physical inactivity
- Tobacco use
- High salt intake

- Stress
- Low vitamin D levels
- High alcohol consumption
- Low potassium intake
- Chronic conditions

According to the American Heart Association, more than 40 percent of non-Hispanic blacks have high blood pressure. African Americans suffer disproportionately from high blood pressure and start showing it earlier in life. There may be a gene that causes people of African ancestry to be hypersensitive to salt, which raises their blood pressure (American Heart Association 2014).

Diagnosis

To be classified as hypertensive, a blood pressure reading of 140/90 mmHg must occur on two separate occasions as recorded by a physician. The top number represents the pressure in the arteries when the heart contracts (systolic pressure). The second number indicates the pressure between beats (relaxation). Physicians may perform a variety of tests using different equipment to assess and measure heart and kidney disease, electrolyte and sugar levels, and cholesterol levels. If there is no health care provider, individuals can invest in a well-fitted blood pressure device to measure blood pressure.

Treatment

The main treatments for hypertension are medications or lifestyle changes or both. Medications attempt to use various classes of drugs to treat blood pressure with such drugs as ACE inhibitors, ARB drugs, beta-blockers, diuretics, calcium channel blockers, alpha blockers, and peripheral vasodilators. These drugs may be used in combination with one another or simply alone, but individual characteristics determine the effects patients receive from the medications.

Prevention

Most effective way to combat hypertension is through lifestyle changes—specifically, by paying attention to foods consumed and participation in regular exercise program. Maintenance of a healthy body weight coupled with reduce intake of salt and alcohol deliver lower blood pressure and improve activities of daily living for patients. More importantly, management of stress and incorporation of relaxation techniques help minimize high blood pressure. Symptoms for essential hypertension rarely appear until patients produce a heart attack or stroke or until kidney failure develops. Regular health checkups are important for early detection of hypertension. Patient education that provides repeated in-depth discussions grouped with counseling that encourage lifestyle modification helps to combat hypertension.

Prognosis and Outcomes

The effects of untreated hypertension affect mortality and morbidity rates. A 30 percent risk of atherosclerosis and 50 percent organ damage appear with 8 to 10 years if left untreated. The mortality rate of ischemic heart and stroke disease doubles for every 20 mmHg (systolic) and 10 mmHg (diastolic) increase BP over 115/75 mmHg.

Future

Hypertension arises from many factors that trigger complications in a multitude of areas throughout the human body. Pharmacologic therapy is one method to control high blood pressure. High blood pressure is considered a modifiable risk factor or disorder. The maintenance of a normal body weight through nutrient-dense food and increased regular physical activity make up the necessary ingredients for improved quality of life for individuals living with hypertension. The adequate intake of vitamins and minerals and the avoidance of illicit drugs, limited alcohol use, and limited (or no) cigarette smoking not only reduce hypertension, but also the increased risk of developing cardiovascular or pulmonary diseases.

Ray Marks

See also: Angina; Arrhythmias/Dysrhythmias; Atherosclerosis; Cardiomyopathy; Circulation Disorders; Coronary Artery Disease; Heart Diseases; Prediabetes; Stroke

Further Reading

American Heart Association. (2014). High blood pressure and African Americans. Retrieved from http://www.heart.org/HEARTORG/Conditions/HighBloodPressure/UnderstandYo urRiskforHighBloodPressure/High-Blood-Pressure-and-African-Americans_UCM _301832_Article.jsp#.VtdcBeba5Bk.

Cunha, J. P., & Marks, J. W. (2012). High blood pressure (hypertension). Retrieved from http://www.medicinenet.com/high_blood_pressure/article.htm.

MacGill, M. (2015). Hypertension: Causes, symptoms, and treatments. *Medical News Today.* Retrieved from: http://www.medicalnewstoday.com/articles/150109.php.

Mayo Clinic. (2012). High blood pressure (hypertension). Retrieved from http://www .mayoclinic.com/health/high-blood-pressure/DS00100.

U.S. National Library of Medicine. (2015). High blood pressure (hypertension). Retrieved from http://www.ncbi.nlm.nih.gov/pubmedhealth/PMH0001502/.

HYPOGLYCEMIA

Often called low blood sugar, hypoglycemia occurs when the glucose level in the blood is abnormally low. Glucose is absorbed into the bloodstream from foods rich in carbohydrates, including bread, rice, and potatoes, as well as fruits, milk products, and sweets. The hormone insulin helps convert it to energy before it enters the cells. Excess glucose gets stored in the liver and muscles, where it will be broken down later and used as energy. Usually, when the glucose level starts to drop, more is released into the bloodstream, and it rises to a normal level. But for those with hypoglycemia, it can remain dangerously low, leading to hunger, trembling, weakness, nausea, pale skin, or sweating.

Rather than a disease itself, hypoglycemia suggests other problems. People with diabetes, including teens, are at risk because their bodies do not produce enough or respond properly to insulin. But hypoglycemia can affect people who do not have diabetes, too.

Symptoms

Individuals react differently to the symptoms of hypoglycemia, which are wide and varied. Common symptoms include heart palpitations, weakness, fatigue, paleness, anxiety, sweating, hunger, anxiety, nightmares, trembling, mouth tingling, and irritability. Signs of worsening hypoglycemia are confusion, impaired vision, seizures, or losing consciousness or appearing intoxicated.

Causes

Diabetes is a common cause of hypoglycemia, which happens when someone with this condition takes too much insulin to regulate blood sugar levels.

In people who do not have diabetes, other conditions or illnesses can cause a drop in blood sugar, resulting in two types: reactive hypoglycemia, which takes place a few hours after eating, and fasting hypoglycemia, which often points to a disorder or disease.

While definitive causes of reactive hypoglycemia are under debate, research suggests that some people exhibit hormonal sensitivity or deficiencies. Uncommon but recognized causes include stomach surgery and rare enzyme deficiencies.

Some underlying causes of fasting hypoglycemia include medications (including those for diabetes); alcohol, especially excessive amounts; serious infections or liver, heart, or kidney illnesses; hormone deficiencies; and tumors in the pancreas, the organ that produces insulin.

Diagnosis

A rapid diagnosis is recommended for all types of suspected hypoglycemia, and the only accurate way a health care provider can make one is with a blood test that measures glucose levels at the time symptoms are present. If it indicates low blood sugar, additional lab tests may be used to determine diseases or other reasons for the symptoms.

A full physical exam—including medical history, medications, and alcohol use—will contribute to the diagnosis. Specific hypoglycemic symptoms will also be examined for frequency and severity, as well as their timing, particularly if they occur after meals high in sugar or if they disappear quickly after ingesting sugar. A rise in glucose that occurs after eating confirms a diagnosis of reactive hypoglycemia. A blood sample showing low glucose after fasting, between meals, or following physical activity diagnoses fasting hypoglycemia.

Treatment

The underlying cause of hypoglycemia determines what kind of treatment will be effective, but it is necessary to get treatment no matter the cause. Immediate treatment addresses the symptoms that come on quickly. For people with diabetes, eating something with sugar or drinking fruit juice, then ingesting cereal, bread, rice, or other carbohydrate food usually helps stabilize glucose levels. If necessary, someone can apply honey or jam inside the cheeks of a person having a hypoglycemic attack. Relief usually occurs within 20 minutes.

When another underlying cause is at work, such as in fasting hypoglycemia, treatment will be focused there. Depending on the cause, it could mean changing medication, surgery, or hormone therapy. Reactive hypoglycemia can be relieved by eating a little every few hours, including a wide variety of foods except those high in sugar, and engaging in physical activity.

Prevention

People with diabetes can prevent the onset of hypoglycemia by careful management of their insulin and medications, as well as by following an eating schedule, adding exercise, monitoring glucose regularly, and staying within the limits of alcohol consumption set by a doctor and eating after consuming alcohol. For those who do not have diabetes, prevention calls for identifying the underlying cause and getting the appropriate treatment. Other measures involve a regular eating routine, including small meals throughout the day and eating carbohydrates before exercising; measuring glucose regularly to learn the signs of a possible impending attack; and avoiding excessive alcohol, which can be a trigger.

Medical experts recommend carrying identification that lets emergency personnel, health care providers, friends and family, colleagues, and others know about the condition so they will be able to care for a person who is experiencing an attack.

Prognosis

If untreated, hypoglycemia can cause serious and permanent neurological damage and even become life-threatening, particularly for people with diabetes. But the underlying cause as well as its severity and duration determine the prognosis.

An inoperable pancreatic tumor indicates poor long-term prognosis, even if it is slow-growing. Prognosis is excellent, however, if the cause is less serious and it is identified so treatment can start early, as with fasting or reactive hypoglycemia. Changes in diet improve the condition long term, and although symptoms may be uncomfortable, they do not generally worsen the condition. One scientific study suggests that hypoglycemia associated with medications may indicate a co-occurring disease, but it did not pose a greater risk of death (Boucai et al. 2011).

Jean Kaplan Teichroew

See also: Diabetes, Type 1; Diabetes, Type 2; Diet and Nutrition

Further Reading

American Diabetes Association. (2015, June 1). Hypoglycemia (low blood glucose). Retrieved from http://www.diabetes.org/living-with-diabetes/treatment-and-care/blood -glucose-control/hypoglycemia-low-blood.html.

Boucai, L., Southern, W. N., & Zonszein, J. (2011, November). Hypoglycemia-associated mortality is not drug-associated but linked to comorbidities. *American Journal of Medicine*, *124*(11), 1028–1035. Retrieved from http://www.ncbi.nlm.nih.gov/pubmed/22017781.

Hormone Health Network. (2013, October). Fact sheet: Nondiabetic hypoglycemia. Retrieved from http://www.hormone.org/questions-and-answers/2013/nondiabetic-hypogly cemia.

What is hypoglycemia? What causes hypoglycemia? (2014, September 9). Retrieved from http://www.medicalnewstoday.com/articles/166815.php.

HYPOTENSION (LOW BLOOD PRESSURE)

The term *hypotension* is the same as the term *low blood pressure*. This is a health condition in which the pressure in the blood vessels is less than what is desirable; thus, organs such as the brain, kidneys, and heart may not receive enough blood after each beat of the heart. The normal range of blood pressure is from 90/60 millimeters of mercury to 130/80 milliliters. If there is a significant drop in a person's normal blood pressure, this may be problematic for them, and they may be diagnosed with low blood pressure if this is less than 90/60, but may vary depending on age, activity level, medications, and underlying medical conditions. Some people routinely have blood pressures 90/50 with no symptoms.

Categories of Hypotension

There are three hypotension categories: orthostatic hypotension, neutrally mediated hypotension, and severe hypotension.

Orthostatic hypotension can be brief in terms of time and is commonly a response to a sudden change in posture, such as moving from lying to sitting. If this type of hypotension occurs after eating, it is termed postprandial hypotension. Neutrally mediated hypotension occurs mostly in children and adults, who commonly grow out of this response, which usually occurs if they stand for a long time period. Severe hypotension can be caused by a sudden loss of blood, an allergic reaction, or infection.

Signs and Symptoms

Signs and symptoms include dizziness, chest pain, lightheadedness, weakness, nausea, confusion, blurry vision, fainting, fever, shortness of breath, thirst, and having an irregular heartbeat.

Causes

Some forms of hypotension are caused by the use of certain drugs, such as diuretics, and/or excess alcohol use. Other causes include heart problems, diabetes, hormone problems, nervous system problems, neurological disorders, nutrient deficiencies (such as folic acid), age, anemia, liver disease, severe inflammation, and dehydration.

Diagnostic Tests

Medical examination and blood pressure checks will reveal if there is a problem. The physician might review the patient's health and medical history. He or she might order chest or abdominal x-rays or heart ultrasound tests, electrocardiograms, and blood tests to check for infection, blood electrolyte measures, blood and urine cultures, and complete blood cell counts. Tilt table tests can be used to examine a persons' reaction to postural changes. Holster and event monitors are devices that are portable and can be worn to record the heart's electrical activity.

Treatment

If the person is healthy, no treatment may be implemented. If treatment is required, it will depend on the cause of the problem. Some forms of treatment include stopping certain medicines; changing medicines; use of fluids, diets, and electrolytes to promote hydration; and restoration of blood levels if there has been extensive bleeding. Medicines may be used to treat underlying disorders or the hypotension in severe cases. Treating shock in severe cases is also indicated.

Prevention

Individuals who develop low blood pressure because they stand a lot should try to reduce the time period for this. If individuals have a tendency to be dehydrated, they should drink plenty of fluids and may need to increase their salt intake. Avoiding alcohol, getting up slowly from a lying to a standing position, and using compression stockings to aid blood flow of the lower limbs may be helpful. Eating small, low-carbohydrate meals may reduce postprandial hypotension symptoms.

Prognosis or Outcome

Chronic low blood pressure that produces no symptoms is usually not serious. It becomes serious if blood pressure drops suddenly and deprives the brain of the appropriate amount of oxygen.

Ray Marks

See also: Blood Pressure; Heart Diseases; Hypertension

Further Reading

Cunha, J. P., & Marks, J. W. (2012). Low blood pressure. MedicineNet.com. Retrieved from http://www.medicinenet.com/script/main/art.asp?articlekey=1950&p.

Mayo Clinic. (2014, May 2). Low blood pressure (hypotension). Retrieved from http://www.mayoclinic.com/health/low-blood-pressure/DS00590.

National Heart Lung and Blood Institute. (2012). What is hypotension? Retrieved from http://www.nhlbi.nih.gov/health/health-topics/topics/hyp.

HYPOTHYROIDISM

Hypothyroidism, a common endocrine disorder, arises from a deficit in the production of thyroid hormone by the thyroid gland, a butterfly-shaped gland in the front of the throat area. This can occur either as a condition on its own, known as *primary hypothyroidism*, or as a result of other health conditions that affect thyroid hormone secretion, where it is known as *secondary hypothyroidism*.

Hypothyroidism affects about 3.7 percent of the United States population, or 25 million people, and is more common in women than men, especially women with a small body size both at birth and during childhood. Whites and Mexican Americans are most commonly affected, and the condition is more common among the elderly than the younger population.

If hypothyroidism occurs in the newborn child, this is referred to as congenital hypothyroidism; it affects 1 in 4,000 newborns in the United States per year.

Because the thyroid hormone is very important for a large number of metabolic processes to function normally, and because it controls how your body—including your heart and brain—uses energy, as well as how cells, tissues, muscles, and organs work, this is an important health condition to rectify where possible.

Symptoms

There may be no symptoms (as in silent hypothyroidism) or very severe symptoms, depending on the nature of the condition and the health status and age of the affected individual.

Some, more severe, changes that occur are decreases in the function of the heart, enlargement of the heart, fluid collection around the heart, a decreased pulse, and diminished output of blood by the heart. In the gastrointestinal tract, decreased intestinal movements can occur. An increase in cholesterol clearance and an increase in insulin resistance can also occur if the amount of thyroid hormone is decreased.

People with this condition may feel weak and sluggish because their bodies produce less energy than they require and because body processes slow down.

They may also experience constipation, increased sensitivity to cold, fatigue, heavier menstrual periods, joint or muscle pain, dry skin or paleness, depression or sadness, and brittle, thin hair and nails.

They may gain weight and experience cold intolerance, decreased sweating, depression, decreased concentration, memory loss, and puffiness if the face.

Other, later symptoms may involve a decrease in taste and smell; hoarseness and slow speech; puffy face, hands, and feet; skin thickening; and eyebrow thinning.

Causes

Most cases of hypothyroidism in the United States are caused by Hashimoto's thyroiditis or chronic lymphocyte thyroiditis, an inflammation of the thyroid gland, which is an autoimmune condition in which the body produces antibodies that attack and destroy the thyroid gland. Thyroiditis may also occur as the result of a viral infection.

Other cause include exposure to neck or brain radiation therapy, in the case of certain cancers; excessive radioactive iodine treatment applied for hyperthyroidism or having an overactive thyroid; certain medications, such as those used to treat heart problems and cancer; and thyroid surgery.

Having too little iodine in the body, pregnancy complications, having other autoimmune diseases, a genetic disorder affecting females called Turner syndrome, and having thyroid problems at birth are other factors.

Diagnosis

In addition to the medical history and physical examination, thyroid function tests, blood tests, tests to examine liver function, and cholesterol level tests may be performed.

Treatments

Synthroid is a medical remedy that can help replace the thyroxine needed to function optimally. The dosage can be determined by the physician according to the extent of the problem.

Prevention

There is no form of prevention for hypothyroidism, but the signs of the disease can be treated, and those who are at risk can be tested to see if they have this condition. The American Thyroid Association recommends all adults be tested at age 35 and above that age routinely every five years. Older adults, especially women older than 60, with a family history of hypothyroidism, and those with rheumatoid arthritis, Type 1 diabetes, pernicious anemia, or Addison's disease should be tested.

Screening tests in newborns can help to establish if the child has congenital hypothyroidism, and people with high cholesterol should be tested for hypothyroidism. Children need to be treated because even mild cases can lead to severe physical and mental retardation.

Although hypothyroidism rarely occurs in severe form, untreated hypothyroidism can lead to a state of myxedema coma, where there is a slowdown of the body that can threaten life, and this requires immediate treatment.

Prognosis and Outcomes

Death from hypothyroidism is uncommon, but untreated hypothyroidism can lead to having a goiter or enlarged thyroid gland that can affect swallowing or breathing.

It can also lead to heart problems, mental health issues, peripheral neuropathy or nerve damage that results in pain, numbness, and tingling in the area of nerve damage. It may also cause weak muscles or loss of muscle control, infertility, and birth defects.

Children and teens who develop hypothyroidism may experience growth retardation, delayed puberty, and poor mental development in addition to adult-like symptoms.

Future

Animal studies show thyroid function can be restored, even if the thyroid gland has been destroyed, through the use of stem cells. That is, stem cell–derived thyroid cells were able to form follicles of functional units similar to those found in the healthy thyroid gland. The researchers grafted the follicles into the thyroid glands that had been altered from a normal to a hypothyroid state. In eight of nine cases, normal thyroid function was observed.

Ray Marks

See also: Autoimmune Disease; Hashimoto's Disease; Thyroid Disease

Further Reading

Cleveland Clinic. (2016). Hypothyroidism. Retrieved from https://my.clevelandclinic.org /health/diseases_conditions/hic_Hypothyroidism.

Mayo Clinic. (2012, June 12). Hypothyroidism (underactive thyroid). Retrieved from http:// www.mayoclinic.org/diseases-conditions/hypothyroidism/home/ovc-20155291.

New York Times online. (2016). Hypothyroidism in-depth report. Retrieved from http://www .nytimes.com/health/guides/disease/hypothyroidism/print.html.